The Business of Building and Managing a Healthcare Practice

Neil Baum • Marc J. Kahn
Jeffery Daigrepont

The Business of Building and Managing a Healthcare Practice

Going Beyond the Basics

Second Edition

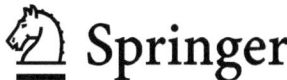 Springer

Neil Baum
Urology
Tulane Medical Center
New Orleans, LA, USA

Jeffery Daigrepont
The Coker Group
Alpharetta, GA, USA

Marc J. Kahn
Kirk Kerkorian School of Medicine
University of Nevada, Las Vegas
Las Vegas, NV, USA

ISBN 978-3-031-37622-1   ISBN 978-3-031-37623-8   (eBook)
https://doi.org/10.1007/978-3-031-37623-8

This Springer imprint is published by the registered company Springer Nature Switzerland AG
The registered company address is: Gewerbestrasse 11, 6330 Cham, Switzerland

Paper in this product is recyclable.

The authors dedicate this book to their teachers, patients, and their students.

Foreword

Working with physicians to address the business of medicine over the past 35 years has proven to be both rewarding and challenging. Balancing the business of medicine with the tenets of patient care is difficult under the US healthcare system. Physicians are tasked with the expanding burden of understanding new technology for clinical care, dynamic treatment guidelines, and coordinating care with other providers which demands time and effort to provide quality patient care. The clinical aspects of healthcare and a commitment to stay abreast of latest clinical information are typically addressed in medical school. The physicians I have worked with have embraced this lifelong learning commitment and, on most days, enjoy the work required.

The business of healthcare is a very different but necessary part of a career as a physician and not a part of the standard medical school curriculum. Physicians have many choices of where and under what circumstance they will practice medicine. The American Association of Medical Colleges estimates there will be a shortage of 37,800 to 124,000 physicians by 2034.[1] The shortage will give physicians more opportunities to choose where and how they want to practice. From the entrepreneurial solo practice to a corporate payer-provider organization, the business of healthcare is the underlying driver of clinical care. In the US healthcare system, money determines the ability of an organization to provide staff, equipment, location, contracts, and marketing to support each practicing physician. Making an informed choice about how you want to practice medicine will require consideration of a myriad of issues, one of the most important is understanding the business relationship between you and your practice choice.

The effect of the pandemic on the practice of medicine has been profound. The number of physicians practicing medicine as an employee of hospital or large corporation jumped from 62.2% in January of 2019 to 73.9% by January of 2022.[2] Regardless of where a physician has chosen to practice or for whom they work, the business basics of building and maintaining a healthcare practice require each physician, as the manager of each healthcare interaction, to

---

[1] AAMC (2021). The Complexities of Physician Supply and Demand: Projections From 2019 to 2034. *AAMC*. https://www.aamc.org/media/54681/download?attachment.

[2] Becker's Hospital Review (2022). 74% of physicians are hospital or corporate employees, with pandemic fueling increase. *Becker's Hospital Review*. https://www.beckershospitalreview.com/hospital-physician-relationships/74-of-physicians-are-hospital-or-corporate-employees-with-pandemic-fueling-increase.html.

understand the relationship between clinical care and the goals of the practice.

The practice of medicine has changed dramatically in my lifetime. As the son of a Urologist in a mid-sized Colorado town, I watched my father, M. Ray Painter, MD, FACS, establish a solo practice which quickly grew to four physicians and expanded to cover underserved areas requiring travel of up to 6 h. My father communicated his services with simple, understandable language, and his patients worked with him to cover the fees. He was able to practice medicine and learn the business requirements of his practice by gleaning information from his staff and from other physicians. He actively participated in his local, state, and national medical organizations. Through his experiences, he was able to anticipate significant changes due to increased reliance on health insurance and the introduction of managed care.

Between college and my planned start in medical school, I worked with him to update *Relative Values for Physicians*, then published by McGraw-Hill. The experience changed my life path. He and I started Physician Reimbursement Systems, Inc. (PRS) in 1989. The goal of the company was to educate physicians on the increasing complexities of the business of medicine. Medicare and other payers were quickly transitioning from a payment system based on Usual, Customary, and Reasonable (UCR) charges to relative value-based fee for service loosely based on cost. It was clear that in association with this foundational change in reimbursement, computer-driven payment would see a marked increase in rules governing how much and under what circumstances each clinical service would be paid for by the third-party insurance. This increase in rules would then drive an increase in the review of medical documentation as support for services provided by physicians.

The initial focus of PRS was to educate physicians about essential requirements to appropriately document care to adhere to clinical and business rules. Over decades, our purpose expanded to general business support for physicians. We have enjoyed national exposure to many physicians and other individuals in different roles and business models of the healthcare practice. One of the greatest privileges of this exposure is the people we have met.

On several occasions, PRS has partnered with one of the primary authors, Neil Baum, MD. Dr. Baum's insights on people, opportunities, and problem solving have been an invaluable asset to PRS and to physicians across the country. He is a tireless champion of physicians and the practice of medicine.

One of Dr. Baum's many talents is his ability to identify people that can further his commitment to continually support his medical colleagues. His co-authors Marc J. Kahn, MD, MBA, Dean of the Kirk Kerkorian School of Medicine at UNLV and Jeffery Daigrepont, senior vice president at Coker Group, are two of the many associates he has identified over the years.

The Second Edition, *The Business Basics of Building and Managing a Healthcare Practice,* is an understandable and comprehensive summary of the requirements for running and supporting a successful healthcare practice, written by physicians for physicians. With new chapters addressing topics such as telehealth, navigating the internet and social media, new business models, and adapting to market trends, the second edition is an excellent tool for any physician.

PRS Managed Services, LLC, Denver, CO, USA   Mark N. Painter

Physicians Reimbursement Systems, Inc.,
Thornton, CA, USA

PRS Consulting, LLC, Gainesville, GA, USA

Relative Value Studies, Inc., Thornton, CA, USA

Contents

About the Authors

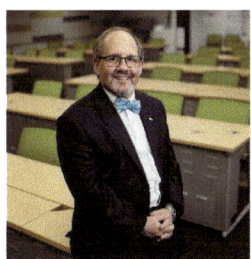

Marc J. Kahn, MD, MBA, MACP, FRCP is the Dean of the Kirk Kerkorian School of Medicine and Vice President for Health Affairs at the University of Nevada Las Vegas where he is also a Professor of Medicine. After completing his undergraduate, medical school, and post-graduate training at the University of Pennsylvania, Dr. Kahn began his faculty career at Tulane in 1994 as an academic hematologist/medical oncologist and internal medicine residency director. He subsequently served as Sr. Associate Dean for Admissions and Student Affairs at Tulane University School of Medicine where he was also the Peterman-Prosser Professor of Medicine in the section of Hematology/Medical Oncology. In 2010, Dr. Kahn received his MBA from Tulane's Freeman School of Business with concentration in both International Business and Finance.

Dr. Kahn is a Master in the American College of Physicians and a Fellow of the Royal College of Physicians, London. Dr. Kahn's research interests include non-malignant hematology, medical education, and the business of medicine.

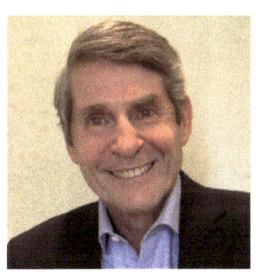

Neil Baum, MD is a Professor of Clinical Urology at Tulane Medical School and Louisiana State University School of Medicine, in New Orleans, LA. Dr. Baum is a Board-Certified Urologist with a successful practice for 30 years.

Dr. Baum has written over 350 peer-reviewed articles and 10 books on men and women's healthcare issues. He is the author of *ECNETOMPI-Impotence It's Reversible* and *What's Going on Down There-Improve Your Pelvic Health,* for women.

Dr. Baum was the columnist for *American Medical News* for more than 20 years. He also focuses on patient education and has written extensively on enhancing communication with patients and their families. He has created a software program that provides customized consents for nearly every medical specialty.

Doctor Baum writes a regular column in American Urological Association News and is the section editor for Practice Tips and Tricks. He provides a weekly video for Medical Economics on improving the efficiency and productivity of medical practices.

Dr. Baum is an amateur magician and uses magic to explain the dangers of drug and alcohol abuse to high school students.

Dr. Baum is married to Linda, has three children, Alisa, Lauren, and Craig, and six grandchildren.

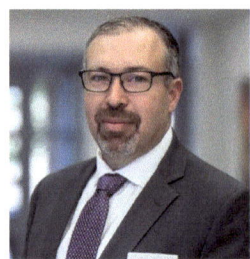

Jeffery Daigrepont senior vice president of Coker Group, specializes in healthcare automation, system integration, cybersecurity, operations, and deployment of enterprise information systems for large integrated delivery networks and medical practices. A popular national speaker, Jeffery is frequently engaged by highly respected organizations across the nation, including many non-profit trade associations and state medical societies.

Mr. Daigrepont authored a top-selling book, *Complete Guide and Toolkit to Successful EHR Adoption*, published by HIMSS in 2011 and was a contributing author to Coker's book, *The Healthcare Executive's Guide to ACO Strategy*, published in March 2012. Mr. Daigrepont is often interviewed by various national media outlets and is frequently quoted in publications.

For FY09, Daigrepont chaired the Ambulatory Information Systems Steering Committee of HIMSS. In addition, as the Ambulatory Committee liaison for FY09 to the ACEC planning Committee, he represented the HIMSS Ambulatory and AISC members. Daigrepont is credentialed by the American Academy of Medical Management (AAMM) with an Executive Fellowship in Practice Management (EFMP).

Mr. Daigrepont also serves as an independent investor advisor to many of the nation's top healthcare venture capitalist firms such as Kleiner Perkins Caufield & Byers (KPCB) and Silver Lake Partners.

May you always have work for your hands to do. May your pockets hold always a coin or two. Irish Blessing

Physicians who aren't good at business won't survive. Russel J, *Washington Post*, May 10, 2010

Good medicine is good business, but not necessarily the other way around. Bill Evans, MD, Pediatric Cardiologist

Case Sally

Sally, a PGY-3 internal medicine resident, spent a rotation with an internist in private practice. She often accompanied him to the doctor's dining room. She heard many doctors complain about decreasing reimbursements, rising overhead, additional government regulations, increasing paperwork, learning to use another electronic medical record program, the issue of burnout, and a host of other complaints. She seldom heard doctors talk about the joys and benefits of becoming a doctor. She started second-guessing her decision to become a physician. This book is not meant to discourage you but to reassure you that you have made an excellent decision to join one of the greatest and most enjoyable professions on this planet. However, to have that enjoyment, it will be necessary to have a modicum of business skills that you probably didn't receive as a medical student.

Let's begin with the topic of becoming a doctor to achieve wealth. Achieving wealth is probably the worst reason to select medicine as an occupation. If you compare the incomes of United Parcel Service (UPS) truck drivers and physicians, you will see that achieving wealth is not a viable reason to become a physician. This very revealing graph (Fig. 1.1) shows that a UPS truck driver enters the workforce and begins to earn money at age 18. However, a physician usually incurs debt for 8–10 years and only enters the workforce around age 30. Therefore, it takes a physician nearly 17 years to equal the accumulated wealth of a UPS truck driver.

Now consider if the UPS truck driver worked the same hours as a physician, 60–70 h a week, and received overtime pay, it would take nearly 24 years for the physician to equal the income of a UPS truck driver.

Any downsides for a doctor? The UPS driver is unlikely to get complimented about the delivery they just completed! Whereas the physician is likely to receive multiple warm fuzzies (compliments) nearly every day in practice.

The UPS driver who drives and delivers packages 6–8 h a day is probably bored after a few hours in the truck. However, a physician has a variety of activities, and no day or patient is ever the same. Boredom is never an issue in healthcare.

The UPS driver is lifting heavy boxes all day and is at risk of early onset back pain because of

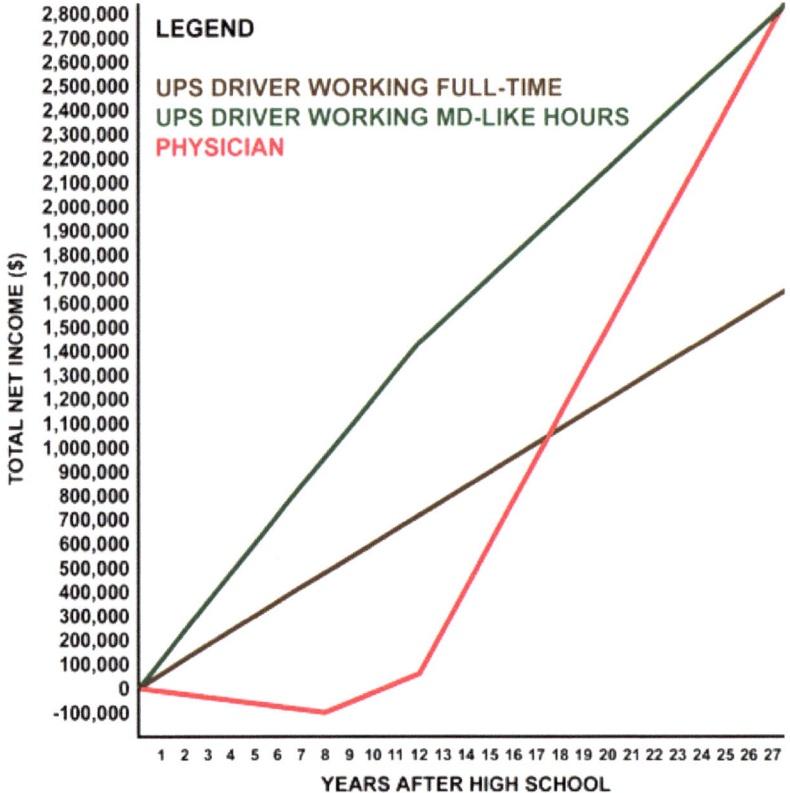

Fig. 1.1 Salary of UPS truck driver (brown line and green line) versus physician salary (red line)

the heavy lifting they must do daily. Back pain is usually not considered an occupational hazard for physicians. (Exceptions are back and neck pain in interventional radiologists and cardiovascular surgeons).

Take it from the experience of the doctor versus the UPS truck driver can readily see that men and women do not decide to become doctors for financial reasons. If we wanted to become wealthy quickly, we might consider becoming UPS truck drivers!

Nearly every physician who decides to become a doctor knows that they will have over $200,000 of debt that will have to be repaid with interest [1]; and that they will have to get up in the middle of the night to go to work to care for the sick and ill patients; that they risk litigation and lawsuits during their career, and that will defer gratification and accumulation of wealth for many years.

Yet, thousands of bright, talented young men and women will enter the healthcare profession, and applications to medical schools are at an all-time high. We become doctors because we truly have a calling. We want to help people not only get well, but now we are interested in helping patients and the public stay well and avoid getting sick and going to see the doctor. We become physicians because we enjoy the gratification from patients who thank us every day for all that we do to make them better or keep them well. We don't believe there is another profession that offers that kind of daily feedback from their customers or clients.

For the most part, physicians love what they do, and money is not the primary driver for joining the exclusive club of healthcare providers. However, this choice of profession does not negate the fact that we are small businessmen and women and must be concerned with the business aspect of our practices and be good clinical doctors.

You will seldom find a doctor who went into medicine to become a businessman or woman.

But nearly all doctors say they need practical, real-world guidance to run the business side of their practice. This book is written for medical students, residents, fellows, and newly minted doctors to fill the void in most medical training programs. That void consists of providing business skills necessary to become complete doctors.

Why Do We Become Physicians?

Doctors are in a field with growing demand, a declining supply of physicians, and formidable barriers to entry, with more applicants to medical school every year [2]. Every other industry or profession would be envious of this economic advantage. If you believe healthcare is difficult, imagine working in an industry such as digital cameras or print newspapers. Can you imagine working in a profession for which demand is declining, where there is an over-supply of competitors, or if almost anyone can gain access to the field with minimal or no barriers to entry? The dynamics in our profession assure us that there will always be work and future employment.

Doctors have instant status as soon as the initials M.D. or D.O. appears after their name. With these two initials following your name, you have credibility immediately accepted by your patients. Doctors should never take this instant status for granted. For example, if a patient sees a doctor they never met, they will divulge the deepest secrets of their medical history, including menstrual history, bowel habits, and even their sexual history. No other professional guarantees its young members such instant credibility. Doctors must always uphold a high standard of confidentiality and ethical behavior and should never take our lofty status with our patients for granted.

Medical doctors are in the top 5% of wage earners in the United States. If we compare the average physician's salary with those of other jobs, our salaries are at the top of the income chart. Also, most of the others in that rare top 5% do not have the same upside potential that we do.

Many successful physicians earn two to three times more than the average physician [3].

Physicians are fortunate not to be compelled to retire at a certain age. Because the practice of medicine is not physically demanding, many physicians can work into their 80s if they so desire, as most hospitals and groups do not have mandatory retirement. Only recently have older doctors, especially aging surgeons, been asked to submit voluntary evaluation and consider accepting an assistant for certain surgical procedures [4].

Doctors, compared with many other professionals, have a wonderful lifestyle. The practice of medicine allows most men and women to spend time with their families, taking 2–4 weeks of vacation each year and having an option of working 8- to 10-h days. This book will provide numerous examples of becoming more efficient and productive so that doctors can be home for dinner with their families. Except for the hours when physicians are on call, they have reasonable lifestyle choices. Younger physicians today are opting to work fewer hours per week, even if it means a lower income. Doctors also can select a geographic location and the kind of practice they wish to have, a choice that is not as readily available to other professionals. Many career choices have geographic limitations regarding where employees can live or are at risk of suddenly being transferred anywhere at the whim of a superior. Still, physicians can work almost anywhere they choose. They can determine where they would like to live before starting their careers.

There are more opportunities for physicians than in other professions, especially for those entering practice within 7 years of graduation from training programs. Doctors can elect to work for themselves, join a large group practice, or be employed by a hospital or academic healthcare center. Although an employed physician must answer to a boss, starting salaries for employed physicians have increased, and these doctors function relatively independently compared to other types of professionals employed by a large group, company, or organization [5].

Using examples, we show how young doctors can sculpt the kind of practice they wish to have. Doctors can carve out the exact type of practice that makes them most comfortable. If a doctor is interested in seeing only patients with specific diagnoses or providing only a limited number of treatment options, they can easily do so. This can be done if a doctor only wants to see certain kinds of patients (e.g., older, geriatric patients, or pediatric patients). If the doctor wishes to see patients who speak only another language besides English, this can be easily achieved. If you want only patients who pay cash or want to have a concierge practice, where a limited number of patients pay an annual fee to have 24/7 access to your practice, then this is also within the realm of possibility.

There isn't a day that goes by that most physicians don't receive a compliment or accolade about the care they provide. Most physicians are told almost daily how terrific they are, unlike the UPS driver. If ego satisfaction and gratification are your drivers, you have selected the right profession.

The practice of medicine provides job security and a future of guaranteed employment. Everyone who graduates from medical school and a training program can find a job. It may not be a perfect job, but it is a profession in demand and will undoubtedly provide a future of job security. It is a sad commentary that so many graduating lawyers cannot find a job practicing law and have thousands of dollars of debt [6].

Even though we face the challenge of declining reimbursements and higher overhead costs, a different career track wouldn't have eliminated these detractors. These same challenges exist in every industry and every profession. These challenges in other industries have resulted in extinction because competition has created ways to do the same things, either better or less expensive. Companies, organizations, and practices have done so because they have found ways to be more efficient and productive. Ultimately, they have done things better. Healthcare is one of the industries that have focused on creating greater efficiencies and lowering operating costs, becoming more efficient and more productive, preserving patient satisfaction, and improving clinical outcomes. This presents an opportunity for improving quality, maintaining patient satisfaction, and, yes, improving the bottom line (i.e., increasing productivity).

Despite all the hardships and detractors associated with modern healthcare, doctors have much to be thankful for. Those working in other industries have their lists of complaints, but they are often powerless to make changes because they are neither owners nor partners in the business. If they are members of a large organization, many layers of bureaucracy must be overcome to make changes. Doctors enjoy the opportunity to have significant control and the tools to implement change and tweak our practices to improve the services that we provide for our patients. If we put our problems and complaints with modern medicine on a scale and then weigh those issues and concerns against the benefits of being a doctor, we will find that the scale weighs heavily on the pluses, and we should be thankful to be a member of this wonderful club.

Why Do Doctors Need to Understand the Basic Principles of Business?

Most physicians will earn $10–12 million over their practice lifetime. However, physicians will control that amount multiple times by directing healthcare for their patients. With the mere signature of a physician, they control almost 100% of all healthcare expenditures, yet physicians receive only 18% of the total $3+ trillion in healthcare expenses [7]. Using basic business skills and outstanding clinical management, individual physicians or groups must understand that to be successful, the physicians must prove that they can deliver a better product at a lower cost than their competitors. This is the direction of the future of American healthcare. That may be why 40% of the enrollment in US business schools are physicians [8]. The authors don't believe that an MBA will be necessary for new physicians to survive in the future. However, we think that a minimum knowledge of the business will be required, and we believe that is the purpose of this book: to help young doctors cross the bridge between practicing medicine and running a business. How doctors understand the business of medicine will determine their future success.

Few of us have any training in the business of healthcare. Our training teaches us how to diagnose and treat medical conditions. We must understand and accept that healthcare is a business. It is no different than Coca-Cola, Microsoft, or Apple but on a much smaller scale. Those companies must be concerned about profit and loss and expenses, including overhead, just as a medical practice must monitor regularly. One big difference is that healthcare is a very regulated industry. We have laws established by the federal and state governments that we must adhere to closely or face fines and penalties.

The nature of medical practice has placed a price tag on nearly everything a doctor does or orders. The patient in this millennium often has high deductible insurance, expensive premiums, and often co-pays, making the patient have skin in the game. The days of transparency have arrived, and when a patient asks how much a CT scan is or what the cost of a BRCA gene test is, the doctor needs to know the answer or be able to provide it quickly for the patient.

Back to the Case

Sally was despondent about her experience after her rotation with the internist in private practice. She discussed her experience with the medical school dean and recommended that other students not be assigned to a physician harboring such negative attitudes about the medical profession. The dean placed Sally in touch with a more encouraging and constructive physician. Sally also decided to try to understand the role of business in medicine. Out of her negative experience, she understood that becoming a complete physician means being a good clinician and becoming knowledgeable and competent in the dollars and cents of the practice of medicine.

Bottom Line

The importance of business in healthcare can be stated by the title, A Doctor by Choice, a Businessman by Necessity, which appeared in the New York Times by Dr. Sandeep Jauhar [9]. It will be necessary for all physicians to have a basic understanding of the basics of business to have a successful practice. This book will provide those basic business principles and metrics that will put you on the road to practice that you will enjoy and will ensure your productivity.

References

1. Rajapuram N, Langness S, Marshall MR, Sammann A. Medical students in distress: the impact of gender, race, debt, and disability. PLoS One. 2020;15(12):e0243250.
2. Weiner S. More students are entering medical school. AAMC. 2020. https://www.aamc.org/news-insights/more-students-are-entering-medical-school.
3. Conover C. Are U.S. doctors paid too much. Forbes. 2013. https://www.forbes.com/sites/theapothecary/2013/05/28/are-u-s-doctors-paid-too-much/?sh=23f7b51ad525.
4. Span P. When is the surgeon too old to operate? The New York Times. 2019. https://www.nytimes.com/2019/02/01/health/surgeons-retirement-competence.html.
5. Physicians Practice. Physician compensation: employed vs. practice owners. Physicians Practice. 2017. https://www.physicianspractice.com/view/physician-compensation-employed-vs-practice-owners.
6. Choyke B. ABA legal education section releases employment data for graduating law class of 2016. Chicago: American Bar Association; 2017. https://www.americanbar.org/content/dam/aba/administrative/legal_education_and_admissions_to_the_bar/statistics/2017_employment_data_2016_graduates_news_release.authcheckdam.pdf.
7. Martin A, Hartman M, Washington B, Caitlin A. National health spending in 2017. Health Aff. 2019;38(1):96–106. https://www.healthaffairs.org/doi/10.1377/hlthaff.2018.05085.
8. Viswanathan V. The rise of the MD\MBA degree. The Atlantic. 2014. https://www.theatlantic.com/education/archive/2014/09/the-rise-of-the-mdmba-degree/380683/.
9. Jauhar S. A doctor by choice, a businessman by necessity. The New York Times. 2009. https://www.nytimes.com/2009/07/07/health/07essa.html.

Time Value of Money, or, What Is the Real Financial Value of an Opportunity?

2

Case Martika

Martika graduated college 5 years ago and took a job with Bond Enterprises, a holding company, as her first job. As an economics major, Martika always envisioned a career in business. After her mother's death from breast cancer 2 years ago, Martika began to have doubts about her career choice and volunteered at the hospice that cared for her mother prior to her mother's death. After speaking with friends and doing some research, she began to explore medicine as a potential career. She took premedical science classes at a local college, did well, studied for the MCAT, applied, and got accepted to her state medical school.

Because of her business background, Martika wondered if medical school would be a good move financially. Her current job at Bond paid well. Going to medical school would involve borrowing money for tuition and living expenses and she would not be able to work while a student. Although she would be paid for residency, her salary would be significantly less than that of a practicing physician. Over her lifetime, would her eventual salary as a physician compensate for her medical school debt and lost income? Would she be able to practice the specialty of her choice or would she be limited to higher-paying specialties? Is medical school worth it?

One of the most basic principles of finance is the time value of money. Conceptually and simply, money is worth more now than at some time in the future. Stated another way, given the choice, you want your money sooner rather than later. This is because invested money earns interest and because you can use the money you have now for things that may not be available later. As an example, the time value of money dictates that if you are lucky enough to win the million-dollar lottery, you want the million dollars now, not 250 thousand dollars a year for the next 4 years. Why is this so?

Money has an opportunity cost. For example, suppose you want to buy an antique clock. If you have the money now, you can successfully negotiate the price and buy the clock. But, if you don't have the money now, you would have to wait until later to purchase the clock and the clock may have already been sold to someone else and no longer be available. Similarly, if presented with an investment opportunity, having money on hand allows you to make an investment that may disappear at a future date. Obviously, having money on hand provides a financial advantage for the holder to use the money for purchases, to lend, or to invest.

In addition to opportunity costs, money has more value in the present because most of us do not hold our money in a basket under our beds. Rather, we either put the money in the bank for safe keeping or invest the money. Either way, our money can earn interest. Interest is the money

© The Author(s), under exclusive license to Springer Nature Switzerland AG 2023
N. Baum et al., *The Business of Building and Managing a Healthcare Practice*,
https://doi.org/10.1007/978-3-031-37623-8_2

paid for the use of your cash. When you borrow money from a bank, or through your credit card, the bank charges interest, a fee for the use of their money. Similarly, if you put money in a bank, or lend money by purchasing bonds, you are compensated with interest payments for the use of your money.

Interest can be simple or compounded. As an example of simple interest, if you invest $100 at 6% annual interest, at the end of the year, you will have $106. Compounded interest allows for you to effectively earn "interest on your interest." When Benjamin Franklin died, he left approximately $5000 to each of the two cities Philadelphia and Boston. He required that the money be invested and that there would be two withdraws, a partial withdraw at 100 years and a final withdraw at 200 years. Because of compounded interest, at 100 years each city received a payment of $500,000 and at 200 years, each city received approximately $20 million. Franklin described compounded interest as, "Money makes money. And the money that makes money makes money" [1].

Going back to the example of a $100 investment at 6% interest, if the interest was compounded monthly, at the end of the year, you would not have $106 but $106.17. If interest was compounded daily, at the end of the year, you would have $106.18. The extra 17 or 18 cents arises by earning interest on interest. Although a mere 17 cents may seem trivial, suppose your initial investment were $100 million. Now your compounded interest would be over $6,170,000—a substantial sum indeed!

Compounding can also be illustrated by the following fable:

A peasant shepherd comes upon a young girl who has become ensnared in a bear trap. He hears her cry out and frees her. The young girl is so thankful that she promises the peasant a large reward as her father is King of the empire. Upon meeting the King, the peasant is offered 100 lbs. of wheat. Noticing that the King has a chessboard displayed on a table, the peasant offers an alternative reward. The peasant suggests that the king put one grain of wheat on the top left square of the chessboard and then doubles the number of grains successively throughout the 64 squares of the chessboard. The King quickly agrees to this

alternative assuming that the uneducated peasant has made a silly concession. Understanding compounding, the wise peasant has actually struck a great deal. If the number of grains of wheat doubles on each successive square, then the sum of grains is $1 + 2 + 4 + 8 + 16 + \ldots, + 2^{64}$ for a total of over 18×10^{18} grains of wheat which would weigh more than 1645 times the global production of wheat in modern times! The amount of wheat placed on an individual square is "compounded" by the amount on the previous square. Certainly, compounding is important if you are borrowing or lending money. For the borrower, compounding costs money and for the lender, compounding allows money to grow.

In addition to the interest rate, the number of times compounding occurs in a given period can also affect the total interest. The more compounding periods there are, the greater the total interest. For example, $1000 borrowed at 6% annual interest would cost $60 of interest if the interest were simple or not compounded. If the interest were compounded monthly, the total interest payment would be $61.68, daily compounding yields a total payment of $61.83 and we can even calculate continuous compounding meaning that the compounding is continuous and ongoing which would yield a total annual payment of $61.84.

Many commercial loans including credit cards display interest as APR (annual percentage rate). For example, if you were considering taking out a business loan of $300,000 with an interest of 6%, your annual interest payment would be $18,000 or $1500 per month. However, the actual payments on such a commercial loan are typically higher as they include not only the cost of interest but also the additional fees attached to the loan. The APR includes these extra costs. In the above example, if the loan also includes closing costs, insurance, and origination fees totaling an additional $5000, then your original loan amount would be $305,000. At 6% interest, the new annual payment would be $18,300 for an APR of 6.1%. The APR gives a better estimate of the actual cost you pay to borrow money because the APR includes the cost of interest plus the cost of additional fees. When shopping for loans, the APR gives a good sense of the monthly costs of borrowing money and can be used to compare loans. However, borrowers need to be cautioned that it is not only the APR that is important in choosing a loan, but also the duration of the loan. A 10-year loan spreads out the additional fees associated with the loan over a much longer time period than a 24-month loan lowering the APR substantially. However, a borrower would pay more total interest on a longer loan. Therefore, when borrowing money, it is important to consider not only the APR but also the total number of payments to determine the better loan for a given situation.

In addition to interest (also called the cost of capital or discount rate) understanding a business opportunity requires understanding of present and future value of money which is intertwined with the time value of money. As is now obvious, the future value of money is greater than the present value because of opportunity costs and the cost of capital. Put mathematically, Future Value (FV) = Present Value $(PV) \times (1 + r)^t$ where r is the interest rate or cost of capital and t is the number of pay periods between the present and the future.

Net present value is a business tool used to determine the financial benefit or detriment of business opportunities and it relies heavily on the concept of the time value of money. Essentially, if costs or payments occur in the same time period, they can be simply added to or subtracted from each other. However, because of the time value of money payments or costs accrued at different time periods cannot be simply added or subtracted because their true value depends on when these transactions occur. To calculate net present value, all costs or payments are brought to the present value, using the present value equation, and can then be summed. In general, from a business perspective, any opportunity presenting positive net present value is beneficial, whereas any opportunity with negative net present value is not advisable.

Going back to our introductory case with Martika, the financial value of an MD degree can be summarized as:

Value of MD = total change in salary with an MD less the cost of medical school attendance less the wages lost during training. These costs and payments must all be corrected for the cost of capital and calculated at the present value.

Using several assumptions in our model including an annual interest rate of 3%, a cost of medical school attendance of $70,000, a salary increase of $130,000 after residency with 3% growth per year, and a 4-year residency duration, the net present value of Martika's MD is over $1.7 million [2]. Certainly, this is a hugely positive net present value making the decision to go to medical school financially advantageous and something that Martika should do from a financial perspective. Obviously, the above analysis does not begin to take into account career satisfaction, self-actualization, social status, and other non-financial gains that Martika might derive from a long career as a physician. In fact, there is probably no more valuable degree in the world than a US MD degree.

Back to the Case
Martika met with her friend, a banker, and referred back to notes she had taken for a Finance class in college. She realized what a great financial deal getting an MD would be and compounded with her interest in healthcare, decided to pursue medical school at a school that offered a combined MD/MBA degree.

What We Have Learned
1. You want your money sooner, rather than later.
2. Early investing can compound earnings leading to a greater net value.
3. Getting an MD is a terrific financial investment.

References

1. Malkiel BJ, Ellis CD. The elements of investing: easy lessons for every investor. Hoboken: Wiley; 2013.
2. Kahn MJ, Nelling EF. Estimating the value of medical education: a net present value approach. Teach Learn Med. 2010;22(3):205–8.

.

Case Bryce

Bryce is in his second year of faculty at an academic medical center. He was asked to serve on the Board of Directors of his school's faculty practice plan, a role he desired because of his interest in practice management and because of his desire to become involved in academic leadership. When it came time to present the financial statements, Bryce felt at a loss. What is EBITDA? What is AR? Why are there multiple statements distributed to the group, rather than a simple table? Why does it appear as if there are different ways to account for the same transaction? Bryce wonders if anyone, other than the business folks in the room, really understand what these statements mean. Bryce wishes he took an accounting class in college or at least paid more attention to his roommates who were business majors.

Basic Accounting

Basic accounting is predicated on the simple equation that *assets = liabilities + equity*. In simple terms, looking at personal wealth, this means that your total wealth, your equity, is equivalent to what you own less what you owe (rearranging the equation: assets − liabilities = equity (see Fig. 3.1). When balancing our own bank account, we typically perform this arithmetic automatically. Each month we have an account balance (equity) to which we add our monthly paycheck (asset) and subtract our payments (liabilities) such as mortgage payments or car expenses. Such a system of bookkeeping may be fine for an individual with a few transactions per month but makes error detection difficult. Suppose you entered the wrong payment or the wrong salary amount? Would your account be overdrawn?

Double-entry accounting, which dates back to the eleventh century, is a system of bookkeeping where every entry into one account requires an opposite, yet equal, entry into another account. These two entries, termed debits and credits, allow for error detection as the sum of all debits must equal the sum of all credits for all accounts. The terms "debit" and "credit" are not foreign as we are used to have debit and credit cards in our wallets. A *credit* card allows us to make purchases that are later paid for, whereas a *debit* card represents a bank account from which funds are drawn. For the bank issuing the card, the credit card payments are recorded as credits as they increase the fund balance of the bank once paid, and the debit card payments are recorded as debits, as they create a negative fund balance in the bank when paid out. The system of double-entry accounting gives the two cards their respective names.

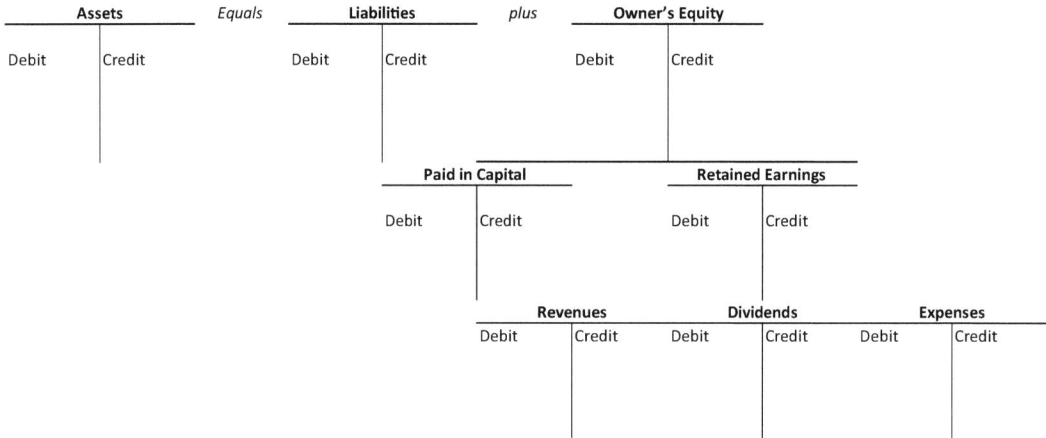

Fig. 3.1 Basic T-accounting

As a simple example of double-entry accounting, say an ophthalmologist's office sells a pair of glasses for $250. This could be recorded both as a debit of $250 to an account named "assets" and a credit of $250 to an account named "revenue." This is because the glasses represent an asset to the ophthalmology office that is lost during the sale, whereas the payment for the glasses represents a gain in revenue for the office. Generally, from a bookkeeping perspective, there are five types of accounts: assets, liabilities, income (revenue), expenses, and capital accounts. Each of these has subaccounts that are recorded as a series of debits and credits.

Bookkeeping using the principles of double-entry accounting results in financial statements that are used daily in all businesses. The three basic financial statements used by businesses are (1) The income statement, also called the profit and loss statement or P&L which demonstrates the "bottom line" of net gains or losses; (2) The balance sheet which uses the basic accounting equation and lists assets, liabilities, and retained earnings (equity); and (3) The cash flow statement that shows the outflow and inflow of cash related to operations, investments, and financial transactions. Sometimes a fourth statement is produced called the equity statement which represents changes in the retained earnings (savings) of the company. We will not be discussing the equity statement further. Analysis of financial

statements can provide an estimate of the financial health of an organization and can be used in planning future business strategies.

The main financial statement of interest to most physicians, and the one distributed on a monthly basis, is the income statement that typically covers a range of time such as the previous month, the fiscal year to date, the previous quarter, or all three time periods. The "bottom line" of an income statement is the net profit or loss for the given time period. Typically, income statements include information for the preceding period and the previous year for comparison. Income statements usually include entries for both budgeted and actual revenues and expenses. Figure 3.2 shows the income statement for Bryce's academic group practice.

From the income statement, looking directly at the bottom line, we can see that for August 2019, the group practice is "in the black" by $14,706, meaning they have income that exceeds expenses by that amount. Looking further at the income statement, in spite of a small positive bottom line, the practice is behind budget by $184,850. This may be of concern if such a trend continues. Looking at both expenses and revenue, the income statement tells us that the practice is behind budget due to both low revenue and increased expenses. Certainly, were this to continue, this would be a problem as the practice may not be able to pay its bills. From a historic

BRYCE'S MEDICAL GROUP
STATEMENT OF ACTIVITY
Aug-19

| 1-MONTH (MTD) | | | | | DESCRIPTION | 2-MONTHS (YTD) | | | |
BUDGET	ACTUAL	FAV (UNFAV)	Jul-18	Aug-18		BUDGET	ACTUAL	FAV (UNFAV)	Aug-18
4,647,325	3,966,168	-681,157	4,109,613	3,898,084	SITE A INCOME	8,890,534	7,864,252	-1,026,283	7,736,099
258,703	152,674	-106,029	118,978	115,425	SITE B INCOME	517,405	268,099	-249,307	209,341
3,009,639	1,905,153	-1,104,486	1,924,358	3,101,420	SITE C INCOME	6,019,278	5,006,572	-1,012,705	4,444,469
808,428	620,808	-187,620	100,230	95,308	SITE D INCOME	1,616,857	716,116	-900,741	281,561
445,608	657,427	211,819	546,321	632,577	SITE E INCOME	891,217	1,290,004	398,788	1,033,651
29,917	32,108	2,191	1,036	21,875	OTHER INCOME	59,833	53,983	-5,850	3,650
9,199,620	**7,334,338**	**-1,865,282**	**6,800,537**	**7,864,688**	TOTAL INCOME	**17,995,124**	**15,199,026**	**-2,796,098**	**13,708,770**
-7,834,158	-6,058,899	1,775,259	-5,520,796	-6,679,667	LESS: Practice -REALTED COSTS	-15,525,502	-12,738,566	2,786,936	-11,674,289
1,365,461	**1,275,439**	**-90,022**	**1,279,740**	**1,185,022**	NET COST OF PRACTICE ASSESSMENTS	**2,469,622**	**2,460,460**	**-9,162**	**2,034,481**
					COST OF PRACTICE:				
538,291	601,893	-63,602	539,745	515,602	NET SALARIES & WAGES	1,076,582	1,117,494	-40,913	954,284
143,535	162,839	-19,304	166,758	133,518	FRINGE BENEFITS	287,070	296,357	-9,287	295,592
7,519	7,515	4	6,544	4,455	OPERATING SUPPLIES	15,038	11,970	3,068	9,041
246,905	244,385	2,521	281,058	220,831	PURCHASED SERVICES	493,811	465,215	28,595	500,977
12,873	15,223	-2,350	72,045	13,704	UTILITIES & POSTAGE	25,747	28,927	-3,180	74,257
44,652	33,740	10,912	31,368	39,009	OTHER EXPENSE	89,304	72,749	16,555	55,607
85,417	74,070	11,347	85,400	82,470	FACILITY FEES	170,833	156,540	14,293	164,730
1,079,192	1,139,665	-60,473	1,182,918	1,009,588	TOTAL OPERATING EXPENSES	2,158,384	2,149,253	9,132	2,054,489
					NON-OPERATING EXPENSES				
125,858	133,316	-7,458	124,691	128,771	MALPRACTICE EXPENSE	251,717	262,087	-10,370	249,317
-39,145	-12,248	-26,897	-28,248	-68,042	LESS: RECOVERIES	-78,290	-80,291	2,001	-56,848
86,713	121,068	-34,354	96,443	60,728	NET MALPRACTICE EXPENSE	173,427	181,796	-8,369	192,470
1,165,905	**1,260,733**	**-94,827**	**1,279,361**	**1,070,316**	TOTAL COST OF PRACTICE EXPENSES	**2,331,811**	**2,331,049**	**762**	**2,246,958**
199,556	**14,706**	**-184,850**	**379**	**114,706**	NET EARNINGS	**137,811**	**129,412**	**-8,400**	**-212,478**

Fig. 3.2 Income statement

perspective, the practice is doing better financially than the previous month where the net earnings were only $379, but the practice is not doing as well as the previous year where net earnings were $114,706. From a year-to-date perspective, the practice is $129,412 in the black, but is still below budget, but much better than this point last year, where the practice was "in the red" for $212,478. Bryce practices at Site E. Looking at the top of the income statement, Bryce can see that his site is doing the best of all of the sites financially and is above budget. This may mean a bonus for Bryce in the future! Certainly, looking at just a few areas of the income statement, we can learn a lot about Bryce's practice.

The balance sheet, unlike the income statement, represents a snapshot in time. The balance sheet provides information on how assets are funded: through debt, equity, or other capital. Assets are generally listed in order of how easily they can be converted to cash, also known as liquidity. Liabilities are listed in the order that they need to be paid from first to last. Accounts receivable refers to money owed to the practice by patients and insurers that have yet to be paid. It is an asset as it provides positive value to the practice. Accounts payable represents money that the practice has to pay out. This may be due to patients that were overcharged or for patients who were charged for a service that was later paid by an insurance company. Accounts payable is a liability because it is money that needs to be paid out. Again, for the balance sheet, from the basic accounting equation, *assets = liabilities + equity*. Equity is that money left over which adds value to a company. Let's look at the balance sheet for Bryce's practice in Fig. 3.3. First, the balance sheet must obey the accounting equation, or assets must equal liabilities plus equity.

BALANCE SHEET
31-Dec-19

ASSETS			LIABILITIES		
Current Assets			**Current Liabilities**		
Cash	$	2,100.00	Notes payable	$	5,000.00
Petty Cash	$	100.00	Accounts payable	$	35,900.00
Temporary investments	$	10,000.00	Wages payable	$	8,500.00
Accounts receivable	$	40,500.00	interest payable	$	2,900.00
Supplies	$	34,800.00	taxes payable	$	6,100.00
Prepaid insurance	$	1,500.00	unearned revenues	$	2,600.00
			total current liabilites	$	61,000.00
Total Current assets	$	89,000.00			
			Long-term liabilites		
Investments	$	36,000.00	notes payable	$	20,000.00
			bonds payable		$ 400,000.00
Property, Plant & Equiptment			Total long-term liabilites		$ 420,000.00
Land	$	12,000.00			
Buildings		$ 180,000.00	**Total Liabilities**		$ 481,000.00
Equiptment		$ 201,000.00			
Less: depreciation		$ (56,000.00)	**OWNER'S EQUITY**		
P,P,E net		$ 337,000.00	Retained earnings		$ 280,000.00
			accumulated other income		$ 9,000.00
Other Assets		$ 308,000.00	total equity		$ 289,000.00
Total Assets		$ 770,000.00	**Total liabilites & Equity**		$ 770,000.00

Fig. 3.3 Balance Sheet 2022

For Bryce's practice, this is the case. He has both assets and debt plus equity of $770,000. Sometimes, the financial health of an organization can be determined by the debt-to-equity ratio. This gives us a measurement of risk as it can tell us how well debt is managed. Lower numbers are better. For Bryce's practice, this ratio is calculated as total liabilities divided by equity, which gives a ratio of 1.66. This is not very high, suggesting that the practice is prudent in its borrowing practices. Another thing to look at is how equity has changed over time. Looking at balance sheets for the past several years can show whether the business is growing or contracting. Finally, return on equity (ROE), defined as net income divided by equity, can give a sense of how well the equity is being used to produce income. For example, if the practice purchased colonoscopes with their equity, the ROE could be an indicator of the success of that strategy.

The cash flow statement shows where cash comes in and goes out of a business in three areas: operations, investments, and financing. As an interesting example, let's look at Ford Motors. We may logically assume that Ford Motors is in the business of making cars. However, looking at the cash flow statement for Ford Motors on yahoo finance for 12/31/21 [1], we see that the total cash flow for Ford from operations was $15.8 billion, the total cash flow from investments was a $2.7 billion, and the total cash flow from financing was $23.5 billion lent out. Based on an analysis of cash flows, Ford Motors is as much a lending company as they are a car manufacturing company!

In addition to the basics of the three financial statements that we have discussed, there are other terms and additional information that can be derived through analysis of financial statements. One commonly used line item in an income statement is EBITDA. EBITDA stands for "earnings before interest, taxes, depreciation, and amortization." EBITDA is sometimes used as an alternative to net income. EBITDA is used in income statements as it eliminates the effects of financing (interest) and capitalization (depreciation and amortization). Do not let this term confuse you. EBITDA and net income are very closely related.

Additionally, analysis of financial statements can help us know how well the practice is doing at collecting owed money. This refers to "days in AR." Although not specifically spelled out in financial statements, this can be calculated if you know the charges for the past year and divide that number by the days in a year. Because most health expenses are discounted by insurance companies and other third-party payors, charges are very different from revenue in healthcare so in addition to the income statement, you would need to know total charges to make this calculation. Additionally, many third-party payors will not pay bills that are older than 180 days. Days in AR is an important number to know!

Finally, the health of a practice can be assumed by the *liquidity* of the practice which gives an impression of the amount of money the practice has on hand in case of emergency. This can be presented as "working capital" which is the difference between current assets and current liabilities. For Bryce's practice, his working capital, from the balance sheet, is $89,000 minus $61,000 or $27,000. A company with negative working capital could not pay off short-term debts if required to do so and would be considered "illiquid." Another commonly used indicator of liquidity, or ability to pay debt, is the *current ratio*, the ratio of current assets to current liabilities.

Although there are many other calculations based on financial statements used by businesses, these are the major ones used and understanding these will go a long way towards being able to analyze financial statements.

Back to the Case

Bryce went to the business manager of his practice to learn more about the data presented. His manager was quick to point out that she worked for Bryce, and not the other way around. She explained the accounting used in his practice and gave him a much better understanding of the financial well-being of his practice. Bryce was satisfied that he was working in the right place and also felt more confident the next month when the group's financial statements were presented. He even knew enough to ask about days in AR and was pleased that it was only 28 days and improved from last year. Bryce wondered if getting an MBA would be valuable in the future.

Bottom Line (No Pun Intended) on What We Have Learned About Accounting and Financial Statements

1. Assets = liabilities + equity
2. There are three basic financial statements: the income statement, balance sheet, and cash flow statement
3. Understanding basic principles of accounting allows physicians to understand the financial health of their practice and allows for strategic planning.

Reference

1. Yahoo. Cash flow. Yahoo. https://finance.yahoo.com/quote/F/cash-flow?p=F.

Case Marcus

Marcus, a pediatrician practicing in Atlanta, Georgia, comes in on a Saturday to get caught up on documentation and notices no one picked up the mail from Friday. Normally mail is processed by her staff and distributed accordingly. The stack of mail is generally a mixture of correspondents, junk mail, and checks from insurance companies. Out of curiosity, Marcus opens the mail and was shocked to see so many claims being denied due to careless mistakes. There were over ten rejected claims for missing modifiers.[1] Several more were rejected due to the patient ID missing. Some claims were deemed not medically necessary due to a lack of supporting documentation. The most unsettling part was knowing that Friday's mail was only a tiny portion of her total volume of claims. On Monday, she called an urgent staff meeting to investigate why so many claims were being denied and discovered there was a major disconnect between the front office and the back office. Most of these denials were avoidable processing errors, but no one was addressing the root cause. As a result, checks and balances were immediately created and a claims scrubber position was created for quality control. Revenue cycle management (RCM) monitoring reports and a key performance indicator (KPI) dashboard were also set up to give Dr. Marcus better insights in real-time. To this day, Marcus is now responsible for processing her mail as a final line of defense.

Revenue is the lifeblood of every business. Most hospitals, health systems, or physician groups under-collect because the rules are so complicated and difficult to understand. Getting paid can be akin to doing your taxes: one honest mistake can trigger an audit or a denial. Even worse, once the denial occurs, you only have so many days to appeal before the claim is considered past the filing timeline. And if that was not unsettling enough, too many denials and appeals might catch the attention of an auditor looking for fraud and abuse.

---

[1]Modifiers are added to the Healthcare Common Procedure Coding System (HCPCS) or Current Procedural Terminology (CPT®) codes to provide additional information necessary for processing a claim, such as identifying why a doctor or other qualified healthcare professional provided a specific service and procedure.

Healthcare margins are tighter than many other service-oriented businesses and, arguably, hampered by stringent regulations. Given the narrow margins in healthcare, the importance of the revenue cycle is no less valid in the operation of hospitals, physician groups, or health systems that employ physicians. Unfortunately, institutions continue to underinvest or underestimate the significance of diligence in revenue cycle management and its accompanying components. Through inactivity or neglect, the monitoring of the revenue cycle can often become a low priority in the operations of the business. In most cases, these issues surface after the fact and are usually compounded by a backlog of claims needing to be reworked. We cannot stress enough how critical it is to put all the effort into the front end of this process to ensure the claim gets sent out correctly. This extra effort will save countless hours on the backend and will dramatically increase the odds of getting paid on the first pass. The remainder of this chapter will address how we make this happen.

The revenue cycle ecosystem is complex and with many moving parts. Each part must be flawless, or it can cause a cascading series of issues. Take, for example, something as simple as entering the patient's date of birth (DOB) correctly. The payors use IT platforms to electronically process claims. These computer systems are used to lock on multiple patient identifiers to prevent fraud and abuse. So even if you have all the information entered correctly, but miss just one digit on the DOB, the claim will be rejected. So, as they say, the devil indeed *is* in the details. And let's be honest: this level of scrutiny is also built into the design as a way to delay payments to providers. Moreover, figures and reports do not always tell the entire story. More scrutiny may be necessary to determine an accurate picture. Further, if data reported to the executive suite and governance boards are inaccurate, miscalculated, or outright corrupt, the C-suite may not learn about the issues until revenue declines.

What may look like a sound days-in-accounts-receivable (AR) measurement (e.g., 30 days) can mask systemic problems in processes and procedures. For example, what if the days in AR look

great because someone is writing off claims as opposed to appealing them? **Important Tip:** Always prohibit write-offs without the approval of an owner no matter how small. These add up and should be investigated. Once you understand the reasons for the write-offs, you can develop policies to manage the prevention of having one in the first place. For example, if we know Blue Cross will only cover one wellness visit per year, you can develop a policy to prevent scheduling this type of visit more than once annually unless the patient wants to pay out of pocket. Or maybe the patient has other issues, and we need to code it accordingly and not default to a wellness visit unless it is truly a wellness visit. Most electronic health records (EHRs) can look for past visits and notify the scheduler if the visit type is approved based on the policy of the payor. The key here is to ALWAYS require these write-offs be approved by the owner of the practice. The owner will have the opportunity to not only have awareness but also adjust policies to prevent it from happening. Having knowledge and awareness is 90% of the battle.

As collecting and accurately tracking revenue grows increasingly complex, the need for monitoring and tracking becomes essential to remain financially viable. This is especially true as we move away from fee-for-service (FFS) and into value-based medicine.

Here are some proven methods for monitoring revenue performance:

- Auditing should NOT be a one-time annual activity. It needs to be done daily, weekly, monthly, quarterly, and yearly. This may sound excessive, but payors have designed denial policies that exploit our ability to act quickly. They know it can take weeks, if not months, before we can identify and respond to mistakes. Therefore, we must structure our efforts and policies to be as error-free as possible on the front end. Here are some key performance indicators that can help reduce mistakes.
  - Daily
    Daily reconciliation of patient to charges. Simply put, did you see a patient? Did the patient get charged?

Did the claim get billed? If you do not have a way to automate this, you can compare the sign-in sheet to the super-bills[2] at the end of the day to make sure each patient was charged for an office visit. This audit is also a great way to prevent fraud and abuse.

Knowing what collections are complete and what has and has not been billed

Compiling a list of prior past due balances before the patient arrives for their appointment.

Audit the deposit slips. This one is critical. The deposit slip will show all the money the office collected for the day. It should always match what is posted in the system. (You will most likely need to add the credit card totals to the deposit slip to get it to balance.)

– Weekly

Payment and procedure code analysis by the payor. This will tell you if the payor paid the charge in accordance with the contract.

Insurance aging report. This report shows you unpaid claims, by age, and by payor.

– Monthly

Patient statements. Just like the aging reports stated above, statements should be run monthly or bi-weekly.

Accumulative totals for major key performance indicators. Totals patients seen, total money collected, adjustments given, total bad debt write-offs, and charges/procedures posted. We recommend looking at this as a month-over-month trend and comparing it to the prior year.

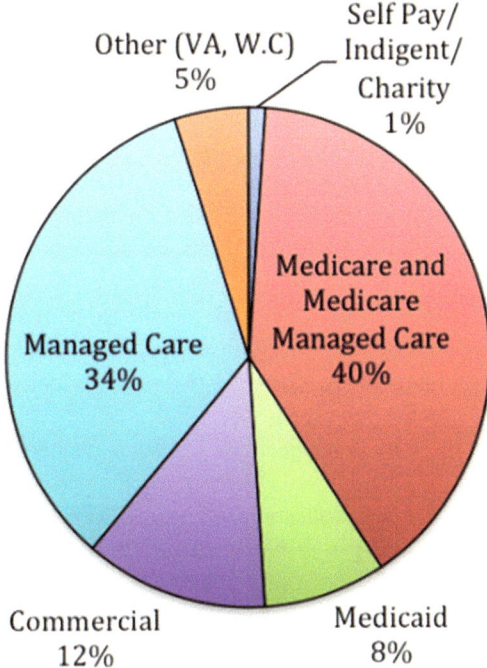

Fig. 4.1 Example payor mix

Report by procedure by every procedure code you billed during whatever time frame you are running it for. This will tell you how many you billed for and what the total charges are. The last page of the report gives you totals for all charges, payments, and adjustments.

– Accounts receivable and accounts receivable aging report by payor. We recommend two views of this report. The first is payer responsibility and the second is patient responsibility.

– Insurance analysis is one of the most important areas to monitor. We recommend organizing by payor mix to have insights into the revenue sources. If 80% of the revenue is coming from a single payor, this may be an indication the practice needs to diversify its income sources. Likewise, if you have too many plans, you may be missing an opportunity to compress into only participating in plans that are more provider-friendly. Fig 4.1 is an example of a payor mix chart.

___

[2]A superbill is a **detailed charge slip used to capture important billing information during a patient visit that is either given to the billing department or the patient so they can bill their insurance company.** It includes information similar to an insurance claim form, such as the date of the service provided, procedure codes, and a total balance due.

- Collections ratios are another key performance indicator that must be carefully monitored and managed. Practices that obsessively track their collection ratios can even predict seasonal trends. For example, collections are known to dip in the first quarter of each year due to deductibles starting over or patients changing health plans through their employers. This is when the front desk needs to increase efforts to verify insurance and collect deductibles. There are two ways to look at collection ratios:

    Gross Collections = Total Payment/ Charges × 100% for a specific period
    Net Collections = Total Payment/ Charges − Contractual Adjustments × 100% for a specific period

The net collection helps to reveal the amount of income your practice is collecting from the payer. But the gross collection rate only shows what your practice is allowed to collect. For example, you may have charged $200 but you only collected $175 from your insurance payer due to the agreement/contract. Here, the $175 is below the gross rate. Most practices look at net collections since it plays a major role in medical billing as it is the only way to calculate net income from various sources/payers. As a general rule, you should always look at collection ratios over a period of 90–120 days to get an average. Looking at one month alone can be misleading and may even appear grossly inaccurate. Keep in mind, payments received today were likely generated from charges in prior months, so to get a clear picture, this needs to be done over several months. According to Medical Group Management Association (MGMA), any ratio over 95% is considered best practice [1]. If collections appear off, do not panic: there could be a simple explanation. The most common cause happens when a provider is extremely busy for one month, then takes an extended vacation or leave the following month. Again, doing this over several months will average this out. The other causes could be more concerning and would require some investigation. In most cases, it would be caused by delays in reimbursement or a denial. If you see a major dip after hiring someone new for charge entry, this would be a major red flag. You can also expect dips in collections anytime you do a major IT upgrade or change billing platforms. You especially want to monitor carefully after any changes with an IT system that manages revenue.

- Having a paybook of the practice's financial transactions and accounts. An example of this would be a list of action items based on the age of the account. Examples include the following:
    - 0–30 days monitoring only
    - 30–60 days follow-up and investigate why payment has not arrived
    - 60 days start calling the patient or payor
    - 90 days appeal letters or collections

In medicine, the value of accounts receivable (AR) will dramatically decline over time. The cost to keep AR on the books can add up. Each time someone has to touch an account, there is a labor cost associated with that. There is also the cost of filing a claim, mail statements, and paying processing fees. In fact, you can even reach a point of diminishing returns if not resolved quickly. Again, monitoring and aggressive intervention are key.

- Performing full micro-level reviews of the revenue cycle. If a central business office (CBO) is involved in an employed model, we review both the CBO and front-end processes at the ambulatory practice level. A missing patient ID is clearly associated with careless registration. Considering how humans can make honest mistakes when it comes to accurate registration, many practices now rely on system-generated rules[3] to enforce the collection of data needed for getting paid. For example, the registration system can be configured

---

[3]An example of a system rule: Social security numbers must be 9 digits or the system will not advance to the next field.

in such a way that the end user cannot skip required fields. If they do, the system will know to suspend the claim until the information is entered. These required fields can dramatically decrease rejections. You can also set up rules that will alert a provider when a modifier is necessary to get paid and/or if a referral is needed. Practices that create these system-generated rules have far fewer denials.

- Reviewing data and providing analysis to benchmark to best in class. Did you know organizations such as MGMA and other trade associations track provider compensation and patient collection rates? These benchmarks can be useful tools for comparing performance. (Payor mix can throw off benchmarks, so you will want to make sure you are being compared to a similar-size practice, in the same market.)
- Identifying revenue opportunities due to lag days, charge capture, coding, inflated write-offs and accelerated accounts receivable capture. Example: Providers who do not capture charges on the same day of the visit will cause the lag time to increase. This is also referred to as the "days in AR," which measure the number of days to receive payment from the date of service. This is an important key performance indicator (KPI) because it will indicate how much cash on hand you will need to float all the expenses until you get paid for the services performed. High-performing practices will typically run for 30–40 days in AR. Entering and submitting charges on the same day of the visit will dramatically reduce your days in AR. It will also improve collection because it will be easier to address any billing issues before the patient leaves the office. It is also recommended to collect co-pays and co-insurance before the visit to avoid any unforeseen issues with collections once the services get rendered.
- Periodic examination of processes, policies, and procedures. RCM requires ongoing adaptation to new policies and payor rules necessary to get paid. Some of these policies such as the adoption of international classification of diseases, tenth revision (ICD-10) guidelines may require new rules for clinical documentation as well. If a provider is participating in shared savings or risk-based[4] contracts, the payor will likely require the submittal or data necessary to measure outcomes and quality improvement.

- Considering the interworking between practices and a CBO[5] model to ensure continuity, communication, and feedback.
- Reviewing staffing, staff fit, and management span of control. Did you know many people are NOT comfortable asking patients for money? You may have a staff member who is uncomfortable in this situation and would need to be utilized in a different role or helped with overcoming these feelings. The right person matters. This should be obvious but hiring inexperienced employees can be very costly. Practices not willing to pay a little extra to have someone with strong experience usually end up spending a lot more on missed opportunities and write-off mistakes.
- Knowing how to prioritize critical tasks is also key. For example, practices that perform a same-day charge entry usually have much lower days in AR because they do not wait to file the claim. This also allows them to resolve any billing issues on the day of the visit as opposed to waiting until later when the information is not as available. Providers must also be willing to enter their charges on the day of the visit. Here is little that can be done to improve collections if a provider is holding onto charges.
- Perform your own self-assessment on the following:
  - Revenue cycle management overview (policies, procedures, patient access management, RCM organizational structure, etc.)

---

[4]Risk-based **contracting** for population **health management is grounded in simple math. Healthcare** organizations that **exceed total medical spending targets for** these **contracts effectively absorb a** penalty. Those that keep expenses below these targets create savings they can keep. (Source: Health Catalyst).

[5]Central Business office allows for the consolidation of back-office functions such as payment posting, appealing claims, working denials, and patient collections.

- Clinic management structure
- RCM operational assessment

    Pre-visit functions (scheduling, pre-registration, patient financial clearance, insurance eligibility, and prior authorization, etc.)

    Patient visit/encounter functions (check-in, check-out, patient collection process, time-of-service collections, financial counseling, etc.)

    Post-service functions (charge capture, office, and outpatient services, hospital and facility services, charge lag, coding, claim submission, third-party insurance follow-up, etc.)

    Remittance processing, rejections/denial management (payment posting, employee metrics, rejections, denial management, credits/refunds, patient collections/statements/bad debt/collection agency, etc.)

- Practice technology (PMS, electronic medical record (EMR), etc.)
- Fee schedule/CDM (Industry average is 2× the Medicare allowable). For example, if Medicare reimbursement for a procedure is $100, the fee schedule is typically set at $200 (Double). This will increase write-off amounts, but it will ensure your fees stay above the allowable as some payors are allowed to pay the lesser of the two.
- Payor reimbursement tracking reports. These reports can determine if the level of payment matches the contracted rate down to the E&M[6] code.
- Mix Match Report will determine if a payment has been misapplied or posted to the wrong account. Most modern billing systems can automate this at the time of payment posting. It will alert the practice if a payment falls below the contracted allowable.[7]

- Audit payors and be aware of their tactics used to deny claims or lower reimbursement. One tactic is called "silent PPOs/HMOs." The payor will process a claim under whichever plan pays the provider the least. This happens when a provider is participating in several plans with the same payor. (e.g., BlueCross health maintenance organization (HMO), BlueCross, preferred provider organization (PPO), BlueCross Commercial, BlueCross High Deductible). The patient may have BlueCross PPO, but the claim is paid under the HMO contract (hence the name, silent HMO). This can be detected by running reports and comparing payments to the contracted rates.

Here are several examples of red flags that should trigger additional investigation:

- *Days in accounts receivable* are declining, even though there are *a significant number of claims pending release to a specific payer.*
- *Lack of validation that claims are being paid* based on current negotiated contracts or allowable schedules.
- Inability to *reconcile services rendered to charges entered* and claims released.
- The claims clearinghouse reports *a significant number of paper claims* submitted.
- Claim denials are increasing, particularly due to *exceeding timely filing limits.*
- Lack of a system *super-user* to keep current on updates and provide staff orientation and ongoing training.

Red flags that may be a sign of fraud:

- **Important:** The patient seen does not match the patient sign-in sheet or schedule. This could be an indication of fraud.
- **Important:** End-of-day receipts do not match the bank deposit slip, including credit card totals. Only the owner of the practice should be taking the deposits to the bank.
- **Important:** Patient was seen, but the charge ticket is missing. This could be another indication of fraud.
- **Important:** Invoices from unknown vendors may be fake. Office managers have been

---

[6]Evaluation and management (E/M) coding is the use of CPT® codes from the range 99,202–99,499 to represent services provided by a physician or other qualified healthcare professionals.

[7]The allowable is the amount the payor has agreed to pay for a service per the contract.

known to create fake vendor invoices as a method of fraud.

- **Important:** Patient who is using a stolen insurance card. These patients are usually unwilling to provide a photo ID.
- **Important:** Patient asking you to go to a website to download their insurance information. This is likely a cybercriminal looking to trick the front deck into downloading a virus.
- **Important:** Staff members who never take any time off work and/or is overly protective about sharing information or control. The practice should always set up checks and balances. For example, you should never allow the same person to check-in and check-out the same patient. Separating these duties will prevent fraud.
- **Important:** Taking insurance only from a Medicare patient is considered fraud.
- **Important:** Doing a professional courtesy discount or write-off is frowned upon by most payers. Medicare considers it fraud.
- **Important:** Do NOT unbundle charges that are approved by one procedure.
- **Important:** Billing a Medicare patient for non-covered services without a signed waiver.
- **Important:** Not collecting co-pays is usually a direct violation of the payor contract.

Back to the Case

Marcus realized that paying attention to the revenue cycle was a critical component to running a successful practice. He decided to hire a management company to assist with billing, collection, and HR. Although this would cost money, Marcus realized that this move would create a significant return on investment.

The key to revenue cycle management is having strong controls and monitoring. The management of claims and receivables is the lifeblood of a practice and is often the leading cause of why some practices end up in the red having not been managed properly. All of these opportunities described are interrelated, and it can be challenging to determine how to prioritize, quantify, and address multiple issues. This is where it can pay off to seek out professional guidance and support from an outside expert to gain more knowledge on how to manage the practice. Unfortunately, day-to-day operations, personnel/provider management, and addressing patient issues often can distract or take priority over a thorough operational performance review. Gain, we would encourage you to hire highly qualified staff and/or a management company that can provide this support. The extra investment in this area will generally yield a strong return on investment of time and money, but more importantly, it will usually flag the gaps that may have hindered your deserved success.

Reference

1. MGMA. Unlocking and using practice performance intelligence. Medical Group Management Association. 2018. https://www.mgma.com/event-registration/mgma18-the-financial-conference/session-handouts/con501-unlocking-and-using-practice-performance-in.

Case Sherri

Sherri is in her final year of her Maternal Fetal Medicine Fellowship and has received her first job offer in a large inner-city Obstetrics and Gynecology Practice. Sherri first learned of this position through a recruiting firm that sent her an email 3 months ago. Sherri spoke on the phone with the recruiter who connected her with the Medical Director of the practice. Following her interview, Sherri felt that this practice was a good fit for her; it was large enough that call would not be onerous, the patient population included medically underserved patients who she like to care for, she liked the other physicians and office staff and had a good vibe about the work environment, and the practice was in a city where she had friends and family. In reviewing her job offer, she was a bit overwhelmed. Although the salary was more money than she thought she would ever earn, was it fair? Sherri had over $300,000 in educational debt and there was no provision to help her pay for some of her loans, a benefit that she knew others in her fellowship program had been offered with other practices. There was no provision for continuing medical education (CME) and license expenses.

Sherri wondered what was negotiable? She was not really comfortable asking for more money. Should she hire an employment lawyer? Sherri wished she were in the where at least she would have an agent to help her negotiate.

Contracts

A contract is a legal agreement, typically between two parties. Although contracts can be verbal, they are almost always written such that all parties in the contract are protected legally and so that there are no misunderstandings between the parties of the contract. The parties of the contract are the entities involved in the agreement. The Terms and Conditions of the contract spell out the rights and responsibilities of each party in the contract. Terms and Conditions often include legal remedies that parties can use if there is a suspected breach in the contract.

Basically, a contract has three parts: offer, acceptance, and consideration. An offer is a promise to provide something to a promisor, acceptance is an agreement by the promisee to abide by the contract, and consideration is a legal concept that involves the bargaining for a quid pro quo that provides a benefit to the promisee and a detriment to the promisor. For example, if I tell you that I am going to give you $100 and then renege, this is not a contract as there is no consideration. There is no exchange of promise. On the other hand, if I tell you that I will give you $100 for cleaning my gutters and you accept my offer, then this is a contract. If you do not provide the services agreed upon, then I have legal recourse. In this example, there is the offer to clean gutters; acceptance of my proposed fee; and consideration, the exchange of fee for services.

Very few physicians enter solo practice nowadays. Because most physicians are employed by a group, hospital, or educational institution, most physicians receive and negotiate an employment contract. Physician employment contracts are both similar and different from other employment contracts. Because most physicians have limited experience with contract law, it is always prudent to have employment contracts reviewed by a legal expert who is representing your best interests. This is firm advice and hiring an attorney is money well spent. In many academic practices, an "offer letter" is substituted for a formal contract. From a legal perspective, assuming verbiage in the offer letter spells out that the letter is binding, offer letters are really a type of contract. Academic practices sometimes use offer letters because of the assumption that they are less formal and less subject to close legal scrutiny. Be careful, however, with offer letters and make sure that as with an employment contract, you do not agree to something that you will later regret. Alternatively, some offer letters may not be binding and are sometimes more like "letters of intent" that merely propose initial terms for the eventual formal contract. In this case, physicians should use caution in accepting the offer prior to seeing the formal contract.

Employment contracts should stipulate a start and end date and should specify the renewal process. The process for terminating the contract should be clearly articulated. Provisions for malpractice insurance after the physician have left the practice should be clearly articulated. This is called *gap* or *tail insurance*. Sometimes this type of insurance is provided by the employer, sometimes it requires the physician to pay out-of-

pocket for such coverage. In any rate, it is important for physicians to understand how they are covered for possible malpractice cases arising after the employment term has ended.

The major focus of a physician employment contract is the stipulated compensation. Compensation takes the form of salary, benefits, and incentive pay. Physician salaries depend on specialty, location, experience, demand, and a host of other factors. This makes comparison between offers difficult and may limit the ability to negotiate a salary. Typically, after the first year of employment, physician salaries include some portion that is "at risk" in the sense that it is related to productivity. This at-risk portion is typically dependent on work relative value units (RVUs), charges, and/or collections. Because collections depend on a number of variables including payor mix, ability of the practice to bill and collect for services, and contracts signed with third party payors, incentive pay based solely on collections may not accurately reward hard work. As such, inventive pay that also includes work generated (RVUs) is preferable. Benefits typically include health insurance, vision and dental insurance, malpractice insurance, money for CME and licenses, vacation, sick leave, and disability insurance. Additionally, maternity and paternity leave may be offered as a benefit. More recently, because of the student debt that young physicians have acquired, loan repayment can be benefit. Many practices also offer a signing bonus and money for relocation. Because this money may be considered salary, there may be tax implications that should be understood prior to signing the contract.

One peculiarity of physician employment contracts is the issue of *restrictive covenants*. These are also called non-compete clauses and are used to prohibit a physician from practicing in a certain geographic area for a set period of time in the case of termination or separation. Restrictive covenants are important to a group practice because they prevent a former employee to leave and take patients away from the practice to then compete with the original group. Restrictive covenants can be difficult to enforce in some jurisdictions as they represent restriction of trade. It is important to have restrictive covenants closely reviewed by an employment lawyer and if part of the final contract, the geographic limitation should be limited in radius and the time restriction should be as short as possible.

Another issue specific to a physician employment contract is the issue of partnership. Partnership is a commitment to partial ownership of the practice. Unlike having equity in a commercially traded company, partnership is illiquid in that it is difficult to value, nearly impossible to sell, and may carry the obligation on part of the physician partner to cover any shortfalls in practice income with personal income. Typically, partnership is a benefit offered after several years of employment and typically becoming a partner involves a series of payments or salary offsets over several additional years until partnership is achieved. Another complication of partnership is the distribution of ownership. Is it equal across the group, or is the majority of the ownership held by those who entered the partnership first, the senior partners? The compensation differences, and distribution of equity in the partnership between junior and senior partners should be clearly articulated prior to signing a contract.

Finally, the employment contract should specify what happens if the group is acquired by another party or in the event of a merger or consolidation. This type of clause is called "assignability." If the employment contract remains in place after merger or acquisition, then it is assignable. If the contract is null and void in case of such an event, then it is non-assignable. The contract should offer a remedy to the physician in the case of non-assignability. This could include release from the non-compete clause or a financial pay out to the physician whose contract was voided by change in ownership.

Negotiation

Most physicians have had little training in the art of negotiation. Some physicians assume that nothing is negotiable and accept an initial contract as is, whereas some feel that everything is negotiable. Basic negotiation skills are obviously

important, especially when negotiating your starting salary as this is the amount that all future increases will be based upon. A 3% increase on $300,000 is more money than a 3% increase on $200,000.

More than anything else, a successful negotiation depends on having *information*. If you know what others are getting paid for the same job, you know your negotiation point. Luckily, especially in academic medicine, salary information is available. The Association of American Medical Colleges (AAMC) publishes annually salary information divided by specialty, geographic region of the country, public/private medical school, and faculty rank. This data is not self-reported but is gathered from business offices of medical school ensuring its accuracy. Additionally, many states such as Nevada have sunshine laws making all salaries of public employees available to the public. As such, the salary of any faculty member at a state school may be available online. For non-academic jobs, Medscape publishes salary information that is gathered from survey responses. Other survey-derived data comes from the American Medical Group Association (AMGA), the Medical Group Management Association (MGMA), Merritt Hawkins, and the US Bureau of Labor and Statistics Occupational Employment Statistics. Care should be used when interpreting self-reported data as physicians who report salaries are more likely to be those on the higher end of the spectrum. Obviously, this type of salary information is absolutely critical at the beginning of any salary negotiation. It is also important to gather other information about the practice prior to negotiation including the degree of competition for patients from other groups, the patient payor mix, and expected work schedules including call.

A successful negotiation involves give and take on both sides and results in an outcome that is usually not perfect for either side but is mutually beneficial to all parties. As such, be prepared to make concessions and when asking the other side to do so, treat people with respect, be patient, and have logical reasons for your requests. Again, use the information you have gathered before the negotiation to make your points. When you are negotiating, set priorities. Identify your limits and identify those things that you could concede if necessary. Develop a strategy. What could you give up and in exchange for what else? Start off with an easy issue, like office space. Then build up to harder negotiating points such as salary or partnership. Finally, return to issues that are likely not to be contentious like vacation time so that both you and your employer can feel good about the negotiation. After most of the bargaining is done, return to those last unresolved issues like restrictive covenants. These trickier issues will be easier to negotiate once both sides have a feeling for each other and both sides have a vested interest in a successful resolution.

Lastly, in the interest of all parties, get your final negotiated contract in writing including all concessions on both sides. Although both sides may negotiate in good faith, anything not written is difficult to prove, especially if there is a change in personnel in the group.

specialty society about benefit packages offered to new graduates. Sherri was not able to negotiate her starting salary but was able to negotiate a signing bonus. The practice had never offered a loan repayment program and was uncomfortable about the tax ramifications of such a benefit. Sherri conceded this issue but was able to negotiate a more generous family leave arrangement, important to her as she thought about starting a family. When Sherri reviewed the contract, she realized that little things like money for CME and licenses were included. She got her contract in writing and hired an attorney friend to review it. Sherri really wanted the job offered as it met so many of her personal and professional needs, so she was less in charge of the negotiation, but in the end, she felt satisfied and comfortable that her first job would be a good fit.

Back to the Case

Sherri gathered information including the salaries offered by other practices to the three other fellows completing her program. She was able to find cost of living conversions for different cities in the United States and was able to derive a fair range of salary for a starting Maternal-Fetal Medicine specialist in her new city. She also was able to get information from her

Bottom Line

1. A contract is a legal document. Get everything in writing and have a legal professional review prior to signing.
2. Do not be afraid to negotiate. Gather information, stay calm, and have a rationale for your asks.
3. Negotiations involve compromise. Identify your limits from the onset. Use your ability to compromise to get the things you really need.

Case Mendel
Mendel was a fellowship-trained surgeon. He was negotiating to join a large multi-specialty practice. The sticking point in his contract was the restricted covenant. The covenant prevented him from practicing within 50 miles for 5 years after leaving the practice, if he decided to leave. Mendel wasn't sure what to do.

Restrictive covenants, or non-compete clauses, are commonly found in contracts and are legal in most states. Restrictive covenants protect the practice that hires a new physician from financial loss. The covenant seeks to prevent the loss of patients from the practice if the newly hired physician should leave the practice but remain in the area. Nevertheless, restrictive covenants should be avoided since they can produce considerable hardship, including financial loss. This chapter will provide an overview of restricted covenants and the options if the clause can't be removed from the contract.

Almost every physician will sign an employment contract in their career. And those contracts include all confusing language, legal jargon, and specific terms, most of which a practicing physician can't decipher.

Physician contracts include details on salary, benefits, and the physician's responsibilities. Most physician employment contracts also include restrictive covenants.

What are Restrictive Covenants?

Restrictive covenants impose restrictions upon the doctor\employee to protect the employer's business interests. These are common in employment agreements and contracts in various industries, including medicine and healthcare.

The restrictive covenant often includes:

- Non-compete clauses.
- Geographical restrictions limit where the doctor leaving a practice is allowed to work.
- Protection of confidential information.
- Non-solicitation agreements.

The U.S. Supreme Court interprets Article IV of the Constitution as giving all citizens the right to travel. They also side with an individual's right to practice their trade or profession.

Where you live and practice medicine can significantly affect the enforceability of the restrictions your employer may impose on you. Nine states have near or total bans on restrictive covenants, spurred, in part, by the Supreme Court's interpretation. However, in some places, they are enforceable through state laws.

We suggest that young physicians understand restrictive covenants while still training. By knowing about these restricted covenant clauses, the doctor protects themselves when it's time to sign that first employment contract.

Restrictive covenants allow medical practices and hospitals to protect their interests. These covenants can help the employer retain patients and key relationships. The purpose of a restricted covenant clause is to protect the employer's financial interests. Also, they can prevent physicians from taking patients with them when they leave. These covenants do not benefit the physician or the employee. They exist only to benefit the employer.

Types of Restrictive Covenants

The four most common restrictive covenants are:

Non-Compete

The non-compete clause is the most common type. The non-compete is a way for your employer to ensure that you will be loyal to them. If you see this term in your contract, it usually means that you are not allowed to work for anyone else while you work for this employer.

This clause restricts you from working for other practices or other medical systems at the same time. It ensures that your entire focus will be on their hospital, their patients, and their interests.

The non-compete clause is standard in contracts for hospitals and large medical groups.

A cardiologist, oncologist, or obstetrician may have a loyal group of patients who want to follow their physician wherever they go. Your patients will probably be willing to see you wherever you work.

Geographic Limitations

Your patients may be loyal, but if you move from New York to Oregon, they probably won't fly across the country to see you. But if you transfer to a hospital only a few miles away, they likely will.

For this reason, many physician contracts prohibit you from working within a radius of a specified number of miles from where the doctor was previously employed for a specified period.

Depending on the stipulations in your contract, you could be looking at a lengthy commute or moving to a new town.

Non-Solicitation

No employer on earth would be happy if you left them, went to work for a competitor, and took your clients/customers/patients with you. Hospitals and healthcare systems are no different.

Many physician contracts include a non-solicitation agreement. These usually say that you cannot take your patients or employees of the practice\hospital with you if you leave. The contract may also prohibit you from soliciting referrals from referring physicians.

If this covenant is enforced and the doctors leaving are prohibited from taking patients with them, it means starting and building a new roster of patients that you don't know and that don't know you.

Non-solicitation restrictions have their limits. They prevent you from trying to convince or coerce patients to move with you to your new hospital or medical practice. But they don't restrict a physician's right to retain patients that seek them out on their own.

You can still advertise and employ general marketing strategies to create new business. If your old patients choose to follow you, they may.

But you might not have access to patients' medical records. However, the patients may access their medical records, take them with them, and select any physician they choose.

Without-Cause Termination

For cause termination of a physician employment agreement means the employee breached the agreement. An employer could terminate the agreement for cause if the other party didn't do what it was supposed to do or did something it wasn't permitted (see Chap. 5 on contracts). The restrictive covenant that can have the most immediate and damaging effect on your career is the without-cause termination of employment.

Without-cause termination means you can be fired or removed from your position for any reason or *no reason*. You don't have to break any rules or violate your contract to be terminated. Your employer has the sole discretion to let you go at any time.

If your contract includes this restrictive covenant, ensure it consists of a few specific details. We suggest you not sign a contract unless it specifies how many days in advance you need to be notified of your termination.

If your contract includes a without-cause termination agreement, it might also have a non-compete clause that says you can't work within a 20-mile radius of the former employer for 2 years. To not violate a non-compete clause, you'll need your without-cause termination agreement to provide you with plenty of advanced notice.

You don't want to find yourself in a situation where the employment relationship ends at a moment's notice. If you are terminated *and* prevented from practicing within your geographic area that can be a double whammy.

Leverage Your Experience to Eliminate Restrictive Covenants

Like all elements in your contract, restrictive covenants are negotiable. But you may be able to negotiate new ones if they still benefit the employer. For example, knowing what triggers those restrictive covenants to go into effect is essential. Ideally, you only want them to go into effect if you are terminated *with cause*.

For example, if a hospital hires you and then experiences a decline in patient volume, the hospital may let you go. This situation might not be your fault, and you shouldn't be penalized or prevented from practicing elsewhere.

There could also be circumstances where your hospital no longer provides the services you specialize in. In that situation, your non-compete should not apply.

For example, if you are an obstetrician and your hospital no longer offers obstetrical services, it is not your fault. Make sure your restrictive covenants have limitations that protect you from unusual occurrences.

With experience and strong negotiation skills, it is possible to make your covenants less restrictive. Few physicians have contract negotiating skills, and you can avail yourself of a contract attorney who specializes in healthcare contracts and is knowledgeable about employment laws in the state where you work. We recommend that a professional review it before signing an employment contract. Contract review specialists will do much more than look at your restrictive covenants. They'll look at all aspects of your physician employment agreement, including salary, benefits, and on-call responsibilities. Once you sign an employment contract, it will be too late to negotiate terms and make changes.

The American Medical Association (AMA) and Restrictive Covenants

The American Medical Association (AMA) says in its code of medical ethics that:

"Covenants-not-to-compete restrict competition, can disrupt the continuity of care, and may limit access to care."

They recommend that physicians be cautious of restrictive agreements that unreasonably restrict:

- Periods of time
- Geographic scope
- Reasonable accommodation of patient choices

The best way to protect yourself from restrictive covenants is to hire a contract review specialist. They will review all the details of your contract before you sign it. A contract review specialist will know if your restrictive covenants are legitimate and common in your state. If they are excessive, they will know.

In addition, a contract review specialist can identify if anything is missing from your contract. For example, non-competes and geographical limitations should only go into effect for with-cause termination. A contract specialist can quickly identify if those clauses and terms are missing.

Back to the Case

Mendel obtained the services of a contract employment specialist. Mendel was asked to sign an employment contract with a geographic limitation of a radius of 25 miles from the address of his employment. Mendel agreed to the stipulation, but he would be able to allow patients to follow him to any new location.

Bottom Line

Restrictive covenants are typical in employment contracts, especially physician contracts. You must understand what they are and know how they will affect your future career.

Look for physician non-compete clauses, geographic limitations, non-solicitation agreements, and without-cause termination agreements. One or more of these clauses can significantly impact your career and cause long-term damage to your career and your reputation.

Case Chris

Chris has been Chair of the Department of Radiology at a community hospital for the past 3 years. When the former chair retired, Chris was considered the best candidate to become chair. Chris had the ability to get along with others, had excellent leadership skills, and had seniority in the department. Although Chris has always prided herself on her interpersonal skills, shortly after assuming the role of Chair, she began to have problems with two of her junior colleagues who both started in the department 2 months prior to Chris' appointment as chair. The two junior associates graduated from the same residency program and had been friends for several years. Chris' difficulties began with the holiday schedule during her first year as chair. Neither of the associates agreed to take call during Christmas, a role typically reserved for junior members in the group. Chris ended up covering the Christmas holiday herself, but problems escalated. Chris finds her decisions continually questioned and feels that she is not respected by the two junior associates. She is worried that her role as chair will be undermined and concerned that her position may be in jeopardy. Chris has discussed her feelings with the two junior physicians, but there was no resolution. She prefers not to terminate them, but is having second thoughts about renewing their contracts for the upcoming year. What should she do?

Leadership is often discussed but rarely taught during a physician's educational journey. Although there are people who are naturally skilled at being leaders, many aspects of becoming a successful leader can be taught and reinforced even for people who are naturally good leaders. It is our experience that most physicians have modest (?) leadership abilities that they have used to their advantage to get into and succeed in college, and medical school, and successfully complete post-graduate training. However, many physicians are uncomfortable taking charge of personnel issues, especially when they pertain to disciplining and terminating an employee.

The primary driver of effective personnel management is the strength of the leader. Although there are many leadership styles described in the business literature, we suggest some common leadership principles that are necessary regardless of an individual manager's style. We suggest that effective leaders possess the following four attributes: integrity, accountability, vision, and communication skills.

Integrity implies that a leader acts ethically, fairly, and consistently. An effective leader is aspirational and someone who others want to emulate. Many of us entered the medical field inspired by people like Albert Schweitzer, C. Everett Koop, William Osler, Benjamin Spock, or even Marcus Welby. Part of integrity is the ability to provide the sense that a group is better with the leader in charge than without. Those who lead with integrity allow others to feel important; they do not abuse power. They allow others to receive rewards and do not hoard accolades. They are not capricious; they make calculated consistent decisions that are considered fair.

Accountability assumes that the leader not only takes responsibility for their own decisions but also takes responsibility for any consequences that their decisions produce. Effective leaders not only hold themselves personally accountable but are also able to instill a sense of accountability in their communications to the group or the organization. This includes motivating others to complete projects on time, maintaining respect for timelines, and working for the betterment of the team, not merely for the benefit of the leader.

Accountability is well demonstrated by the following example: In previous times, while playing poker, a knife with a buckhorn handle was often used to indicate whose turn it was to deal the cards. A player had the option, to "pass the buck" if they wished to pass the deal to the next player at the table. Passing the buck subsequently became a metaphor in international politics when countries refused to address a threat or concern with the hope that another country would deal with the problem. "The buck stops here" is a phrase attributed to President Harry S. Truman who kept a sign on his desk with this motto. Truman would refer to this motto often: "You know, it's easy for the Monday morning quarterback to say what the coach should have done, after the game is over. But when the decision is up before you—… the buck stops here."

Vision is the ability to develop and articulate goals and a plan for reaching them. Vision implies a balance between what is possible and what is practical. To quote Eric Hoffer, "The leader has to be practical and a realist, yet must talk the language of the visionary and the idealist." Truly visionary leaders are unusual and not always effective, especially if they are thought to be unrealistic. An example of a visionary leader is Steve Jobs whose vision for Apple computer was at times unrealistic and unmanageable, but whose vision leads to one of the most successful companies in the history of humankind.

Communication is essential in a leader who hopes to capitalize on the collective wisdom of the team. Seldom are leaders successful in isolation. Rather, in order to be effective, leaders need to develop teams that share information and learn from each other. Effective leaders foster communication, encourage dissent and discourse, and empower others to feel comfortable about contributing ideas for the betterment of the group. Effective leaders know how to listen and are consistent with their message. In the world of social media, there are now multiple avenues for effective communication. The use of social media will be specifically discussed in Chap. 21. Effective leaders use a palate of tools to communicate a consistent message.

Jack Welch served as CEO of General Electric (GE) for many years and his communication skills are legendary. Welch believed that if his company could not be number 1 or number 2 in any product line, that they should get out of that market space. A great example of Welch's ability to communicate this vision is the story of a consumer survey asking who made the best gas ovens. The survey revealed that GE came in second, although they did not even make a gas oven! Welch's communication skills put GE in everyone's mind when thinking about appliances, regardless of whether or not they were even in that market space. Welch's ability to communicate and articulate what GE was as a company created a halo effect whereby consumers were so impressed with their electrical appliances that they felt that they must also make great gas appliances even though these were not in their product line.

Medicine is practiced in teams, and in addition to having an effective leader, effective teams need to work together. The first part of working together is for the team to trust each other. Trust implies a sense of openness among team members and the lack of any one member feeling vulnerable. If a team has a culture of trust, then the team will embrace conflict. Conflict is not always a bad thing in that discourse leads to better decision making through the generation of diverse opinions and ideas to better solve problems.

A great example of the value of diverse opinions is the story of Tabasco hot sauce. Allegedly, the executives at Tabasco were trying to increase their market share. Ideas from the group included marketing Tabasco in Asia where spicy foods are appreciated, or creating a Tabasco cookbook, and even creating new products such as corn chips that contained Tabasco sauce. Apparently, one executive thought differently and offered the idea that to sell more hot sauce, the company should double the width of the bottle opening. The rest is history. This simple idea of increasing the diameter of the bottle opening significantly increased sales.

Trust and welcoming conflict allow teams to feel a sense of commitment to the organization. Committed groups act to the betterment of the organization. Commitment leads to accountability, whereby all members act to further the mission of the group and call out those individuals who are not acting in the group's best interests. Accountability leads to achieving collective results which do not benefit any one person, but work to improve the final product of the organization.

In managing people, the above steps are a necessary progression to achieve buy-in and to obtain the best results. But what do you do when people do not behave?

The first step is to listen. Listen to the employee in question. Listen to other employees who have complaints. Listen to patients. Through listening, you will gather information to help you better understand the situation. The fault may be with the employee or it may be a structural problem. Physicians who do not complete medical records on time are not bad people, rather, this is typically the fault of a faulty system or an electronic health record program that is cumbersome to use or does not provide feedback that charts need to be signed.

Next, give clear feedback. Feedback is best when it focuses on behaviors rather than results. This prevents subjectivism. For example, rather than complaining that an employee always comes in late for work, focus on the behavior and mention that when the receptionist comes in late, phones are not answered, and patient problems are not addressed in a timely manner, the daily schedule may be delayed, and morale among the other employees declines. Feedback should also focus on the impact the negative behavior has on the organization. In the above example, that impact would be bad customer service which impacts patient satisfaction, and ultimately patient outcomes. Finally, effective feedback should focus on the consequences of the deviant behavior. "When you don't complete your medical records in a timely fashion, we don't get paid." For effective feedback, *focus on behaviors, focus on the impact these behaviors have, and focus on the consequences of the behavior.* In addition to these three primary features, feedback should be specific, accurate, unbiased, usable, timely, and welcomed (perhaps replace welcomed with understood) by the recipient.

Always document the problems you are having with an employee. A record of bad behaviors is essential if your actions may result in dismissal. Careful documentation may prevent a costly lawsuit for wrongful termination.

Be consistent. Set policies and hold everyone accountable for these policies.

Set consequences and timelines. Make it clear to a poorly performing employee that there are consequences to behaviors. Set limits on when you expect improvements and set milestones for improvement.

Take action. Sometimes, as unpleasant as it might be, an employee may not be right for your organization. It is better for the whole team to replace that individual. Typically, other employees speak negatively about the errant employee. The leader should avoid at all costs talking adversely about another member of the staff or another physician even if the employee was terminated. This makes the leader look weak and creates distrust among other employees who fear that you may be talking badly of them to other staff members.

Back to the Case

Chris met with her two junior associates. She clearly articulated what the group's expectations were for them. She listened to their opinion on the situation regarding the two junior associates. She recognized that she was not communicating well. She explained the history of the department and the fact that junior associates were not only respected but were an important part of the team and that the practice always required that junior associates take call on holidays. Ultimately, the junior associates would eventually benefit from fewer calls on holidays as they matured in the department. Chris agreed to have more regular meetings with the department to articulate strategy and vision and to allow a forum to voice complaints. Unfortunately, over the next 2 years, her two junior associates became less and less willing to work as a team. They eventually decided to start their own practice. Fortunately, the "divorce" was mutual and collegial. Their departure did save Chris from the uncomfortable situation of having to fire them directly.

Bottom Line

1. In managing people, first develop your own leadership skills
2. Conflict can be used to make better decisions
3. Sometimes, an employee has to be terminated. This may be best for the employee, the group, and patients. (The concept of firing an employee will be discussed in greater detail in Chap. 15 regarding legal requirements for terminating an employee or a partner.

Case Jamal

Jamal is 40-years old and about to complete his neurosurgery residency. Jamal was a non-traditional medical student, starting medical school after working for a start-up in the biotech industry for nearly a decade. During medical school, his wife worked as a labor and delivery nurse. He and his wife had a baby daughter when medical school started. Although Jamal has medical school debt of nearly $300,000, he does have $40,000 saved in a 401 K from his previous employer. He already signed a contract for a job with a large multispecialty group practice. His contract includes a signing bonus of $50,000 along with $10,000 to be used towards moving and other related expenses. His initial salary is guaranteed for one year at $550,000. After one year, and for the next 3 years, his salary includes a $400,000 guarantee and bonus to be paid based on his clinical productivity. Although his employer will not be contributing towards his retirement for the first 2 years, however, after 2 years, his employer will match his contributions up to 10% of his take-home pay to a retirement plan. The benefit package provided by his employer includes life and disability insurance, health insurance for him and the ability to purchase health insurance for his family at a reasonable cost, and an allowance for CME. Jamal is happy to be finally finishing residency and earning real money. He is concerned that he has not really paid attention to things like life insurance and how to put money away for retirement and wants to make sure that he can retire by age 65. He is anxious and in need of advice.

Physicians are typically in the top 5% of wage earners in the United States and physicians in specialties like neurosurgery can easily be in the top 1% of wage earners. Despite this fact, many physicians find themselves ill-equipped to manage their money due to lack of expertise and training. It is very prudent, if not essential, for physicians to solicit the help of a financial planner. The earlier a physician establishes a relationship with a financial planner, the better because of compounded interest that was discussed in Chap. 2. In addition to a financial planner, it is also important for a physician to have an accountant. Even though doctors can do their own taxes, the time spent doing this is probably worth more than an accountant will cost. Additionally, an accountant signature on a tax return is reassuring. Even with a financial planner, understanding some basic investment strategies will allow for a more fruitful relationship with a financial planner.

One of the fundamental tenets of investment is the relationship between risk and reward. This means that the *greater risk an investor is willing to take, the higher the potential reward, and the higher the potential loss.* An example of the relationship between risk and reward is the story of the Beardstown Ladies who were featured in both the lay press and television[1]. This group, composed of older women in Illinois, formed an investment club known formally as the Beardstown Business and Professional Women's Investment Club in 1983. This group achieved notoriety for its returns on investment of over 23% per year for their first 10 years of activity, greatly exceeding average market returns. These women even wrote a book titled, "Beardstown Ladies' Common-Sense Investment Guide." Based on the concept of risk and reward, returns this high would suggest that this investment group assumed a high level of risk, or that they were extremely lucky. However, neither explanation appeared to be the case in a review of their portfolio. Rather, when audited, it appeared that the group did not properly account for returns, as they included new contributions to the fund by members in the group in their calculation of total return on investment. When properly audited and accounted for, the group was found to have a rate of return of only 9%, which is nearly 5% less that the return on the S&P for that same time period. This finding is consistent with another investment concept which asserts that the average investor will earn an average rate of return. This means that the only way to consistently beat the market average in an investment portfolio would be to either have unusual luck, to have improperly accounted for earnings, as in the case of the Beardstown Ladies, or to have insider information which will land you in jail. In fact, in a perfect market, factors affecting stock prices are already figured into its cost. When Amazon first started operations, the financial benefit to FedEx who shipped their products was theoretically already accounted for in the FedEx stock price. For those who have trouble believing that over time, they cannot beat the market average,

because they have a "better broker" or because they are a "better investor," Consider 100 people standing in a room each holding a penny. They flip their coins in unison and sit down when the flip landed on tails. At some point, someone is left standing. Are they a "better" coin flipper than all of the others? Certainly not!

Another important tenet of investing is the concept of diversification which can help to mitigate risk. For example, consider an investor who owns stock in an airline company. This investor is at risk if oil prices rise, because then his stock will lose value since the major expense of an airline is its fuel costs. To diversify, this investor may want to also purchase stock in an oil company. This will provide a hedge against rising oil prices, thus decreasing the value of his airline company stock. If he invests in oil companies, he will be financially protected due to the increased value of his oil company stock. Similarly, if oil prices fall, the value of his oil company stock will decrease, but his airline stock will provide a financial hedge against such a rise in oil prices. Diversification can be accomplished by owning stocks in multiple economic sectors, or by owning stocks in different areas of the world.

We have spent time using stocks as examples, but what exactly is stock? Simply stated, stock represents ownership or equity in a company. Suppose your family owns a company that makes chocolates. The shareholders in this family business are you and your relatives. Suppose further that the chocolate business is becoming increasingly successful such that the company wishes to expand to a national market. This is going to require a significant amount of cash for additional equipment, supplies, employees, and marketing. Where can you obtain the additional funds? You could ask the shareholders to contribute personal money towards the expansion. Alternatively, you could sell part ownership in the company to investors. This part ownership is stock and when companies do this on a large scale it is known as going public. Shareholders are able to vote on company policies as they are part owners.

Stock price is dependent on many variables but because stocks are traded publicly, there is a market that determines the stock price. The return on investment for a stock purchase is related to the riskiness of the stock itself with the rate of return being the same for all stocks of equal risk. Owning stock carries financial risk because if a company goes bankrupt, the stock may be worth nothing. Some stocks pay dividends which are periodic cash payments to shareholders. Some stocks never pay dividends. As with all stock prices, the value of a stock that pays dividends is incorporated into the stock price. This particular type of stock is known as common stock. There is another type of stock called preferred stock, which obtains its name because in case of bankruptcy, preferred stockholders are paid before common stockholders. However, unlike common stock, preferred stockholders do not really have equity (ownership) of the company and do not have voting rights. As such, preferred stock can be thought of as a type of debt. Because preferred stock is less risky, its rate of return is generally less than common stock.

Generally, if a stock is undervalued, you should buy it. On the other hand, if a stock is overvalued, you should sell it. But suppose we believe the stock is overvalued and we do not own it? A short sale refers to selling overvalued stock that you do not have at a later date. This type of investment is legal but risky because if you are wrong, and the stock price increases, you have to provide the stock at the higher price even though it was priced lower at the time of the transaction. The finance pages often include stories about people who made money in the stock market in the face of a steep decline. Typically, these people are said to have shorted the market. What they did was to sell stock that they did not own at an inflated price only to later purchase the stock at a discounted price, then sell the stock to the buyer at the higher price, and pocket the difference as a profit. As an example, in 1992, George Soros was said to have made $1 billion in one month by shorting the British Pound or betting that it would decrease in value.[2]

Most investors diversify their stock portfolio through the purchase of mutual funds or exchange traded funds (ETFs). Mutual funds are companies that pool money from many investors and purchase many stocks to make up the fund. This allows the investor to have a diversified portfolio without having to personally purchase many individual stocks. There are several indicators (indexes) of the strength of the US economy based on stock prices. The Dow Jones Industrial Average (DJIA) which is calculated as the sum of 30 representative stocks divided by a number called the Dow Divisor. The Dow Divisor is formulated such that stock splits or other structural changes do not alter the DJIA. The divisor also corrects for inflation. Another commonly used index is the Standard and Poor 500 (S&P 500). The S&P 500 is a weighted sum of the prices of 500 large common stocks actively traded in the US. Index funds are mutual funds that follow a given index. These are also called ETFs. An ETF is like a mutual fund but typically includes all of the stocks contained in an index. Owning ETFs is like owning a piece of the Dow or a piece of the S&P. ETFs are diversified due to the varied industries and economic sectors represented in the index.

Another way that your family chocolate company could raise capital to expand would be to borrow money from the public. This type of business debt is called a *bond*. Bonds are less risky for investors than stocks because in the case of bankruptcy, debt holders are paid first. Based on what you have learned, it should not come as a surprise that bonds generally have a lower rate of return than stocks as they are less risky. Bonds typically pay interest on the borrowed money several times a year. These payments are called coupons. Bonds are also sometimes called fixed income investments because their value is predetermined at the point of sale. Bonds have a maturity date that designates the date when the bond principle is to be paid. Bonds also have a face value dictating the payment due at maturity, and bonds have a coupon rate. As an example, a 10-year $10,000 US Treasury Note with a 6% coupon rate. We know that this bond will mature at 10 years at which point the holder is entitled to full payment of $10,000. The bond holder is also entitled to two $300 coupon payments per year for the life of the bond. Many of us have received US savings bonds as gifts from an aunt or uncle.

These are called zero coupon bonds as they do not have biannual interest payments. Rather, they are discounted at the point of sale. For example, currently you can buy (online) a $100 US savings bond for $50. The bond reaches face value at 20 years and will continue to earn interest for up to 30 years. Aunt Sally purchased that bond for you for your first birthday because it only cost her half the face value and she wanted to provide money for you when you reached 21 years of age. Your aunt also felt good about contributing to the US economy and she knew that savings bonds carry no risk as they are backed by the US government.

Another major type of financial instrument includes derivatives or options. Derivatives are investments whose value depends on the value of an underlying asset. Fire insurance is an example of a derivative. If you purchase fire insurance for the total value of a $400,000 home, the insurance policy is worth nothing unless your house burns to the ground at which point it is worth $400,000. Fire insurance can therefore be considered a derivative investment on your house.

Generally, there are two types of options called "puts" and "calls." A put is the right to sell and a call is the right to buy. Physicians are familiar with options without realizing it. Take a salary structure that includes a salary guarantee and a salary cap. The salary guarantee is an option provided that is a derivative of your salary. A salary cap is a benefit to your employer and is also an option. In the above example, the salary guarantee is a put because it protects against low earnings, whereas the salary cap is a call as it sets an upward limit. The value of options can be calculated where the value of the put is set to be equivalent to the value of the call. In options lingo, this is called a zero premium collar and such a strategy may be better at setting physician salary caps and guarantees than trial and error.[3]

Options are traded on the Chicago Board Options Exchange. For example, on December 14, 2018, an investor could purchase a call option on Apple stock for $5.25 for a strike price of $165 with an expiration date of Dec 28. At that time, Apple stock was trading at $167. This means that any time prior to December 28, the holder of the call option could purchase a share of Apple stock for $165. Obviously, this option is worthless at the point of purchase because the option costs over $5 so the holder would have to spend $170 for something worth $167. Suppose the price of Apple stock rose to $175 prior to December 28th? Then the option would be profitable as the holder could purchase for $170 something worth $175. Puts work the same way but are a right to sell so are profitable when a stock price falls below a certain value.

Why are options important? Obviously, they are speculative investments as they require some prediction of the future and they are zero sum as for every seller, their needs to be a buyer so someone always wins and someone always loses in an options transaction. Stock purchase, in contrast, can provide a net gain for both seller and buyer if the stock price goes up after purchase.

Like fire insurance, options can be used as insurance for stock purchases. Say you purchased 100 shares of Apple stock at $165. You would be out of pocket $16,500. If you wanted to reduce your out-of-pocket expenses, and have an immediate return on investment, you could sell call options on your stock. Let's say you sold 100 calls for $5 each with a strike price of $170 and an expiration date in 6 months. You would immediately receive $500 for the options sale. Assuming the stock price prior to expiration was $175, you would be forced to sell your shares at the strike price of $170, and would receive $170 × 100 = $17,000. Your net profit on the transaction would be $1000, $500 from the option sale and $500 from the $5 increase in price per share. On the other hand, if the stock price never went above $160, the options you sold would be worthless, but you would still have the $500 from the sale and would effectively recoup the money lost on the stock price drop. This investment strategy is called selling covered calls. The calls are covered because you own the underlying stock. There is nothing illegal about selling calls on stock you do not own (uncovered calls), but this is extremely risky because there is theoretically no upward limit to the stock price and if the stock price increases you would have to provide the stock at the strike price regardless of the cost. For example, if something remarkable happened to Apple and the stock price went to $1165, and you owned no shares, you would have to provide 100 shares for this price even though at the time of the option purchase, shares were trading for $165. You would have to pay $116,500 for stock that was only worth $16,500 at the time of the option sale for a net loss of $116,000!

Another way to use options as an insurance policy on a stock is the concept of a protective put. In this instance, you buy a put to protect you against an unexpected drop in stock price. Using the above example, suppose you bought 100 puts on your Apple stock that you bought for $165 a share. Suppose the puts cost $5 and suppose the expiration date is in 6 months and that the strike price is $160. This strategy would mitigate any drop in stock price that is more than $5 because if the price drops to say $150, you still have a right to sell it at $160.

These examples show how options can be used to protect stock investments, but also show how selling uncovered calls can be quite risky indeed.

What gives US currency value? Many physicians are shocked to learn that US currency is not backed by gold or silver since 1933. Currency backed by gold or silver is called commodity currency. A great example of the definition of money and the concept of commodity currency occurred on the tiny island of Yap in the South Pacific (Yap is also known for being the highest per capita consumers of Budweiser beer!). On Yap, instead of gold or silver, several hundred years ago, money came in the form of large limestone discs, often weighing several tons, which were traded in exchange for goods and often transported on small bamboo canoes. Because of the sheer girth of these stones, the concept of money on Yap became abstract and the coins or large stone discs could often not be moved at all.

Interestingly, there is a story about one large stone that ended up on the bottom of the sea due to a huge storm that capsized a canoe. Even though the stone was under hundreds of feet of water, the stone was still considered currency and was traded as any other stone. This abstract notion of money should not be unfamiliar as we never see our money in a bank, but believe that it is there based on pixels that produce account information on our computer monitors. This is another definition of faith.

What gives the US dollar value? The US dollar is fiat currency meaning its value is backed by the US government. One US dollar is valued at the amount of US goods and services that can be purchased for that dollar. A dollar bill in your wallet has the seal of the US Federal Reserve System. The Federal Reserve System is a bank for banks. The Federal Reserve does not print money, that is the job of the Bureau of Engraving and Printing. Rather, the Federal Reserve can loan money to banks. Why would banks need to borrow money? When you deposit $100 into a bank, they do not store the $100 in a vault. Rather, the bank lends the money to others and collects interest on the debt. This greatly increases the total supply of money in the United States. In fact, for large banks, only 10% of deposits must be held in reserve. When banks fall below this level, they have to borrow money from the Federal Reserve. As such, the Federal Reserve controls the economy. Although it does not print money, it sets interest rates for short-term loans to other banks which in turn affect interest rates on car loans, mortgages, and other bank loans. The Federal Reserve can also buy and sell US government bonds. If the Federal Reserve wants to slow the economy, the Federal Reserve will increase interest rates and will sell bonds to reduce the amount of money available for spending. If the Federal Reserve wants to stimulate the economy, it can decrease interest rates to encourage spending and the Federal Reserve can buy bonds to put more money into the economy.

Back to the Case

Jamal took the advice of others and found a financial planner who was highly recommended by his brother-in-law. Jamal and his financial planner discussed his short- and long-term financial goals including providing for his family, providing for his daughter's education, and his desire to retire at 65. Jamal bought additional life insurance and invested in mutual funds and worked out a monthly purchase to dollar average. With dollar averaging, if the market dropped, Jamal' mutual funds were cheaper that month, and if the market rose, his current funds were more valuable but the funds he bought were more expensive. Jamal comfortably invested the most he could each month based on his budget. Jamal also hired an accountant.

Bottom Line

1. Get a financial planner and an accountant.
2. Reward is related to risk. There is no free lunch!
3. The average investor earns an average rate of return.

Case Amber

Amber is in her second year of residency training in physical medicine and rehabilitation at a major academic medical center. Amber became interested in how to better make changes for populations of patients from a policy perspective. Amber has received emails from the American Medical Association (AMA) inviting her to attend an AMA-sponsored meeting in Chicago. Amber has never considered herself much of a joiner. What should she do?

Organized medicine allows individual physicians to join an organization in order to advocate for themselves and their patients. This can be done at the local, state, and national levels. Organized medicine is what gives physicians, medical students, residents, and fellows a voice in policy-making and government. It is through organized medicine that physicians can advocate for the best quality care for their patients while also ensuring that doctors are treated fairly. It is also through organized medicine that young doctors learn about the economics and politics of American medicine. This chapter will briefly discuss the history of organized medicine in the United States and present a case as to why young doctors should participate in organized medicine

and learn about the real world of American medicine.

History of Organized Medicine in the United States

Prior to the establishment of the American Medical Association in 1845, *anyone* could publicly place a sign stating they were a doctor as there was no national standard for physician training.

In 1845, Dr. Nathan S. Davis called for the first national medical convention, which led to the establishment of the American Medical Association (AMA) in 1847. Their first charter was focused on scientific advancement, setting standards for medical education, launching a program of medical ethics, and improving public health. These were the initial goals of the AMA more than 150 years ago and they are still the aspirations of the organization today. The AMA is the first organization of its kind in the world to establish uniform standards for medical education, training, and practice as well as the first to develop a national code for ethical medical practice. Ever since its inception, the AMA Code of Ethics dictates professional conduct for all practicing physicians. The AMA, with the Association of American Medical Colleges, sets the standards for medical education today through the Liaison Committee on Medical Education, the accreditation body for allopathic medical schools in the United States.

The AMA provides health and scientific information to its members and to the public and carries out a broad range of health education programs via mass media and lectures. It keeps its members informed of significant medical and health legislation, and it represents its profession before Congress and other governmental bodies. The AMA sets standards for medical schools and internship programs, and it alerts the public to quack medical remedies, snake oil salesmen, and other medical charlatans.

Publications of the AMA include the highly-rated *Journal of the American Medical Association (JAMA)* and 11 other journals devoted to such medical specialties as internal medicine, psychiatry, and pediatrics. In addition, the AMA publishes the online journal *JAMA Network Open*, which focuses on original medical research in an open-source format.

Just a few decades ago, it was not unusual for physicians to be members of their county medical society, specialty society, state medical association, national specialty society, and the AMA, but physician participation is steadily decreasing. While the practice of medicine seems to be changing almost daily, support for organized medicine as a whole seems to be decreasing during a time at which patients and their physicians need help more than ever. Let us not forget that there is strength in numbers. It would be very difficult for one doctor to create changes in healthcare policy alone. Whereas if doctors join together in support or protest of legislation, it becomes a much more powerful display of force and much more can be accomplished.

Historically, just as the economy expands and grows during war, physician membership in organized medicine usually increases during difficult times—times in which medicine is facing more intrusion by government regulation and restriction on how physicians can and do practice medicine, often without consideration for the protection of patients' rights. In the 1950s, about 75% of all practicing physicians in the United States were members of the AMA. According to

recent statistics in 2019, membership in the AMA is only about 12% of the nation's physicians.

So, where are all the physicians going? Today, there appears to be apathy for participation in organized medicine. Certainly, membership costs are one constraint especially if a physician joins local, state, national organizations plus one or more of the specialty societies. Many practices and hospitals that employ physicians will cover the costs of these annual dues to these organizations. However, this provision must be in the physician's contract. (see Chap. 5). In addition to cost concerns, doctors today have time constraints that might preclude going to additional meetings and time away from their families. Finally, there are concerns as to the actual value of membership.

It has not been easy for organized medicine. Some of the consequences may be worth noting. Physicians are no longer the powerful force in society they once were. Their opinions and recommendations no longer go almost unchallenged. Although the AMA's use of political action committee (PAC) dollars can be used to assure that legislators at least listen to physicians' views, the effectiveness of such a strategy is mitigated by underfunding.

There was a time, more than half a century ago, when organized medicine played a key role in physicians' lives and held enormous sway over US healthcare policy-making. During that time, three quarters of physicians were simultaneously members of their county and state medical societies and the American Medical Association (AMA).[1] Physicians spent many hours of their free time in these three groups, dealing with clinical learning, running for elected offices, holding forums, and hammering out positions on all kinds of issues. For most older physicians, that era is long gone.

In contrast to the AMA, specialty societies enjoy very high membership rates and do not seem to have a problem staying relevant to doctors. However, each specialty society has developed its own particular position on healthcare issues, replacing the once unified voice of the House of Medicine with a chorus of sometimes conflicting views.

Meanwhile, doctors seem to be following the growing trend among all Americans of moving away from groups. The 2000 book *Bowling Alone*, by Robert D. Putnam, demonstrated this trend by showing that even as the number of bowlers continued to rise, the number of people in bowling leagues had markedly fallen.

What Are the Reasons to Consider Joining Organized Medicine?

Organized medicine consists of groups of physicians categorized into three groups: (1) practicing physicians, (2) young physicians, and (3) resident and medical student sections. Each group or section works together to advocate collectively on behalf of the physician-patient relationship, patients' rights, and medicine as a whole. Each individual group also works together to advocate for their section's interests. Giving physicians and medical students a voice in the business of medicine allows physicians to advocate for the best quality of care for their patients and ensures physicians are also treated fairly on the state and national levels.

Organized medicine has been front and center in confronting the problem of physician burnout which is impacting nearly 50% of all healthcare providers (see Chap. 22). Burnout is a complicated issue complicated by physician feeling of irrelevance in a complex healthcare market. Organized medicine has recognized that medicine is a business and doctors are in dire need of guidelines on suggestions for running an efficient, productive, and, yes, profitable practice that is relevant to the care of patients. These organizations are providing young doctors with the necessary tools and resources to run a cost-effective medical practice and to hopefully feel less burned out.

Compliance with national imperatives is major problem that impacts nearly every practice. There are compliance regulations that are onerous, time consuming, and difficult to interpret. Recent reports looking at HIPAA and Meaningful Use audit findings have shown that most organizations do not retain the necessary supporting documentation of completion of core set objectives and measures. This puts the practice at increased risk of decreased reimbursement, costly fines, and prohibition of certain patient populations, such as those covered by Medicare and Medicaid, from using the practice. Many organizations offer audit solutions that help practices verify and validate that privacy and security programs meet compliance and business objectives. Billing and coding have become increasingly more complex. Organized medicine can help physicians understand these complexities and be properly reimbursed for their work.

Organized medicine has been, and will continue to play, a major role in the education and training of young physicians. You can plan on accessing the latest in technology and education through your national, state, local, and specialty organizations.

Our national medical societies and organizations have taken a leadership role in confronting and managing the American opioid crisis. This has been a crisis which the medical community is culpable and we have taken responsibility for solving this crisis and reducing the use of opioids and providing services for those who are addicted to these drugs. Organized medicine, as a national voice, had the clout to affect change through education and through their ability to direct local and national resources towards solving this crisis.

One of the best examples of the effectiveness of organized medicine was a report in the New England Journal of Medicine in 1991 authored by Lucien Leape who reviewed 30,000 randomly selected patients' hospital records. The study shocked the medical profession. This report demonstrated that nearly 4% of patients admitted to a hospital suffered an injury that prolonged their hospital stay or resulted in measurable disability and that nearly 14% of those injuries were fatal. Further, the study found that 70% of those injuries were clearly preventable. The study extrapolated the data of 30,000 patient records to the entire nation and estimated that 120,000 people were dying from preventable medical errors. The study showed medication errors accounted for the largest group of preventable medical errors. Leape estimated that there were one million preventable medical errors in the United States each year and the cost of these errors added to the already bloated healthcare budget by $33 million every year. This report in the NEJM generated front page coverage in nearly every major American newspaper. This was an unacceptable blemish on American healthcare that galvanized organized medicine (AMA) as this was such a large problem that one person or group could not possibly solve. The AMA demonstrated that error prevention systems were in place in other industries such as the airline industry. The AMA recommended that the healthcare profession adapt the same systems that were accomplished in other industries and that errors could be reduced and the quality of medicine improve.

Shortly after the publication of the Leake report, the AMA, Joint Commission on the Accreditation of Healthcare Organizations, and the American Association for the Advancement of Science hosted a conference on errors in medicine where a prevention, education, and research agenda was established. It was through this pioneering work on part of a group of organized physicians that patient safety was recognized as the sine qua non of quality. Thanks to these doctors and organized medicine there were, for the first time, sophisticated and efficient methods of measuring quality that could compare institutions and doctors through the quality lens. The take-home message is that change can occur in medicine, albeit slowly, but when we put the patient first and recognize that we are fallible but that we can correct our errors, we are, indeed, making progress.

Medical associations provide unparalleled networking opportunities, allowing young doctors to connect with their peers, mentors, and other industry leaders. As a member, you are in the unique position to attend conventions, seminars, and other related events with like-minded professionals in the field. Medical associations will provide you with not only clinical collaboration but also socialization with like-minded colleagues.

A medical association's annual meeting represents an incredible opportunity for you to meet and network with the largest gathering of your peers every year. Networking with professionals outside your place of employment can give you a broader perspective on the market and healthcare in general. Listening to the experiences of others may even leave you feeling energized and refreshed with the feeling you are not alone in the fight to change the course of American medicine.

The field of medicine is always in a state of change. Healthcare professionals can keep up with the newest developments and scientific breakthroughs through their associations' seminars, journals, CME courses, and other educational opportunities. Additionally, many associations, especially the specialty societies, offer all of the certification courses you will need throughout your entire career. Your professional organization also provides access to mentors, giving you an opportunity to participate in mentoring others as well. Having a mentor in any field will help your career grow and thrive. As an association member, you are in the unique position to gain a competitive edge by utilizing all of the educational resources and marketing materials available to you.

Associations are always looking for young doctors to help organize their annual meetings, workshops, CME courses, and legislative committees. Helping your organization work to improve your profession as well as to help improve the overall state of healthcare can be a very rewarding opportunity. Working on these projects will also be a great introduction to organized medicine and will often serve as a springboard to reach higher levels in the organization.

To fully receive the benefits of membership, you need to be engaged with the association. With any membership you get what you put into it. Get involved early in your career and as often as possible and you will reap the benefits offered to you as a member.

Healthcare associations are great places to find the latest jobs in your field! Looking for a new position during your training? Most organizations collect positions available throughout the nation and you can submit areas where you would like to work and find available jobs in your specialty and location where you would like to work.

An excellent resource is www.healthecareers. com. This site allows you submit your name and Email and you can be notified electronically as new jobs become available.

There are several special examples of organized medicine besides the AMA, state organizations, and specialty societies that you may consider joining. These include the American Medical Women's Association (www.amwa-doc. org), which is an organization which functions at the local and national level to advance women in medicine and improve women's health.

The National Medical Association (NMA) (www.nmanet.org) is the voice of African American physicians and the leading voice for parity and justice in medicine and the elimination of disparities in healthcare for all Americans regardless of ethnicity.

The NMA represents the interests of more than 50,000 African American physicians and the patients they serve. NMA is committed to improving the quality of health among all minorities and disadvantaged people through its membership, professional development, community health education, advocacy, research, and partnerships with federal and private agencies.

The American Medical Student Association (AMSA) is the oldest and largest independent association of physicians-in-training in the United States. AMSA members are medical students, premedical students, interns, residents, and practicing physicians. AMSA is focused on future physicians who believe that patients and health professionals are partners in the management of healthcare and that access to high-quality healthcare is a right and not a privilege. The AMSA annual convention is the largest gathering of medical students and regularly draws an attendance of more than 1500 physicians-in-training, medical educators, and health policy innovators. AMSA continues to search for new and innovative ways to improve healthcare, healthcare delivery, and medical education.

AMSA remains a leader in the campaign for resident work hour reform—authoring the Patient and Physician Safety and Protection Act of 2003. The passage of this act by Congress limited the work week of residents and fellows to 80 h per week.

AMSA publishes an excellent magazine, *The New Physician*, available to all students and new physicians, which will provide information you need to enrich your medical training and launch your career as a physician.

AMSA local chapters continue to reach out to serve the health needs of their communities. Annually, local chapters contribute over one million hours of community service.

Back to the Case
Amber's trip to Chicago was "mind-blowing," allowing her to serve as an alternate delegate for the first time. Because the AMA trip to Chicago was her first introduction to organized medicine on a national stage, she did not know what to expect, which made for an even better experience. She experienced collegiality of residents from all different walks of life and all different types of programs, from multiple geographic areas all coming together for one specific cause. She decided to become involved in organized medicine because she knew that there were strengths in numbers and that a group of doctors could advocate better for patients than one doctor alone could possibly accomplish.

Bottom Line

Organization medicine has the objective of promoting the science and art of medicine and also to enhance public health. Let us not forget that there's strength in numbers. It is highly unlike that one person can produce significant changes in healthcare policy. However, when we work together through the auspices of organized medicine, we can improve American healthcare. By standing together, united in vision and commitment, we physicians can shape the healthcare system this country needs.

Case Phil the Neurosurgeon

Phil is a fellowship-trained neurosurgeon. He had 13 years of training and is about to finish 5 years of military service, including several tours in Afghanistan and Iraq, to pay back for his education. Fortunately, Phil did not have any appreciable debt upon entering private practice. Phil has expertise in midbrain surgery using stereotaxic localization of brain tumors. He is a highly skilled surgeon, but because of his extensive training and lack of mentors during his military experience, he is at a loss for how to transition into private practice.

Moving from a training program to private practice can be stressful for any doctor. During your training program, you are in a cocoon or bubble and are protected by staff and faculty. There are so many things to consider when making that transition to practice. Balancing your current workload as a resident or fellow and managing family responsibilities while attempting to start your new practice can often lead to mistakes and missed opportunities. This chapter will help make that transition seamless. The following suggestions are a compilation of advice from several young physicians who entered private practice within the past 3 years. They will share what worked for them and what they would do if they had a chance to start again.

Ideally, you would like to have everything in order and ready to start caring for patients the first day you begin your practice. The first recommendation is to start early, which is usually 6–9 months before the end of your training. Starting early will require a significant commitment of time. Everything takes time to prepare for practice and that is often more time than you anticipate. Obtaining a license in another state can take months of correspondence, copying transcripts from undergraduate and medical school, proof of citizenship, and a copy of your medical degree issued by a medical school approved by the state board. This vetting process by state boards of medical examiners can be very frustrating. In training, you are accustomed to having documents and forms regarding patient care available at the click of a mouse. However, working with other people, such as bureaucrats in state medical societies, insurance companies, lenders, real estate agents, lawyers, contractors, third-party payers, and technology firms, can be a source of anxiety and frustration. Because let's face it—no one is as eager to start a practice as are you. Even when everyone is on board, much of the preparation for practice takes time, and there is not much you can do to speed up those processes. For example, the credentialing process for most hospitals requires at least 6 months.

Most physicians who are successful at making transitions use a checklist. An excellent checklist is provided in Fig. 10.1 provided by Physician Practice Specialists (https://physicianpractice-specialists.com/contact/).

The following is an abbreviated list of items for consideration when contemplating opening a new practice. This list is not complete and should be considered to be only a general guide. Actual needs will be dictated by specific markets, programming, and strategic goals of the principal(s) involved.

Planning
1. Select a Qualified Consultant to Develop
    (a) Business Description and Goals
    (b) Market Assessment
    (c) Financial Feasibility Study: Assumptions, Proforma Financial Statements, and Capital Requirements
    (d) Operational and Marketing Strategies

Facilities
1. Select Office Site/Negotiate Lease
2. Design Office Layout/Tenant Improvement Needed/Desired
3. Design Office Signs (Interior/Exterior)
4. Design Employee Workstations
5. Investigate Structural Alterations/Regulatory Issues/Infection Control Issues
6. Address HIPAA (Privacy Regulation) Facility Design Issues
7. Design Patient Flow (Incl. Privacy) Issues
8. Lay Out Exam Rooms/Procedure Room/Public Areas/Staff Areas
9. Select Phone Systems: Design and Layout
10. Plan EHR & EMR system | Billing, Accounts Receivable & Practice Management Information Systems
11. Select Information System Hardware and telecommunications equipment
12. Procure Office and Clinical Equipment
13. Select Supply Vendor and Order Initial Inventory

Practice Management
1. Select Legal Counsel And CPA
2. Develop Legal Structure
3. Create Corporate Documents
4. File Fictitious Business Name
5. Establish Tax ID Number
6. Obtain Business License
7. Obtain Business Liability, Malpractice, And Worker's Compensation Insurance
8. EHR: Selection and Implementation of an Electronic Health Records system (PM and EMR)
9. Prepare for Health Plan(ss) Participation Including Medicare/Medicaid to meet All Relevant Requirements Established in Federal/State Guidelines and Demonstrate Compliance *(Physical Plant, Equipment, Supplies, Written Clinical and Administrative Policies/Procedures, Forms, Staff Qualifications, Traceable Systems, Chart Note Review, OSHA, Etc.)*
10. Negotiate Payor Contracts
11. Identify Clinical Services/Develop Special Program/Services
12. Write Clinical and Operations Policies, Procedures, and Protocols
    (a) Office Systems and Information Flows
    (b) Appointment Scheduling
    (c) Patient Registration
    (d) Check-In/Reception
    (e) Medical Records
    (f) Nursing/Back Office
    (g) Check-out Reception
    (h) Referrals/Follow-Up Care
    (i) Pharmacy
    (j) Supplies (Clinical/Non-Clinical)
13. Conduct a HIPAA Risk Assessment for Privacy, Security and Breach Notification rules
14. Establish Practice Management Benchmarks and Indicators by Which to Judge Success
15. Develop a Medicare Fraud and Abuse Compliance Program and Evidence of Implementation
16. Conduct Ongoing Operational Reviews and Strategic Planning

The following is an abbreviated list of items for consideration when contemplating opening a new practice. This list is not complete and should be considered to be only a general guide. Actual needs will be dictated by specific markets, programming, and strategic goals of the principal(s) involved.

PLANNING
1. Select a qualified consultant to develop:
   1. Business Description and Goals
   2. Market Assessment
   3. Financial Feasibility Study: Assumptions, Proforma Financial Statements and Capital Requirements
   4. Operational and Marketing Strategies

FACILITIES
   1. Select Office Site/Negotiate Lease
   2. Design Office Layout/Tenant Improvement Needed/Desired
   3. Design Office Signs (Interior/Exterior)
   4. Design Employee Workstations
   5. Investigate Structural Alterations/Regulatory Issues/Infection Control Issues
   6. Address HIPAA (Privacy Regulation) Facility Design Issues
   7. Design Patient Flow (Incl. Privacy) Issues
   8. Lay Out Exam Rooms/Procedure Room/Public Areas/Staff Areas
   9. Select Phone Systems: Design And Layout
   10. Plan EHR & EMR system I Billing, Accounts Receivable & Practice Management Information Systems
   11. Select Information System Hardware and telecommunications equipment
   12. Procure Office And Clinical Equipment
   13. Select Supply Vendor And Order Initial Inventory

PRACTICE MANAGEMENT
   1. Select Legal Counsel And CPA
   2. Develop Legal Structure
   3. Create Corporate Documents
   4. File Fictitious Business Name
   5. Establish Tax ID Number
   6. Obtain Business License
   7. Obtain Business Liability, Malpractice, And Worker's Compensation Insurance
   8. EHR: Selection and Implementation of an Electronic Health Records system (PM and EMR)
   9. Prepare for Health Plan(s) Participation Including Medicare/Medicaid to meet all Relevant Requirements Established in Federal/State Guidelines and Demonstrate Compliance (Physical Plant, Equipment, Supplies, Written Clinical and Administrative Policies/Procedures, Forms, Staff Qualifications, Traceable Systems, Chart Note Review, OSHA, Etc.)
   10. Negotiate Payor Contracts
   11. Identify Clinical Services/Develop Special Program/Services
   12. Write Clinical and Operations Policies, Procedures And Protocols
        1. Office Systems and Information Flows
        2. Appointment Scheduling
        3. Patient Registration
        4. Check-in/Reception
        5. Medical Records
        6. Nursing/Back Office
        7. Check-out Reception
        8. Referrals/Follow-Up Care
        9. Pharmacy
        10. Supplies (Clinical/Non-Clinical)
   13. Conduct a HIPAA Risk Assessment for Privacy, Security and Breach Notification rules
   14. Establish Practice Management Benchmarks and Indicators By Which To Judge Success
   15. Develop A Medicare Fraud and Abuse Compliance Program And Evidence Of Implementation
   16. Conduct Ongoing Operational Reviews And Strategic Planning

FINANCIAL PLANNING
   1. Establish And Implement An Operating Budget
   2. Set Up Billing And Collection Protocols/Policies
   3. Open Bank Accounts
   4. Establish Working Capital Line of Credit
   5. Establish Credit Card Processing Capability
   6. Determine Outsourcing Needs/Establish Contracts (e.g., Billing, Payroll)
   7. Establish and Implement Proper Purchasing Policies And Procedures
   8. Establish Accounting And Reporting Systems For Effective Cash Management
   9. Develop Financial Management Policies And Procedures
   10. Establish Proper Internal Control Measures

HUMAN RESOURCES
   1. Develop Personnel Policies And Initial Staffing Plan
   2. Establish Proper Orientation And Training Programs
   3. Establish Internal Safety Program
   4. Set up Payroll And Quarterly Tax Reporting Systems
   5. Post Federal/State Mandated Employee Postings
   6. Develop Position Descriptions
   7. Develop A Compensation and Benefits Plan
   8. Recruit Employees

MARKETING AND REFERRAL DEVELOPMENT
   1. Develop Collateral Material
   2. Establish And Implement A Marketing/Referral Development Plan
   3. Develop A Public Relations Program
   4. Plan and Develop an Online presence program

Fig. 10.1 Healthcare start-up issues

Financial Planning

1. Establish and Implement an Operating Budget
2. Set Up Billing and Collection Protocols/Policies
3. Open Bank Accounts
4. Establish Working Capital Line of Credit
5. Establish Credit Card Processing Capability
6. Determine Outsourcing Needs/Establish Contracts (e.g., Billing, Payroll)
7. Establish and Implement Proper Purchasing Policies and Procedures
8. Establish Accounting and Reporting Systems for Effective Cash Management
9. Develop Financial Management Policies and Procedures
10. Establish Proper Internal Control Measures

Human Resources

1. Develop Personnel Policies and Initial Staffing Plan
2. Establish Proper Orientation and Training Programs
3. Establish Internal Safety Program
4. Set up Payroll And Quarterly Tax Reporting Systems
5. Post Federal/State Mandated Employee Postings
6. Develop Position Descriptions
7. Develop a Compensation and Benefits Plan
8. Recruit Employees

Marketing and Referral Development

1. Develop Collateral Material
2. Establish and Implement a Marketing/Referral Development Plan
3. Develop a Public Relations Program
4. Plan and Develop an Online Presence Program

Checklist for transition from training to practice. (Used with permission from Provider Services Nationwide (providerservicesnationwide.com).

Once you have finished your training program, signed your contract or lease, had business cards and stationery printed, and your name is on the door to the list of doctors in practice, what do you do next?

Credentialing with Insurance Companies

It is to begin the credentialing process early as it may take 4–6 months to obtain permission to see their patients covered by their insurance. We have seen doctors start practicing and have a state license to practice but are not on the insurance plans and cannot be paid for services provided. This can be frustrating to a young doctor starting their practice.

Credentialing is a process used to evaluate physician qualifications and practice history. This process includes reviewing a doctor's completed education, training, residency, and licenses. The process also includes review of any certifications issued by a board in the doctor's specialty. You do not have to be board certified, but if you are going to practice a specialty, you must demonstrate that you are at least board eligible.

Credentialing with insurance companies, otherwise known as provider enrollment or achieving in-network status, can be challenging, especially if this is your first foray into that process. Even with experience and every tool at your disposal, credentialing can be exhausting. Here is a brief overview of how to complete the provider enrollment or insurance credentialing process to become an in-network provider. Keep in mind that each payer may be slightly different [1]. Start with obtaining your CAQH ID. The Universal Credentialing Data Source is designed to make the credentialing process easier for providers by gathering data in a single repository. This data may be accessed by participating health plans and other healthcare organizations. The CAQH ID enables providers to update their information. Commercial payers will require this information for your application. Make sure CAQH has a valid W9 and malpractice certificate uploaded. You can easily register for your CAQH ID online at https://proview.caqh.org/PR/Registration.

Next, request to join the network on the insurance company's website. Sometimes it is not easy to find a network site, so always contact the payer to follow up with your request or call them if you cannot find the join network request. Many insurance companies have credentialing hotlines set up; hence, check out their website for this number.

If the panel is open or the insurance company needs doctors in your specialty or if they need additional primary care doctors, the credentialing process can begin. The panel will request some information such as CAQH ID, NPI, practice EIN. The practice EIN is an employer identification number (EIN) or the nine-digit number assigned by the IRS. The EIN number identifies the tax accounts of employers and others even if there are no additional employees. The IRS uses the number to identify taxpayers who must file various business tax returns each year. You need to be sure that the practice EIN you provide is the same on the W9 that should already be in CAQH.

You must follow up on the material you submitted. Your request may fall through the cracks at the payer level. Information and documents may be lost or misplaced, and it is unlikely that you will be notified that the file is incomplete. Therefore, we suggest that you call the payer frequently and ensure that everything is proceeding correctly. If a document or a form is missing, you can promptly submit or resubmit anything required or missing.

Contracting with Insurance Companies

Once credentialing or primary source verification is complete, you will move to contracting. The contracting phase is the all-important part of determining how much you will get paid for your services to the payers' members. A contracting representative will be assigned to you, and that representative will draft your agreement. Your agreement will be drafted by the payer usually 3 months after you initiated the credentialing process and will move through the contracting department. It is at this time that your fee schedule is created. You will want to follow up every week or two to check the status with the payer regarding your fee schedule. It is critical that you review the fee schedule before signing, as they may submit a lousy initial agreement. The fee schedule is not always included, so you may need

to request a fee schedule and provide the payer with your top 20 codes or the procedures you perform or plan to perform most often. After signing the contract, plan on an additional 30 days for them to load your name, contact information, and the fee schedule in their system. You will be issued a provider identification number (PIN) and a letter of participation that indicates your effective date of having permission to see their patients.

You are still not done! You must verify payer participation and save the email or letter received from the payer confirming participation. Finally, ensure your billing system is updated with payer information (EDI enrollment), and only then can you start submitting claims.

It is now evident why this process takes a long time. Getting credentialed and contracted does take time, and you cannot be paid unless you have a self-pay practice where credentialing is not required.

Use of Technology

Regardless, if you are an employed physician or decide to open your own practice, you will depend on technology to support your practice. Effective use of modern technology will enhance the care of your patients. Great care must be taken in selecting, installing, training, and supporting technology that you use in your practice.

Currently, technology is relatively cheap compared to the cost of employee salaries, which ranges from 18 to 25% of gross income. You need to get comfortable with that technology that is constantly changing. The technology that you purchase will soon become obsolete within a short period. Therefore, your technology selection should include the necessity to upgrade, expand, and replace your existing technology. If you are just starting your practice, you should consider the intended purpose of the technology. Think about the needs and requirements before reaching out to a vendor. We suggest you write your technology requirements and present your desires to a vendor and ask them how their product supports what is essential for your practice.

Look at the reliability of the product you are considering. Nothing can bring your practice to a screeching halt than a power outage, and all of the technology is out of commission. With that in mind, check the performance record of the technology. We also suggest you purchase devices that preserve your data in a power outage. This includes a surge protector and battery backup that powers down to protect hardware, software, and sensitive data.

One size does not fit all. Consequently, you want to ensure that your technology acquisition can be adjusted to your workflow and meets HIPAA regulatory requirements. This means selecting a flexible program that can be adjusted for your unique practice needs. The best example is your electronic medical record program and practice management system.

An essential requirement for any technology purchase is the service reputation of the equipment. It is essential to know about the tech support of the program. You will want to know if help is available early in the day, on weekends, and after your practice closes. Also, you want to know how quickly the vendor's support team responds to problems that you have with their product. It is reasonable to expect that your practice will receive a response in 1–2 h when you reach out for assistance.

You will need to decide whether to have your own insurance billing software program or avail yourself to a service that will do the billing on behalf of your practice. One of us (NHB) has used both methods and the experience with the billing service was abysmal. The billing service doesn't know the patients and can be rude and insensitive to patients when asking for payment for services. Also, most of these services do not have coding experts and will make their collection statistics look favorable by down coding your services. It is true that a billing service means one less employee, but you may be leaving significant amounts of money on the table.

The age of telemedicine has arrived which is one positive side effect of the pandemic in 2020. Now many patients, especially millennials, are expecting to have virtual visits with their physi-cians. For telehealth sessions you will need to select a platform that is HIPPA compliant. (For more information on telemedicine see Chap. 26).

Finally, we suggest you investigate the security of any technology system you decide to use. Sensitive information must be encrypted. A recent concern is the ability of hackers to obtain access to your data and then in charge demanding payment for you to have your data returned.

Our best advice is to obtain references from users of the technology. We suggest that you visit practices that already have implemented the technology and "kick the tires" of the technology, which means watching the program in use in a similar practice. Most physicians and office managers will provide you with their opinion of the program and tell you the benefits and problems with the technology.

Eleven Suggestions for Getting Started

We provide ten suggestions for the transition process to take place. All these suggestions might not apply to you and your practice, but we can assure you that most of the suggestions will be helpful.

Find a Mentor

Your senior partner may not be able to help you—chances are they entered private practice more than 10 years ago. Although the senior partners may be excellent clinicians, we can assure you that their clinical skills probably will not help you in your shift from training to practice. Finding a career mentor is a vital step after finishing your residency. A senior physician who knows the ropes or the politics of the medical community in which you plan to practice can be an invaluable resource. A senior physician will likely be flattered that you have asked them for guidance and counsel. Pick their brains about practice and the realities of the real world of medicine.

For a career mentor, we recommend selecting an older physician who is visible and has status in your medical community. Examples might include an executive in your local medical society, the previous chief of staff at your hospital, or even a family friend in the medical profession. It is not necessary to select a mentor in your specialty. If you are a surgeon, feel free to choose an internist or a medical specialist. If you are in sports medicine, consider selecting a cardiologist or rheumatologist. Your purpose in choosing a mentor is not primarily to develop a referral source but to learn the unique aspects of your medical community. The mentor should introduce you to physicians with whom you have something in common and who would be your future professional allies. Your mentor may also include you in social functions at the hospital that you might not be otherwise invited. Ask to join the mentor at the first few hospital staff meetings, requesting them to introduce you to their friends and contemporaries. You will find that the advice from a mentor is priceless. The mentor will be quite helpful in ensuring a rapid acceleration of your career.

Learn How to Write or Create an Effective Referral Letter

Most residency programs focus on the diagnosis and treatment of disease. They provide little training on the techniques of communicating with other physicians. Therefore, most new physicians unknowingly give the referring doctor too much information. Like you, today's doctors are too busy to read two- to three-page letters. They will be unimpressed by a lengthy letter, and chances are also they will not even read it. Referring doctors appreciate short letters, and those that are to the point and timely. What information are primary care doctors looking for in a letter from a referring doctor? The working diagnosis, the medications you recommend prescribing for the patient, and the treatment plan you wish to initiate are most often cited. (For more information on communicating with referring physicians, see Chap. 13.)

Meet the VIPs

As soon as you begin your practice, you must introduce yourself to several key people in your hospital. They are:

- The medical director
- The hospital administrator
- The chief of staff
- The chief of your department
- The emergency room physicians and staff
- The business/admitting office staff
- The physician services representative
- The marketing/PR staff
- The director of MCE
- The head of physician referral services

Court Other Physicians

You need a core group of physicians to send you patients. Probably 10–15 physicians who will refer to you regularly is all that is required initially. Block out time each week for calling upon doctors you think could send you referrals. Initially, you will find that doctors in practice less than 5 years and older physicians near retirement are the best contact to make. Look beyond your specialty when courting referring physicians. On the other hand, do not neglect your specialty, as you may find colleagues in your specialty do not perform the procedures that you do as a result of your recent training. You might also consider sending a brief letter to a doctor you plan to meet a few days before the scheduled appointment. The letter could mention your training and areas of interest and expertise, as well as why you moved to the community and any personal information that may be of interest to the doctor you are approaching. Sending a brief thank-you letter after the meeting is also a nice gesture. Invite this colleague to assist you. For example, if you are a recently trained plastic surgeon and an older plastic surgeon is not trained in breast reconstruction, then they may be happy to send you their patients. This way, the more senior physician is still involved in the patient's care and assured of getting the patient back.

Remember, you do not always need to meet a potential referral source in the doctor's office. Visit the physicians' lounges and the physicians' dining rooms and attend social events organized by the hospital, such as sporting events and health fairs. Today, it is possible to introduce yourself virtually, however, an in-person meeting is still the best way to start the professional relationship.

The Buddy System

Most medical staff offices have programs to orient new physicians to the hospital. Be sure and find out if the hospital has a "buddy system" in which an assigned physician will be your guide and show you around the hospital and the medical community. Request a copy of the medical directory and names of other new physicians on the staff. Find out when staff meetings are held and which committees you might join. Be sure and contact the chairpersons of committees who are of interest to you or provide opportunities to meet new physicians.

Contact Nonphysicians

Introduce yourself to the nurses in your hospital to discuss your area of expertise and interest. Meeting the community's pharmacists is also a good idea; patients often ask them to recommend a physician. Other worthwhile contacts include podiatrists, chiropractors, lawyers, social workers, beauticians, barbers, and manicurists.

Especially for Surgeons

To have your first cases go smoothly consider the following:

1. Introduce yourself to the operating room supervisor and staff.
2. If you are performing procedures new to the staff, offer an in-service program to the operating room nurses.

3. Before leaving your residency, obtain copies of your instrument cards to present to the operating room staff to have the appropriate instruments on hand for your first cases. This measure will ensure that all the instruments needed, sutures you require, intraoperative medications on hand, and any additional equipment you need for your surgical procedures will be available for the early cases you schedule in the hospital.

Before starting your first few cases, meet with the scrub nurse and the circulating nurse and indicate your plans, wants, and needs—including your glove size. Educating the operating room personnel before surgery begins is the best way to succeed for your first few cases. Your first few cases must be seamless. There will be people looking at your behavior, skills, and outcomes, so be sure that the early cases represent your personality and your talents.

Keep in Touch

There are those who state the Rolodex cards are a thing of the past. Yet, we notice that many offices still collect cards of colleagues, pharma, device companies, and other important contacts and use a Rolodex file. Address/file cards are an effective method of keeping your name in front of the physician and the staff. A good card will contain not only your name, address, and phone number but an email address, a direct line to your cell phone, and even your home number. Additionally, you can include your office hours, answering service, professional information number (PIN), partners, and names of your office manager, secretary, and nurse. Also, add any other information you might feel is helpful such as the insurance plans you are on. For those who are more technologically savvy, consider using one of the electronic file card apps. CamCard (https://www.camcard.com) is a business card reader which uses a smartphone's camera to capture, store, and edit business cards using optical character recognition.

Pharmaceutical Contacts

Physician services departments will have the names and telephone numbers of the contacts who can help you. Knowing pharmaceutical representatives and medical manufacturing companies can also be helpful. Pharmaceutical representatives have the materials and resources to assist new physicians set up their practices. Some pharma companies even have divisions for the sole purpose of helping new physicians begin their careers.

Setting Fees

Lastly, you will want to consider how much to charge for your services. Few areas will impact your practice more than the fees you decide for your services. Most studies indicate that few patients select doctors based on fees alone. If you join a group or have partners, this task will be easy as their fees are your fees. Occasionally, a colleague will share this information with you. Another technique is to use the relative value unit. These values are located in "Relative Values for Physicians" [2].

Take a Vacation

And our final piece of advice—do not go to work the day after you complete your training on July 1! Why? There will never be a time when you will be able to have a long vacation with very little responsibility. We understand that you may have significant debt and are eager to lower your financial obligations (see Chap. 11 on debt reduction). We suggest that you consider, at a minimum, a 4- to 6-week hiatus between ending your training and starting your practice. If the practice or hospital you are joining managed without you for months or years, a few additional weeks will not make a difference. Yes, they may be eager to begin, but you should take advantage of this hiatus and take a long vacation with your significant other and family. We can assure you that you will not have 6 weeks off from your practice until 35–40 years later when you retire. We have never seen or heard of a doctor who has regretted this decision.

> **Back to the Case**
> *Phil went online and obtained a checklist for the process of licensing and credentialing. He spent nearly 6 months to prepare for the transition to private practice. He joined a single specialty neurosurgery practice and had partners help with the hospital credentialing process. Phil admits that there was nothing easy about the move from training to practice but starting early was his best advice. He also took a much-needed vacation after being discharged from the service and was delighted that he did.*

Bottom Line

It is true that medicine has undergone significant changes since the first day you started medical school or even began your residency. Many young physicians are discouraged at the future prospects in healthcare or find starting a practice daunting and will opt for becoming an employed physician. However, there are still wonderful opportunities available to every physician regardless of the length of practice. The transition from residency to private practice can be less daunting by knowing and implementing the right steps for success.

References

1. For practice start up and credentialing. https://www.providerservicesnationwide.com.
2. Hall D. Relative values for physicians. https://www.optum360coding.com/Product/47867/.

Case Dimitri

Dimitri is a fourth-year medical student who is about to graduate from a private medical school in the northeast. Dimitri has borrowed money to cover his medical school expenses and has additional loan debt from college. His total educational debt is over $300,000. Dimitri is fortunate to have matched into his first-choice spot for his Family Practice residency. He is going to a small town in the southeastern United States. He has just met with his financial aid counselor to do his exit interview to review his total debt, and is astonished by the amount of money he will be expected to repay. What are his repayment options?

In 2021, the mean and median indebtedness of all medical school graduates was $203,062 and $200,000 respectively, with debt being higher for graduates of private medical schools when compared with public medical schools [1]. Nineteen percent of medical school graduates reported debt of over $300,000, and 73% of graduates reported some medical education debt. Certainly, Dimitri is not alone. The cost of attendance at US medical schools has increased at a pace surpassing that of inflation, with a median 4 year cost of attendance for private schools for the Class of 2021 at $357,868 [1].

Despite the high cost of attendance, going to medical school is financially advantageous with a net present value of over $1.6 million [2]. This means that someone would have to give you $1.6 million prior to starting medical school for you to be in the same financial position at retirement as if you went to medical school! A medical education is an investment with an excellent return. Even for students planning careers in lower-paying primary care specialties do well financially as physicians. A recent study investigated whether or not students could afford a career in primary care using financial planning software [3]. The authors concluded that a primary care field remains financially viable for medical school graduates with median levels of debt. The study further concluded that graduates with high levels of debt needed to consider extended payment plans, loan forgiveness programs, or living in a lower cost area of the country in order to cover their educational debt.

In spite of the fact that going to medical school is a good financial move, the amount of debt accrued by graduates can be onerous, and because physicians have a high earning potential, they have little choice but to pay back their loans. They cannot default. Generally, monthly loan repayments include both a portion of the amount borrowed (principal), and a portion of the interest accrued over the life of the loan. Remember, you have to pay for someone to lend you money. For new graduates, or in the case of financial hardship, most loans allow for a period of forbearance where payments can be suspended or delayed with the accrual of additional interest. Again, if a physician delays paying their loans, they will be penalized with additional interest payments. As such, it is generally not advisable to delay the start of educational loan repayment.

Basically, there are three types of traditional loan repayment models for physicians: (1). Standard Repayment; (2). Extended Repayment; and (3). Graduated Repayment. Standard repayment requires the borrower to make fixed monthly payments that include both principal and interest. Typically, the borrower is required to pay off the principal and interest in 10 years. Of course, if a borrower has multiple sources of loans (federal government and private loans), all of the loans can be consolidated through a third party who basically "buy" the individual loans and package them as one larger loan. Typically, consolidated loans are paid off over a longer period of time (20 or 30 years). Generally, this reduces the monthly payment, but increases the total amount of interest paid over the life of the loan, raising the overall total amount paid back bay the borrower. Standard repayment is the "default" if no other type of repayment plan is chosen.

Extended repayment, like consolidation, allows the borrower to spread out the payments over a longer period of time (20 or 30 years) with an increase in the total interest accrued. As such, the monthly payments are lower, but the total amount of money repaid is increased due to interest charged on the loan during the extended repayment period.

Graduated repayment allows the borrower to make smaller payments initially, with increases in payments after several years. As with extended payment, the borrower pays for this benefit with higher interest payments.

In addition to the three typical repayment models, borrowers can enter income-driven repayment plans. In each of these, the amount paid per month in repayment is closely tied to income earned. These loans are generally divided into those that are income contingent and those that are income based. Income contingent plan payments are based on the lesser of either 20% monthly discretionary income or a calculated amount based on a 12-year repayment plan and a multiplier based on income. Income-based plans allow borrowers to make monthly payments based on family size and adjusted gross income. Typically, payments are capped at 10% of discretionary income. For a typical resident earning $50,000 per year, the income-based repayment would be about $370 per month. In addition to income contingent and income-based repayment plans, borrowers can enter pay as you earn (PAYE) or revised pay as you earn (REPAYE) plans, both of which require payments that are calculated as a percentage of discretionary income with some consideration for family size. REPAYE plans differ from PAYE plans in limiting interest payments to 50%, if the monthly payment does not cover the entire interest payment. As with all financial decisions, it is best to discuss loan repayment strategies with a financial advisor before making any final decisions. Each repayment plan has its own tax implications including whether or not the payments of principal and/or interest are tax deductible. Additionally, some repayment plans may allow for loan forgiveness after a certain number of payments.

Are there ways to have someone else pay off your educational debt?

In 2007, the College Cost Reduction and Access Act was created to provide indebted college, graduate, or professional school graduates a way to reduce their federal student debt burden by working in public service. Loans considered eligible for public service loan forgiveness (PSLF) included any loan issued under the federal Direct Loan Program including subsidized and unsubsidized Stafford Loans, PLUS loans, and Federal Direct Consolidation Loans. Unfortunately, private loans were not deemed eligible for forgiveness.

To qualify for PSLF, the borrower has to make 120 monthly on-time payments in a qualifying plan and has to work full time for 10 years in a government or not-for-profit (501c) organization. Qualifying repayment plans for PSLF include any one of the previously described income-driven repayment plans (income contingent repayment, income-based repayment, PAYE, or REPAYE). The huge benefit of PSLF is that after making 120 payments, the remainder of the loan balance is *forgiven*. When originally established, there was no cap or maximum amount of loan debt that could be forgiven. As such, under PSLF, it really does not matter how much you owe. Your payment is only dependent on your income. Those with higher debt have a larger amount of debt forgiven at the end of the loan period. Over the past few years, attempts have been made to cap the amount of PSLF at $57,000. More recent proposals include eliminating PSLF entirely. The future of PSLF remains uncertain, but as of the time of this writing, PSLF remains intact under law.

In addition to PSLF, there are several other federally based loan forgiveness programs. All three branches of the military (Army, Navy, Air Force) offer medical school scholarships through the Health Professions Scholarship Program (HPSP) that cover medical school tuition fees and provide a stipend for living expenses for medical students in exchange for military service. What is often not recognized is that the military also offers loan repayment opportunities after graduation from medical school. Loan repayment does require active military duty and/or reserve status in a branch of the US military. The amount of repayment can be substantial (up to $275,000) and may also include sign-on bonuses for practicing physicians that range between $220,000 and $400,000 depending on specialty.

Like the military, the Indian Health Service offers loan repayment, paying up to $40,000 per year for service in Indian Health Service facilities providing care of American Indians or Alaska Natives.

For physicians involved in research careers, the National Institutes of Health (NIH) offers a competitive loan repayment program where successful applicants who agree to a 2-year minimum contract to engage in research funded by a non-profit organization are provided $35,000 per year to repay undergraduate, medical school, or graduate school debt. The NIH also offers loan repayment programs for clinicians from disadvantaged backgrounds or for physicians engaged in health disparity research.

The National Health Service Corps (NHSC) offers loan repayment for those physicians who commit to working at least 2 years at an NHSC-approved site. These are typically in rural communities or in the inner city. Physicians who practice primary care or mental health are eligible for up to $50,000 that is tax free and extendable for an additional 2 years.

In addition to the above federal programs, many states have programs that repay medical school loans for physicians who agree to practice in medically underserved regions or federally designated health professional shortage areas.

Finally, many practices and hospitals offer a sign-on bonus for new hires, if not a direct stipend for loan repayment. For a $25,000 bonus, assuming a 25% tax rate, the signing bonus would net $18,750. That sum could be used to make an extra bonus payment on student loans, saving thousands of dollars in interest over the life of the loan.

In addition to loan repayment, it may also be advisable to refinance debt at a lower interest rate. Depending on the interest rates on loans and interest rates offered by consolidation companies, this may be an attractive way to decrease the total money paid on a loan. As with other decisions, careful consultation with a financial advisor is important before making any decision regarding loan repayment.

Back to Case

Dimitri met with a financial advisor and decided to enter an income-dependent repayment plan during residency. He hoped to be able to use loan repayment during his time spent in residency, in a small not-for-profit hospital, toward qualification for the PSLF program. He planned to remain in the small community and to work for a federally qualified health center. After 10 years, he hoped that the PSLF program would still be in place when he would become eligible for loan forgiveness. Dimitri felt comfortable with the $370 per month repayment schedule. He remained optimistic that as a physician, even one engaged in primary care, that he would enjoy his lifestyle and career and that financially, he would be secure.

Bottom Line

1. Most medical students in the US graduate with educational debt.
2. Physicians will be able to pay back their debt.
3. There are many opportunities for loan forgiveness including federal and state programs.

References

1. Association of American Medical Colleges. Medical student education: debt, costs, and loan repayment fact card. Association of American Medical Colleges; 2021.
2. Kahn MJ, Nelling EF. Estimating the value of medical education: a net present value approach. Teach Learn Med. 2010;22:205–8.
3. Youngclaus JA, Koehler PA, Kotlikoff LJ, Wiecha JM. Can medical students afford to choose primary care? An economic analysis of physician debt repayment. Acad Med. 2013;88(1):16–25.

Case Dr. Davis

Dr. Davis, the managing partner of a large urology group, has become concerned about the changing reimbursement landscape shifting from volume to value. The transition has been the subject of much discussion, but up until now, the new payment methods have largely been optional. Moreover, in comparison to the current structure, it has been challenging to estimate the positive aspects of this change. The practice has successfully operated on a productivity model where provider compensation and incomes are driven by patient volume and procedures. This structure has served the practice well and has been straightforward and easy to both manage and measure. Suffice to say, there has not been a pressing need to alter the current structure. Recently, however, an accountable care organization (ACO) was established in collaboration with the local hospital, which employs all of the primary care providers. In order to stay in the network and continue to receive referrals from the primary care network, Dr. Davis' practice will need to take part in the AOC and accept a value-based medicine reimbursement structure. Additionally, he has been informed that Medicare intends to cut pay-

ments (penalties) to providers who do not take part in at least one advance payment model (APM). To make matters more concerning, one condition for participating in the ACO is the requirement of sharing data with an entity managed by the local hospital that also employs its own urologist. Dr. Davis suddenly finds himself in a difficult position and begins to consider other options, including forming his own ACO with other urology practitioners who may share similar concerns.

A significant emphasis has fallen on primary care for value-based initiatives, as this area can impact the overall healthcare system through coordination of care and preventative measures. As was mentioned in the chapter's introduction, the hospital-owned ACO was pressuring the specialist to join the AOC by leveraging the access to referrals from the primary care providers they employed. A common theme is a fear of being excluded from participating networks. You may recall that this was the exact strategy used when managed care initially entered the market, yet it never produced any major benefits for participation. In fact, many will contend that it increased expenses and layers of bureaucracy without increasing results. The second attempt at this focuses on advance payment arrangements rather than clinical outcomes.

The focus on primary care has led to innovation in the space and investment from nontraditional healthcare sources. There is considerable opportunity for development in the value-based space as many markets are only recently branching into this domain with any degree of significance. The new activity will continue to progress, and private enterprises will innovate to capture market share from traditional healthcare solutions. Thus, it is imperative to think ahead about how patients will access healthcare in the future and to modernize in order to develop solutions they will utilize. Below is an example of an emerging company and its impact on traditional care delivery.

Dr. Davis has good cause to be wary given the difficulty in transitioning to an alternative model. It is said that the best predictor of the future is looking back at past experiences. How will this be different from managed care, which did not produce much value for providers and patients? The short answer is that there are reductions in Medicare reimbursement for not participating starting at 4%, then a gradual increase to a full 9% for not adopting. Margins are already shrinking, and cost is rising, so a 9% reduction would be a significant hit to the bottom line for most providers, especially if the practice has the typical 50% of Medicare in their payor mix. Commercial payors are also following the same guidelines and will be implementing similar reductions in reimbursement for not participating in value-based medicine. But for APMs to be successful, it requires providers, health systems, payers, and patients to adjust economically and operationally to be fully aligned with a single mission. As for outcomes, most providers find it difficult to control patient behavior outside of the clinic, so taking responsibility (or having compensation tied) to outcomes can be unsettling. There is also going to be a need to provide robust data to support these outcomes, which should include tracking patient engagement to prevent providers from getting penalized when patients are not doing their part. Some contend that patients who do not participate in their own qual-

ity outcomes should pay higher premiums, much as how bad drivers pay more for car insurance. Politically this would be difficult to enforce, but employers have already taken steps to pressure their employees to become more engaged with their caregivers.

Since the signing of the Affordable Care Act (ACA) in 2010, value-based reimbursement strategies have demonstrated success as well as failure, with a prevailing theme of uncertainty on both sides of the coin. A variety of programs and incentive structures have been tested by CMS, commercial payers, self-funded employers, and others. From Pioneer ACOs to NextGen ACOs and bundled payments to BPCI Advanced, we are experiencing value-based care 2.0 and should expect to see additional versions in the years to come.

The objectives remain consistent: reduce healthcare costs and improve clinical quality/outcomes while enhancing the experience for patients and providers alike—a worthy pursuit. The Medicare Access and CHIP Reauthorization Act of 2015 (MACRA) was intended to advance these initiatives by establishing the Quality Payment Program (QPP), which replaced the Sustainable Growth Rate (SGR) law that proved, ironically, to be unsustainable. QPP offers two tracks for Medicare clinicians to choose from:

1. **The Merit-Based Incentive Payments System (MIPS)** updates and consolidates multiple previous CMS quality programs such as PQRS.
2. **Alternative Payment Models (APMs)** provide incentive payments for high-quality and cost-efficient care related to a clinical condition, a care episode, or a population.

The year 2017 was the initial year of QPP reporting and was designed to promote success and elicit participation. More than 1 million clinicians participated in QPP, and almost 100,000 of those earned APM participant status, which provided additional financial benefit opportunities. Here, 93% of MIPS participants received a positive payment adjustment (maximum of 1.88%), and only 5% of clinicians received a negative payment adjustment (maximum of −4%). Small and rural practices performed significantly worse, but CMS now offers free support in the form of technical assistance to practices with 15 or fewer clinicians.

Additionally, QPP performance thresholds have increased from 3 to 15 to 30 points in 2017, 2018, and 2019, respectively, and CMS expects to continue increasing targets by 15 points annually. Penalty ranges for low performance also increased to a maximum of 7%, up from 5% in 2018, which will continue to raise the economic stakes for participants. Given the net neutral payment provision, there will be more winners and bigger losers moving forward. It will be interesting to observe how participation is affected by a more pronounced risk-and-reward framework.

The 2019 Final Rule introduced several key changes for MACRA and Physician Fee Schedules (PFS):

- Expanded QPP eligibility to include more provider types as well as an established "opt-in" process for providers who did not meet previous volume requirements.
- Revised interoperability performance category for MIPS.
- Increased PFS payment by 0.25% from 2018.
- Providers can now bill separately for virtual communication with patients such as telehealth visits or reviewing photos and videos.
- Providers are not required to enter redundant information already documented in medical records.
- Delayed the proposed E/M billing code collapse for levels 2 through 4 until 2021.
- Changed fee schedules and added new codes to recognize advances in communication technology and its significant role in the modern patient–provider relationship.
- Created new E/M documentation guidelines to streamline payment and potentially reduce clinician burden.

MACRA is our current vehicle for the journey to value, but time will tell whether its programs and incentives can truly change provider and patient behavior, which is crucial for sustainable success with any model. CMS is taking a step in the right direction to improve access to care and more appropriately compensate physicians and health systems for their work. Technology will continue to play a key role in reporting and monitoring, as evidenced by the increased focus on her interoperability in the 2019 MIPS scoring. Reducing documentation guidelines supports the CMS "patients-over-paperwork" initiative, and providers could potentially increase revenue with more efficient documentation leading to increased availability/access, streamlined coding, enhanced template utilization, and simplified billing processes. Regardless of MIPS participation, it is imperative that providers better understand and prepare for the proposed E/M billing code consolidation which took place in 2021 but is still not fully implemented in some practices.

Proactively Preparing Your Practice for Success:

- Evaluate economic opportunity by modeling financial and quality metric performance.
- Perform a coding audit and establish consistent documentation training.
- Assess the compliance risks and opportunities for your practice.
- Evaluate service offerings such as remote visits to maximize fee-for-service revenue.
- Understand market dynamics and the competitive landscape of value-based care.
- Optimize value-based care infrastructure and operational efficiency to achieve full reimbursement potential.
- Engage providers in operational improvements to drive desired clinical and financial outcomes.
- Utilize the CMS-supported Transforming Clinical Practice Initiative (TCPI) and other free resources to alleviate the administrative burden of QPP participation.
- Take full advantage of all the CMS tools and workbooks for evaluating participation. Refer to the following:
  - MACRA: MIPS & APMs| CMS
  - To check your eligibility, click: The Quality Payment Program (cms.gov)
  - Participation Fact Sheet: MIPS Participation Fact Sheet (cms.gov)

Will MACRA advance us beyond basic data reporting and drive meaningful operational change along with clinical accountability at the provider–patient level? We are poised to take a significant step forward, but the balance of incentives and risk must be more compelling, which cannot be accomplished overnight. Value-based care continues to be a game of timing, and each provider, group, and health system has unique circumstances to consider before participating in QPP or any other value-based programs. Many providers we work with have already engaged in some form of value-based incentives, but strategies are often fragmented with inefficient operational infrastructure. Success is predicated on a proactive and cohesive strategy that explicitly aligns incentives.

Back to the Case
Dr. Davis decided that joining an already-formed ACO would allow him to better position his practice for value-based contracts. He joined an ACO that did not have a downside penalty for subpar performance for the first 3 years. Dr. Davis considered this a good way to learn the principles of value-based care.

Bottom Line:
Value-based care will be the dominant payment model in the future.

Case Omar

Omar is a fellowship-trained urologist who joined an academic practice. His practice consisted of hundreds of patients from the previous urologist. However, he complained of having few physicians in the area refer patients to him. It was a source of frustration. He needed to figure out what action steps he should take to increase physician referrals.

Maintaining positive relationships with patients and colleagues is key to successful healthcare practice. Specifically, establishing and preserving connections with physicians is essential to creating a solid referral network and a steady supply of patients. The mainstay of any successful practice is the patients you already have and the ability to attract new patients, which includes referrals from other physicians. This chapter will discuss methods and techniques to enhance referrals from your colleagues.

Talks on medical marketing often begin with the three A's of marketing: availability, affability, and affordability. Since all physicians probably think of themselves as available, as likable, and as offering appropriately priced services, how do you differentiate yourself from the competition? Using fancy stationery, having a fancy three-colored brochure, a practice logo, or having a slick website will not generate referrals from your colleagues. The last thing to consider is a logo and slick brochure.

One of the biggest misconceptions about marketing is that you must spend lots of money on peripherals and advertising to do it well. The most critical element of your marketing plan is to make your practice user-friendly. Nowhere is this more important than in working with your referring physicians. Many other steps are far more effective and essential to marketing than logos and gifts you send at Christmas.

The traditional methods of obtaining physician referrals usually involve trial and error. These hit-and-miss methods were seldom discussed, and some were almost unquantifiable. Perhaps you went to school with another physician in the area, and later they referred patients to you. Maybe you went to emergency rooms and made yourself available to treat patients who did not have their own physicians. Another source of referrals may occur when you join a group practice and receive overflow patients.

One of the cardinal rules and appropriate advice, especially for new physicians, is to always be available. Suppose a new physician does an excellent job with every new patient referred to them gradually. In that case, the word-of-mouth method will start working, and new patients will be forthcoming. The word gets back to the guiding physician that the new physician is available and is truly competent. The new physician could slowly build a good reputation in this way.

By relying on word-of-mouth and outstanding service, it could take two to 3 years to get a practice up and running. These methods worked in the past because there were enough primary care doctors, enough patients, and enough referrals to go around. Today we are seeing fewer physicians start out by themselves in private practice. Many physicians are opting to join large group practices or are employed by hospitals or are joining with mega groups consisting of large numbers of physicians all in the same specialty and may have physicians who are fellowship trained and are subspecialists with unique, specified areas of medical interest. You must be much more organized about getting those physician referrals.

This chapter will take the concept of physician referrals out of the realm of hit or miss—you will not have to use the shotgun or scattershot approach. Still, you can focus your efforts like a laser to obtain physician referrals. Follow the steps outlined in this chapter. You will have a guaranteed plan for making your name visible and your reputation known within the medical community in a shorter period than it takes word-of-mouth to spread your name and reputation within the physician community. By targeting your efforts, your practice, in essence, will become user-friendly—your colleagues will want to refer patients to you and will enjoy doing so. And as the quote from Aristotle makes clear, this is a deliberate process that requires patience and tenacity over time.

The primary strategy for achieving physician referrals is to have your name cross the minds and desks of referring physicians and their staff members frequently and in a position fashion. If you can do that, physician referrals will come your way. This strategy derives from the tactics of William Wrigley, the chewing gum magnate, who set down this dictum at the turn of the century: "Tell 'em quick, and tell 'em often."

There should be good chemistry between you and your referring physicians. If they have good feelings about you, they want to refer patients to you. You can make yourself more attractive to referring physicians by making it easy to do business with you and your staff. All the 26 techniques outlined in this chapter, from prompt reporting to gift giving, are designed with this strategy in mind.

Almost all the techniques described in this chapter require minimal time, energy, and negligible expense; however, their effectiveness in generating physician referrals is quite significant. Remember, you must have a staff capable of handling patients and ensuring follow-up and excellent communication with referring physicians.

1. Promptly report to referring physicians. The adage for selling real estate is location, location, location. When it comes to increasing your attractiveness to referring physicians, your mantra is communication, communication, and communication. Consider prompt reporting if you are looking for the best way to make yourself accessible to your referring physicians. When primary care physicians were surveyed about why they make referrals, prompt reporting was at the top of the list [1]. It would be best to inform your referring physicians about their patient's progress. It would help if you made them feel that they are the captain of the patient's care ship.

   Nothing is more embarrassing to the primary care doctor than to be in the dark about your opinion or management plan that you have instituted on his/her patient. When you see a patient by referral, follow this cardinal rule: Never allow the patient to return to the referring physician's office or call the referring physician *before* your report has reached the physician's desk. If the patient or the patient's family calls the referring physician before he/she has had a full report, it makes you both look bad.

   The following story is an example of what must never happen: A primary care physician called his patient's relatives at home to tell the family that the grandfather in the intensive care unit was not doing too well. The family said, "Yes, we know he died last night!" This gross lapse in communication resulted in embarrassment for a primary care physician. It would help if you avoided communication failures with your referring doctors.

When a physician sees a patient referred by a primary care physician, it is often seven to 10 days before the primary care physician receives the referral letter. Even with electronic medical records, primary care physicians will only receive follow-up communication for a few days, which increases the possibility that the patient will contact the primary care doctor before the referral letter arrives. The older method consisted of a report dictated, transcribed, and mailed. Frequently the patient will beat the referring letter back to the primary care physician.

How user-friendly are you when a patient returns to their primary care physician, and the referral letter has not arrived? The primary care physician asks the patient what the specialist said or did. The patient responds, "I don't know, but he gave me a large yellow pill, and now I have a rash and am itching all over." Now the primary care physician must ask his nurse to tell the receptionist to call your office, have your receptionist or nurse locate the paper chart or open the electronic medical record, and then track you down if you are not in the office to discuss your management of the patient. That scenario does not endear you to the referring primary care physician as you are wasting the referring physician's time and the time of their staff.

Our solution for avoiding this scenario is to use what we call the "lazy person's referral letter." This is a referral letter that requires absolutely no dictating. Here is how it works: as soon as you have seen the patient, write down, at the end of your office notes, your impressions, the medications you prescribed, and the treatment plan. For instance, if the doctor sees Mrs. Smith for cystitis, recommend that she takes a course of antibiotics and suggest that you see her again in 2 weeks; you circle these three words in the notes or highlight them in the EMR.

When the nurse or medical assistant goes through the electronic medical record after Mrs. Smith's visit, she sees that you have circled or highlighted these words. The nurse uses a boilerplate referral letter with blanks to complete (see Fig. 13.1). The nurse types in the appropriate referring physician's name, the diagnosis, the medications, and the treatment plan. The letter closes with the statement, "I will keep in touch with you regarding her medical progress." We then print out the letter and fax it directly to the physician's office.

This letter delivers the essentials to the referring physician. What are primary care physicians looking for? Most primary doctors will tell you that there are three ingredients of an effective referral letter: the working diagnosis, the medications you have prescribed, and the treatment plan. You can bank money on this one—they are not interested in the depth and detail of your history or the fine nuances you detected on the physical examination. For the most part, they are as

Fig. 13.1 Boilerplate referral letter

Dear [Referring Physician],

[Patient] _____ was seen for a problem of [diagnosis], and he/she is being treated with

[medication] _____ . I recommend that he/she have [treatment] _____ .

I will see him/her again after he/she finishes the medication and will keep in touch with you regarding

their urologic progress.

Sincerely,

Neil Baum, MD

busy as you are and do not have the time to read a lengthy two- to three-page report that you dictated and conduct a treasure hunt to find the diagnosis, prescribed medication, and treatment plan. You can create a user-friendly referral letter that meets the three necessary criteria and lands on the primary care physician's desk before the patient returns for an office visit. If your practice uses an electronic medical record, sending a copy of the EMR notes that can often be coded to an E&M level four or five E&M does not constitute an effective letter. The typical length of these notes—three to four pages—is far too long. Often, the vital information (i.e., diagnosis, medication, and treatment plan) is hidden in the notes and not easy for a busy primary care doctor to locate. Today, most EMRs allow you to create a template with fields that include diagnosis, medication, and treatment plan. Then, with a few mouse clicks or taps on a touch screen computer, you can generate a very effective referral letter that can be faxed immediately to a referring physician while the patient is

still in the examination room. The patient can't be seen by the primary care physician or make a call to the primary care physician before the referral letter arrives. This level of communication with the referring doctors is so effective that if a patient is seen by the specialist and then goes directly from the specialist's office to the referring physician, the letter is in his/her office before the patient arrives. You and your practice become user-friendly by telling the patient that a letter has been sent to the referring physician and that he/she should mention this to the receptionist when they check in with the referring doctor (Fig. 13.2 is an example of a referral letter created on EMR).

Because the letter is sent out immediately, if the patient calls with any questions, the referring doctor can answer any question without contacting the specialist. Furthermore, the letter can usually be generated without any dictating. For those who must dictate the two- or three-page traditional referral letter, consider underlining or boldfacing the essential information, includ-

Fig. 13.2 Example of a referral letter created on EMR

January 22, 2017

Dr. Alfred Colfry
4224 Houma Blvd
Metairie, LA 70006

RE: XXXX

DOB: XXXX

Date of Visit: XXXX

Dear Al,

XXXX was seen for a problem of: XXXX

Chief Complaint: Urinary retention after hernia surgery. The catheter was removed and he was able to void with a weak urinary stream.

Current Impression:

Retention of urine unspecified (788.20; New Without Added Workup)

BPH with obstruction or lower UT symptoms (600.01)

XXXX request transfer of his urologic care to this office because he is elderly, and it is difficult for him to travel to your Metairie office. I told him you have an office on Napoleon Avenue, and he was going to speak with you about those days you are in that office. I also told him that he had to speak with you before he could make an appointment with me, and he told me he would give you a call.

Sincerely,

Neil Baum, M.D.

Fig. 13.3 Stat operative note

Neil Baum, M.D.3525 Prytania, #614New Orleans, LA, 70115 Phone: (504) 891-8454

Date: _____

Your patient _____ had the following procedure: _____

The pertinent findings included: _____

I recommended_____

You will be receiving the dictated operative note. Please call me if you have any questions.

Dr. Neil Baum

ing your impressions, the medications, and recommendations. Nearly all referring physicians prefer a timely computerized referral letter over a delayed three-pager. Doctors may be concerned if referring physicians are upset when they receive a computerized, impersonal form letter. Surveys indicate that referring physicians prefer timely information to delayed personal letters.

Most visits can be handled this way; some of your examinations will uncover a complicated or ominous problem. Suppose your examination reveals a significant finding, or you recommend changing the patient's treatment plan. In that case, you should contact the referring physician by phone and notify them of your findings and recommendations. Failure to do so can potentially result in embarrassment for both you and the referring physician. If the patient calls the referring physician to discuss your suggestions, and you have not yet informed the physician about your treatment plan, it makes them appear uninformed or even uncaring. The referring physician will likely think of you as unprofessional and stop referring patients to you.

Call the referring physician's office immediately afterward if you operate on a patient. Notify the physician's nurse that the surgery went well and everything was successful. A stat operative note that notifies the referring doctor of the outcomes of the patient's surgery, the pertinent findings, and what postoperative treatment will be instituted is very appreciated by the referring doctor. This stat operative note is faxed to the referring physician. It arrives long before the dictated operative note from the hospital or ATC.

(Fig. 13.3 is a sample of the stat operative note.)

Also, notify the primary care physician's office if you realize before or during the procedure that the surgery will be significantly delayed. The doctor will then be up-to-date on the patient's progress if they run into the family on the way to the hospital. However, if a complication develops during surgery or the patient has changed rooms or been sent to the intensive care unit, we suggest you notify the referring physician via a phone call or text the doctor if that is a preferred form of communication. If there is a significant lab or pathology report, call the referring physician and let them know what has been found. In those situations, the patient or the patient's family may contact the physician immediately. If you have not apprised the physician, they will not be well informed.

Other economic considerations are involved in using the lazy person's referral letter. Do you know that the typical referral letter can cost anywhere from $13 to $25 or more every time you pick up the tape recorder to dictate a referral note? How can this be, you ask? Let us do the math: Today, most physician time is valued at $250–$350 an hour. The typical referral letter requires 3–5 min of physician time. So, for your time alone, the cost would range from $7.50 to $16.65. The charges of a transcriptionist, who makes $25,000–$35,000 a year plus benefits and charges you $2–$3 a page, must be added to the equation. Finally, there are costs for stationery and postage. This works out to \$13–\$25 or more per letter. Using the lazy person's referral letter, you reduce your costs to less than \$1 per letter. Plus, it satisfies the needs and wants of your primary care physicians and referral doctors—the letter arrives before the patient returns.

You will find that most of your colleagues will be delighted with the letter and often say they "hoped that our other colleagues would learn to use the same technique." However, if you find a referring doctor who does not wish to receive the lazy person's referral letter, send the more extended version referral letter to one of those doctors. Should you send the longer referral letter, then underline the three necessary areas: diagnosis, medications, and treatment plan. Remember, one size does not fit all.

2. Make your referring physicians look good. Your objective should be to keep the referring physician involved and allow them to function as the captain of the patient's healthcare ship. I am reminded of the story of a patient who went to see an orthopedic surgeon. During the history and physical examination, the doctor asked the patient, "What have you done for your problem?" The patient said, "I've been to a chiropractor." The doctor asked, "What did that fool tell you?" The patient responded, "He sent me to you!"

Whenever possible, compliment the referring physician. Of course, you do not want to appear unnatural or superficial. When the referring physician's name comes up in conversation with the patient, you can comment such as, "He is such a fine doctor and is very knowledgeable about your medical problem," or "She is one of the best doctors in our community."

Often you will receive complimentary notes from patients referred to you by other physicians. These special notes are usually discarded or placed in the patient's charts. Thank you, complimentary notes, placed in a nice scrapbook, can add favorable advantage to the patient's perception of the physician and the office. According to local, state, and national medical societies (including the American Medical Association) that have been contacted, it is stated that there is no violation of patient privacy or confidentiality if you are sure to obtain the patient's permission for placing the letters or notes in your reception area scrapbook.

We also suggest you photocopy each note and send it back to the referring physician with an accompanying note that reads, "Thought you might like to see that your patient had a positive experience at my office." After all, the kind of experience the patient had reflects back on the referring physician.

If a patient tells me, "I sure am glad that Dr. Jones sent me to you," I have a response. "Do me a favor," I say. "The next time you see Dr. Jones, mention that you had a good experience at my office." The patient is more than happy to oblige, increasing the positive feedback the referring physician receives. Also, if the patient gives you a compliment, ask him/her if she would submit that compliment to the online reputation review sites such as Healthgrades.com, yelp.com, or RateMDs.com.

Also, remember that the patient's perception of you is partly determined by the patient's opinion of the referring physician. If you make the referring physician look good, you are also enhancing your image.

3. Vary your referral patterns. Today, the number of patients referred to specialists is decreasing. One of the reasons for this is that certain specialists (for instance, gynecologists and general surgeons) are doing more primary care and keeping the patients in their practices. When patients go to a multispecialty group practice or preferred provider organization (PPO), they are kept there. They do not circulate in the community looking for other healthcare providers. Also, primary care physicians are treating more medical conditions that were once referred to specialists. Finally, an emphasis on cost-containment means that many primary care physicians now treat adult-onset diabetes, arthritis,

benign prostate enlargement, urinary incontinence, and even common dermatological conditions.

Often, referral patterns are cut in stone, and specialists refer to only one or a few groups of primary care doctors. One of the benefits of your marketing efforts will be that patients will come directly to you. As a result, you will become the primary care doctor and control the referrals. For example, if a patient comes to a urologist with urinary symptoms, she needs to see a gynecologist or a cardiologist, and the urologist becomes the referring physician and can direct the referrals.

Specialists must make every effort to send new patients to primary care doctors who have frequently referred patients to them. Now more than ever, it is essential to acknowledge referrals from primary care doctors and other specialists. The best way for you to do this is to take advantage of your marketing and send new patients to your colleagues. They will appreciate new patients more than a fruit basket at Christmas.

4. Provide courtesies to your referring physicians, and do not inconvenience them. One of the best ways to prevent inconveniences for your referring physicians is to assist with the hospital paperwork on patients you share. For example, has your office notified the referring physician when admitting their patient. If you do this, the hospital secretary will only call the referring physician on time, which may require the physician to see the patient later that evening or early in the morning. Likewise, contact the referring physician when you discharge their patient. By doing this, you ensure that the referring physician will not make a needless trip to the hospital to see a patient who has been recently discharged.

You can fill out the prescriptions that apply to your specialty and leave them in the patient's chart or with the patient so that the referring physician does not have to write all the prescriptions.

This also applies to hospitalists who are caring for referring doctors' patients in the hospital. Hospitalists are also marketing themselves to the PCPs and the specialists, and they want to be user-friendly. Hospitalists also need to keep the avenues of communication open between the hospitalists and the referring doctors by ensuring that what was done to their patient was sent to the referring doctor so that continuity of care will occur after the patient is discharged from the care of the hospitalists.

Remember, you want your referring physicians to feel that it is easy to work with you and that you will go the extra mile on their behalf.

5. Recognize your referring physicians' accomplishments and those of their children. There is no better way to enhance your relationship with your referring physicians than to acknowledge their accomplishments. Whenever one of your referring physicians receives an appointment or promotion, acknowledge it with a written note. It is a nice gesture to cut out articles from local newspapers that mention your referring physicians or their families.

A nonmedical story that emphasizes this concept: A doctor's son was 4 years old, and he rescued a bird from the backyard swimming pool. The family took the bird to the zoo, where it was saved. The family's rabbi heard the story and sent the 4 year-old boy a letter:

"I just heard the story of your wonderful, good deed in saving the bird from drowning in the pool. You should be proud of yourself. I am proud of you for doing such a wonderful thing. Whenever you hear the birds chirping to themselves, you can be sure they're singing your praises.

Well done, Craig. Rabbi Cohn."

Can you imagine how much Rabbi Cohn's stock escalated when the 4 year-old boy received that letter? The parents could not wait to contribute to the synagogue's annual fundraising campaign!

Doctors like to hear positive comments about their children. Taking the time to learn about their children is a guaranteed way to let your referring physicians know that you are thinking of them. (This is also a nice gesture to do for your patients.) Send a note if a referring physician's child just received a scholarship or athletic award. Your staff is usually familiar with the names of your referring physicians. They can call them to your attention when reading the newspaper or finding evidence of online accolades. This is a simple little thing to do, but it is universally appreciated.

6. Send birthday cards. Sometimes it isn't easy to find out your colleagues' birthdays. You can try calling their hospitals or the county medical society. Ask for the birthdays, not the birth years. You will not be given the years—that is confidential—but frequently, you will find out the days. You might want to compile a list and ask for all the birthdays at the same time.

7. Do not intrude on your referring physicians' turf. Today, many physicians are trying to generate additional practice income by performing procedures or diagnostic tests in their offices. You need to be aware of who performs which tests. Avoid performing tests or procedures that your referring physicians are equipped to handle. For example, if you plan to admit the patient of a referring physician to the hospital, ask the patient to have the preadmission blood work, EKG, and chest X-ray done in the referring physician's office rather than at the hospital or a third-party laboratory. If blood work is all you request, have your office draws the blood, sends it by courier to the referring physician's office, and asks for a copy of the results for your records. When you use the referring physician's facility or laboratory, you are being considerate and allowing the physician to maximize the use of their equipment and employees.

8. Show an interest in your referring physicians as people/friends in addition to their role as a source of patients. Try to know about your referring physicians' nonmedical interests and hobbies. Whenever you see or read something of interest to one of your referring physicians, take the time to send it to them or call it to their attention. This is one way of saying that you are interested in your referring physicians even when you are not professionally relating to one another. For example, if one of your colleagues is a fly fisherman and you see a book on fly fishing offered in a catalog or on Amazon.com, send him the book, especially if you know he plans to leave for Alaska to go salmon fishing. This simple and inexpensive gesture will endear you to your referring physicians.

9. Invite your referring physicians to participate in support groups or seminars. This increases their exposure in the community and also provides them with an opportunity to attract more patients.

If a referring gynecologic physician is an expert in hormonal issues in menopause, invite him/her to participate in one of your programs on women's health issues. This can be a plus for both doctors in terms of exposure in the community and will likely result in new patients for both doctors.

If you involve colleagues in your specialty, they will be less likely to try to torpedo your marketing efforts. You will create allies, not adversaries, in the medical community.

10. Remember your referring physicians' staff. In addition to building a good relationship with your referring physicians, you must include their staff. Whenever you have contacted with them, make it a point to be pleasant, cooperative, and interested in them as people. Learning their names will go a long way toward building a good working relationship. You will be surprised how many physicians staff have the ability and the permission to make referrals to other physicians.

11. Ensure that you are easy to contact. You can make it easier for your referring physicians and their staff to contact you and your office by supplying each office with a colored

Rolodex card. The card can be made more visible by making it slightly higher than the standard Rolodex card. It should contain your telephone number, including your private line, office hours, answering service number, and the names of your office manager, secretary, nurse, and any other employees who may be requested by the referring physicians or their staff. Most practice management software programs contain physician directories where the contact information is located. You want to be sure that your information is correct in those directories. A nice gesture is to provide referring doctors with your cell phone number so they can easily reach you. Remember, you do not want to make it difficult for a referring doctor to locate you.

12. Start a journal club network. As every physician knows, staying abreast of the medical literature is no trivial pursuit. There are over 5200 medical journals indexed on Medline, and the National Library of Medicine search service now has access to 9 million articles. With the literature doubling or tripling every decade, it is nearly impossible for busy practitioners to read all the journals in their areas of interest and expertise. Fig. 13.4 is an example of a letter for starting a journal club.

By developing a journal club network with your fellow physicians, you maintain an awareness of the literature and help your colleagues at the same time. For example, there were reports in the medical literature on the ophthalmologic side effects of Viagra and other phosphodiesterase-5 inhibitors. If you see articles that might be of interest to your ophthalmologic colleagues, send them copies and also to any other doctors who might be prescribing phosphodiesterase-5 inhibitors.

You can start your journal club network by sending a letter to about ten of your colleagues. Explain what you are doing and what they can gain from participating. Fig. 13.4 is an example of a letter that can be used to start a journal club.

The network is best kept informal—you do not want to add work to your colleagues' loads. The easiest way to accomplish this is to email the articles to your colleagues, and they can read them online or print them if they want a hard copy. Your staff can also be alerted to look for newspaper articles and lay magazines related to your colleagues' specialties. This helps keep your colleagues informed on what their patients are reading.

13. Target your colleagues' reading. As with the journal club network, targeting their reading can facilitate your colleagues' continuing medical education and yours. If you send a referral letter that mentions a new diagnosis or treatment modality, attach an article that contains the latest information. Doing this increases the likelihood that your colleague will read the article. Consider using a yellow highlighter pen and mark the one or two sentences most pertinent to the patient and the referral letter. For example, the use of thiazide diuretics is associated with the side effect of erectile dysfunction. ACE inhibitors or calcium channel blockers are less likely to produce erectile dysfunction (ED). Before a patient starts on one of these antihypertensive drugs associated with ED or stops the thiazides because of the fear or presence of

Fig. 13.4 Example of a letter for starting a journal club

[Date] _____

Dear [Physician] _____,

With the rapid pace of developments in medicine today, it is difficult for most physicians to keep up with the progress. As a way to stay abreast of all the changes, I suggest that you and I establish an informal journal club.

I will be reviewing the urologic literature on a regular basis. If I see articles that are pertinent to [physician's specialty], I will make copies and forward them to you. I hope you will do the same for me. Perhaps in this way we can extend and increase our coverage of the medical literature.

Sincerely,
Neil Baum, MD

ED, make an effort to educate your referring doctors by including a copy of the journal article with the referral letter. To ensure that referring doctor reads the article, underline the one or two sentences describing the efficacy of the medication you recommend.

To further direct a colleague's attention, you can add a note to the article's front page with a message (e.g., "Please see page XX"). Although this might seem like you are setting up a treasure hunt, you can be sure your colleague will appreciate being directed to the appropriate information. You have supplied new information and saved your colleague time.

14. Identify interests that you share with your referring physicians. For example, if one of your colleagues graduated from Notre Dame and was a fan of Lou Holtz when he was the head coach of the football team, and you have a copy of a speech by the famous Coach Holtz, send a copy of the speech or the link of the speech from YouTube. Another way to let referring physicians know you care about them is to send them books, CDs, cartoons, and even nonmedical articles that may interest them.

Suggested books you might send colleagues to include Tim Russert's book, Big Russ and Me, Richard Carlson's Don't Sweat the Small Stuff—and It's All Small Stuff. Rabbi Harold Kushner's When Bad Things Happen to Good People.

15. Hold on to old friends. When physicians retire, their former patients often continue to call them. They still have a lot of clout in the professional community. And, of course, their patients ask them for referrals to primary care physicians and specialists. Acknowledge a colleague's retirement in some way by sending a note of appreciation or taking them to lunch. Then, continue to remember your colleague on the same dates as before. This will help you maintain a referral source even after your colleague's shingle has been taken down.

16. Keep tabs on the movers. When a physician moves to another area of the country, it is essential to maintain communication. If you send a "good luck" letter, cards during the holidays, and your blog/website information, this will encourage the physician to send you patients when someone from the community asks for a referral.

17. Develop intra-specialty referrals. You can do this by finding niches in the marketplace. Even if you are a specialist, you can still get referrals from other doctors in the same specialty. You may be doing procedures or diagnostic tests that they are not doing, and that may be helpful to them. You may have equipment or training that they do not have, allowing you to develop referrals from colleagues in your specialty.

The key to these referrals is to ensure you send the patients back to your colleagues and that you do not operate on these patients for other problems that the original doctors can handle. Treat the patients only for the problems that the referring physicians requested.

Let your colleagues know you are willing to see their patients and send them back. The easiest way to do this and make your colleagues feel secure is to offer to work at their institutions. In that way, the referring physician gets to see the procedure and has the security of knowing that you are not taking the patient away.

Another way to get referrals from specialists in your field is to refer patients who call when you are unavailable. Sometimes patients call with a problem that cannot wait. Rather than have your staff said, "I'm sorry, the doctor is not available," and let that patient go back to the Internet to find a doctor, you can refer them to one of your colleagues. For instance, if you are out of town, have your staff called the covering doctor's office to get an appointment for the patient. Your colleague appreciates getting a new patient and hopefully will return the favor.

18. Develop cooperative projects with referring physicians. For example, a urologist worked with a group of gynecologists interested in treating urinary incontinence. They did a project comparing biological materials to

synthetic materials for vaginal slings. It was a small project, but it created an excellent opportunity to work together and learn what worked best for our patients with this condition. The doctors receive recognition and publicity if they collect the data and write a paper. This collaboration has the potential to bring all the participants, new patients.

19. Personally meet every physician who refers a patient to you. If you do not go out of your way to meet that physician and invite him to your office, somebody else will, and that referral source will soon dry up. You often hear the following remark in the doctor's lounge: "You know, I have a referring doctor down in St. Elsewhere. He's sent me two to three patients a month for the past 5 years, and I've never even met the guy!"

If a physician refers two to three patients a month to you, you need to visit their office and meet him/her personally. Try to make your paths cross. Offer to give a talk at the physician's hospital. Otherwise, that golden goose (your referring physician) will cease laying the golden egg (referring patients to you).

20. Meet all new physicians in your area. Every July and August, when physicians announce they are starting their practices, you will receive announcement cards in the mail, or you will see these announcements in the paper. Most doctors throw those cards away. Some doctors write "congratulations" on the cards and send them back to the sender. It is best to take this gesture one step further.

Write a welcoming letter to each new physician. Offer to get together for breakfast or lunch. Then offer to share resources. If the new physician is in private practice, visit the office with your manager. Indicate that you would be more than happy to have your office manager assist the new physician's office manager.

New physicians frequently will have many questions, even if they join a group or are employed by the hospital. You can offer to be of assistance, and this will be appreciated by your colleagues.

21. Refer patients to physicians new to the area, especially those just starting their practices. Send patients to new physicians as soon as possible. Everyone remembers who their first few patients were. If you are the person who referred those patients, you will be forever appreciated by the primary care doctor. First, patients make an indelible impression.

22. Offer marketing advice to new physicians. In addition to sending new patients to new physicians, refer them to one of the best books on ethical medical marketing, *Marketing Your Clinical Practice—Ethically Effectively, and Economically* Jones and Bartlett, 2010 [2]. This book provides ideas for new physicians just starting their practices, and the marketing chapter discusses ethical but effective methods of practice promotion. Another good resource is the article "Ten Action Steps to Transition from Residency to Private Practice." This article includes a segment on marketing a medical practice, especially for the physician just entering practice [3].

23. Keep your referring physicians abreast of your specialty or practice changes. If you attend a meeting or convention with new information that may interest your colleagues, email a single-sheet informal newsletter about the latest developments in your practice and field. These short newsletters are often much appreciated by referring physicians.

Give your referring physicians valuable and unique gifts. Giving gifts to referring physicians is not the most effective method of generating referrals. If you send wine or a fruit and cheese basket between Thanksgiving and Christmas, it will most likely get lost among the dozens of similar gifts the physician received. However, there are techniques of providing gifts that will make you stand out from the others at holiday time.

If you know your colleagues' reading habits, consider giving them subscriptions to their favorite magazines such as Architectural Digest, Connoisseur, or National Geographic as gifts.

Another nice gift is a Lucite cube that could be used either as a picture holder or as a place for motivational quotes by Winston Churchill ("Never give in, never give up, NEVER, NEVER, NEVER"), Vince Lombardi ("If you strive for perfection, you may not always reach it, but you will achieve excellence."), and Abraham Lincoln ("Success may come to those who wait, but they will receive only the things left by those who hustle."). Then each month, send another motivational message to insert in the cube, as well as a story or comment about the author and how the quote applies to the contemporary practice of medicine. Experience has demonstrated that colleagues really seemed to appreciate this unique gift. You know that this is an appreciated gift. When you visit the referring physician's office, you spot those Lucite cubes with motivational quotes on their desks.

One of the best gifts is laminated and personalized luggage tags. The tags are bright red with the colleague's last name in white type and laminated, with gold-colored plastic cords to attach the tags to the luggage. The luggage owner with these tags will recognize their suitcase when it comes down to the baggage chute at the airport.

By varying the time of year, you send your gifts, you can also make them stand out. For instance, consider sending your gifts and holiday wishes at Thanksgiving instead of during December. People are usually more relaxed at this time, and chances are that they will remember your gifts.

One very generous and appreciated gift is to donate to a charity or civic organization in the name of one of your referring physicians. Of course, it helps if you know your colleague well and choose a charity or foundation they have worked for or supported.

We do not consider gift-giving essential to a successful marketing plan or effective physician referral program, but if you decide to give gifts, make them timely, unique, and one that will last the entire year.

24. Provide suggestions and recommendations to your primary care doctors for referral to your specialty. For example, only some UTIs or enlarged prostates require a consultation with a specialist. Provide the primary care doctor with a short monograph on suggestions for specialist referral. This monograph reviews the most common urologic conditions and gives evidence-based medical guidelines for management and referral.

25. Finally, go the extra mile for your referring physicians. Make it a pleasure for them to work with you. Find the little extras that make it a convenience instead of a chore. These little extras can significantly affect your relationships with your referring physicians.

For example, a referring physician once asked about the office's unique uniforms. The office manager sent the doctor and the doctor and his office manager a copy of the catalog used to purchase the uniforms. Both highly appreciated this gesture, and all it took was a little effort from us.

Facts of Life Discussion

All of us would like to have a bilateral referral arrangement with our colleagues. Have you ever experienced a situation where you send patients to another physician and get no reverse referrals? Of course, you can change your referral source, hoping that the other physician will notice a decrease in referrals and call you to ask what happened, but do not hold your breath. Chances are the physician is busy enough and will not notice the decrease.

A better alternative is to discuss the facts of life with the physician. Ask whether the quality of patients was satisfactory and whether the physician would like to continue receiving your referrals. During your meeting, recall for the physician the number and names of patients you have sent them in the last 6–12 months.

If the physician answers yes to both questions, ask how they feel about your quality of medical care: "Do I enjoy a good reputation in our community? Have the patients I have sent you, as well as any others we may both be treating, been satisfied with my medical services?"

If the answers are yes, it is time to initiate the "facts-of-life discussion." If they disagree, it is time to find another referral source. You should consider seeing some patients in return if you are to continue referring patients to that physician.

Facts of life discussion story: An internist contacted a urologist when one of his patients from the intensive care unit was in urinary retention and needed the insertion of a urethral catheter. For several years, the urologist went to see these patients, often in the middle of the night, hoping to demonstrate that he could provide urologic care for all his patients. However, when this internist had patients with nonemergency urologic problems, the internist referred them to another urologist. After a few years of being inconvenienced in this way, the urologist requested a meeting with the internist. The urologist started the discussion by saying, "I am capable of seeing patients not only in the middle of the night but also between 8:00 AM and 5:00 PM as well!" The urologist did not request all his referrals, but he did ask for a few. If that was not acceptable, the internist should call another urologist to come in the evening to insert catheters. What was the worst that could happen? He would receive no referrals; however, he would have a good night's sleep!

As it happened, this discussion brought about a change in that internist's referral pattern, and the urologist also began receiving a few daytime referrals. This hard-ball approach is only for some and in some circumstances. However, whenever you feel exploited or that referrals are a one-way street consider having a tactful discussion before abandoning the potential referral source. Remember not to go into such a discussion with a defensive attitude. There may be a straightforward reason for the physician's behavior, and you only saw it from your point of view.

If you are worried that marketing will leave you all alone, perhaps even generating contempt from your colleagues, remember that effective marketing includes rather than excludes your colleagues.

Back to the Case

Omar recognized that staying in the office and not trying to meet the potential referring physicians in the area was the best place to start his marketing efforts with his colleagues. He visited all the physicians his age in the community and tried to know their staff. He arranged to give several grand rounds of presentations on his areas of interest and expertise. Omar created an informal journal club with his fellow colleagues. He sent effective referral letters to the local doctors, including articles he authored demonstrating his areas of expertise. Omar made every effort to be available when called for a consult or for a patient in the emergency room. Within a few months, he noted the fruits of his labor and started receiving referrals from the doctors in the area. In essence, he took the advice from Aristotle and recognized that obtaining physician referrals was metaphorically "a slow ripening fruit."

Bottom Line

Marketing yourself to your colleagues does not mean you are trying to take away "market share." When you open possibilities, you increase their business as well as yours. How you do this does not take away, it just adds—to your stature in the professional community, to the respect you get from your peers, and to the bottom line.

References

1. Barnett ML, Keating NL, Christakis NA, et al. Reasons for choice of referrals among primary care and specialist physicians. J Gen Intern Med. 2012;27(5):506–12.
2. Baum NH. Marketing your clinical practice-ethically effectively, and economically. Burlington, MA: Jones and Bartlett; 2010.
3. McGuire P. Smoothing out the transition from residency to practice. Today's Hospitalist. https://www.todayshospitalist.com/Smoothing-out-the-transition-from-residency-to-practice/.

Branding Your Medical Practice: How to Make Your Practice Distinctive and Unique or Branding Your Medical Practice-Going from Tap Water to Evian

14

Case Kaila

Kaila is a junior associate practicing primary care in a multispecialty practice located in a moderate-sized community. Kaila joined the multispecialty group practice immediately after residency and received most of her patients from specialists in her group. Kaila is interested in nutrition and weight loss and chose her residency because of its focus on wellness. Kaila would like to put those skills to use to broaden her referral base. Kaila plans to attend practice promotion and marketing seminars to learn more about branding her practice.

It was not so long ago that the concept of branding referred to using a hot iron to make your cattle look different from all other cattle on the range to distinguish your cattle from others. Today, in the business world, branding is used to create the perception that a product or service is superior to other businesses in the community, the region, and the nation.

How does a passenger train differentiate itself from the behemoth airline industry and keep market share in the transportation market? One distinction is all it takes—Amtrak's distinct competitive advantage against airlines: scenery!

Flying to a distant destination certainly takes less time and may even cost less than taking a train. So why does passenger train travel still exist when an airplane ride takes less time and is cheaper?

One example, the Northern Pacific rail line, has a new "Vista Dome" car, and passengers can marvel at a 360° view from inside the dome. Amtrak carefully schedules its rides so that passengers can see the best vistas during the prime sunlight of the day. Their subtle message is, "You can't see the same scenery from an airplane." This distinctive branding, and their scenery message, cannot be duplicated by multibillion-dollar airlines.

Another example that nearly everyone has experienced is the marketing and promoting of bottled water, i.e., Evian®, Fiji®, and Smartwater®, to name a few of the many bottled water brands. In contrast to many areas of the world, most tap water is free and safe to drink in our country, yet millions of Americans pay $1.69 or more for a liter of bottled water. The price of bottled water is 20% more than the same volume of Budweiser beer, 40% more than the same volume of milk, and three times the cost of gasoline! Now that is the power of branding: motivating people to pay more for water than what is available for free at the tap. Let us provide some examples of how physicians can make their practices the Evian of healthcare.

Most of our choices—from the coffee shop we frequent for our jolt of java to the company that provides the medical supplies for a medical office—are based on a branding strategy. Doctors may not even be aware of it because subliminal suggestions, social media, and word-of-mouth marketing can be as contagious as a multimillion-dollar advertising campaign.

The healthcare profession is late to the concept of branding. Branding occurs in the real world by associating a product or service with a company or organization. If you hear jogging shoes, you think of Nike. If you hear the word "computers," you think of Apple. If you hear "soft drinks," you will likely think of Coca-Cola. What does the public in your community think of when they hear about weight loss, controlling blood pressure, or in-vitro fertilization (IVF)?

If this is not your practice, it is time to think about branding your practice. Brand loyalty does not happen by accident. Practices that cultivate loyalty find ways to connect with their customers and patients. Brands stand for something meaningful to your existing patients and are essential for attracting new patients to your practice and maintaining the loyalty of patients already in your practice.

The healthcare industry can learn invaluable lessons from other industries. Benefits exist at physicians' fingertips if they can effectively leverage the advances in digital technology to market and manage their medical practices. First, the rise of digital technology changes the landscape of the entire healthcare industry, and physicians must build their businesses with an eye toward the future. Second, physicians must create a professional brand, and they must promote this brand where their potential patients are. Patients are increasingly seeking healthcare answers, as well as providers, online. Finally, recognize that digital technology lowers the cost of healthcare, both for doctors and patients.

For a medical practice to thrive, brand recognition helps obtain recognition. If a practice does not take the time to build a unique brand, patients will seek care elsewhere. Perhaps the practice has had the unfortunate situation of just one "negative online review" giving the practice a "one-star rating," or the practice may have a label or reputation that cannot be erased or prevented. Some examples of things that lead to negative reviews include long wait times, unfriendly front desk personnel, and the inability of patients to get through by phone because of the phone tree. As in other businesses, the most successful hospitals and practices usually have a strong brand that differentiates them from others that provide similar services. This chapter will define the concept of branding and show how any practice, regardless of size or budget, can create a brand. This chapter will also discuss creating and establishing a successful brand that brings loyal patients to your office for their medical care.

What Is Branding?

The American Marketing Association (the other "AMA") defines a brand as a "name, term, sign, symbol or design, or a combination of them intended to identify the goods and services of one seller or group of sellers and to differentiate their product from those of other sellers." The act of "branding" is more than that. It is everything you do to attract and maintain quality patients. Branding allows for a practice to emotionally attract the type of patient they want in their practice. Such a "fit" creates patients who choose you over your competition. Branding allows you to differentiate your medical practice from all other practices in the community. Branding takes into account the "look and feel" of your office, your staff, your materials, you, and every other detail that gives your patients clues as to who you are, what you value, and how a patient might receive treatment if they become a patient in the practice.

The business side of healthcare is swiftly changing. Both physicians and office managers are looking for new ways to connect with patients. In the distant past, a new physician would place an announcement in the paper and a listing in the Yellow Pages® of the local phone book, and then she was ready to practice her craft. Physicians would promote themselves by meeting colleagues in the physician lounges, going to the emergency rooms, and waiting for patients to arrive. Today, it is more difficult to build a practice using these antiquated techniques with managed care plans, healthcare reform, the Internet, and social media. Now it is necessary to build a brand for your practice.

Questions you need to ask *and* answer in considering your brand include: What makes your medical practice unique and special? What is your sustainable competitive advantage? Everyone believes that they are members of a unique practice or organization, but how do we convey that to our existing patients and potential new patients? Have you thought of yourself as the best in your field in your community? Or are you the best physician to treat a specific disease or condition? Are you the best surgeon in your area or region? Do your patients see you as the superstar, and, most importantly, do they know about your areas of interest or expertise? If not, you need to build a more cohesive image using branding. Branding is the art of attracting your preferred patients using very specific messaging that will get their attention and motivate them to select your practice for their medical care.

Branding is also an opportunity to create a name, a term, a symbol, or a design that identifies and defines your practice and will differentiate your practice from others. Branding is more critical than marketing or sales. Branding is influencing and changing the way people think. Branding appeals to desire and touches emotions. The goal of branding is to emotionally predispose potential patients into entering into a relationship with you because they believe you are the best choice for them. With more medical information available to existing and potential patients at their fingertips, today's medical consumers are too sophisticated and skeptical about being sold.

They want to arrive at their own decision on their terms. Branding is helping them get there. Branding "presells" your expertise or practice before the patients even meet you or open your office door and enter the reception area. These potential patients call to make an appointment because of the aura or the impression you have created that you are the best at what you do and the best fit for them. Your patients also believe they will receive outstanding care and attention from you and your staff. Branding offers you an opportunity to sculpt your practice exactly as you would like. Your brand can attract only cash-paying patients, patients of a specific demographic such as age or location, patients with the disease or conditions you would like to treat, and patients with the disease or conditions where you are the expert. These are likely patients who provide you with the greatest satisfaction of providing them with your medical care and your medical expertise.

Successful practices and businesses have a mission statement that serves as a road map for employees and guarantees to patients (customers) the excellent service they will receive. A brand is your opportunity to declare your promise to your patients about the outstanding service they will receive when they are part of your practice. Your brand can attract patients to the practice as long as you keep the promise and you deliver on that promise. This ability to find a unique distinction also applies to the healthcare profession and even to a medical practice if the practice can identify its unique distinction in its marketplace.

Benefits of Branding

Branding allows you to become your patient's first choice as their physician even before needing a doctor. Branding can attract and maintain quality patients who have had a positive experience with you and your practice. Attracting and maintaining quality patients happen by promising and then delivering on the promise to give your patients a stellar medical experience. Then, patients return to you repeatedly, and they brag about you and your practice to their family and friends creating invaluable word-of-mouth buzz about you and your practice. If you are in a competitive environment, you need to attract patients by creating visibility for you and your practice. Your visibility brings more prospective patients to you, but your ability to keep them depends on the quality of service you provide them when they are with you and when they interact with your staff. So, your name and your face need to be circulating in the community in a tasteful, professional way that your preferred patient base will see.

Branding is all about perception and visibility, which builds credibility in the eyes of your prospective patients. Patients want to feel comfortable with their choices, and familiarity breeds that comfort. If they see something in the media a few times, it sounds familiar to them, and they get the impression it must be good. When prospective patients recognize you and say to themselves, "gosh, he looks familiar" or "I've heard that name before," you are on your way to developing a brand. All things being equal, the more positive visibility you create, the more likely you will attract patients to your practice.

Your patients' and prospective patients' perceptions are your reality, and they define their decision to go to you versus all the others due mainly to your branding. They have made this decision not based on evidence but on their perception that you are the best choice. They did not get to that choice using logic—they made the decision emotionally and then justified their decision with logic. Perhaps they saw you on the news, your photo in the social column at a fundraiser or their friend passed along the informative newsletter you distributed to your patients. It can be the monthly column you write for a local magazine or publication or your appearance on the local news, including an interview about a new procedure or treatment you offer your patients. Branding also occurs if you sponsor a health-related event such as a walk or run to cure a specific kind of cancer.

Another benefit of branding occurs when your website is at the top of the search engine list on Google, Yelp, or Yahoo. Today it is far too competitive to rest on your laurels. Your name needs to stay in front of your preferred patient base, so they visit you when they have a present medical need now or in 6 months or next year. You cannot assume they will stay loyal to you if you do not keep your relationship current with them. If you are not visible, you allow your competitors to redirect your patients to their practices. Avoid this situation at all costs.

Getting Started to Brand Your Practice

Begin by letting your patients know why you are unique such as your specific fellowship training or advanced medical skills. Inform your patients about what you offer beyond what most of your competitors do not—such as evening and Saturday morning appointments or technology or treatment that others do not have or offer. Do things differently to stand out—provide transportation for your older or housebound patients to and from your office or the hospital (as long as this is legal in your practice area).

Convey your personality in your marketing tools—you can portray yourself as the "Top Doc to the Stars," the professional team in your community as their doctor, or "The Local Neighborhood Doctor."

- Specialize and be selective. It is not possible to be everything to everyone. Instead, select an area of interest or expertise that is unique and special and that makes you and your practice special.
- Be where your prospective patients are—have offices in various parts of the community or region where your preferred patients live. Having multiple offices makes it convenient for your patients to become part of your practice without traveling a great distance to receive medical care.
- Build rapport and trust with every patient—use the patient's name when speaking to them in person or over the telephone. Make the patient feel special and not just a diagnosis or a medical condition. When a patient calls for

an appointment, your receptionist should conclude the phone call by stating the patient's name at least twice before terminating the call: "Mrs. Smith, it is nice to speak with you. Dr. Strangelove looks forward to meeting you a week from now at 2:00 P.M. Do you have any questions before that appointment?"

- Stay in contact with your patients throughout the year—send them a practice newsletter, birthday cards, and thank you notes when they refer a patient to you.
- Refine your patient relations processes—have your staff introduce themselves by name to new patients and then walk all new patients from the reception area to the exam rooms. Of course, make sure you see them on time!
- Stay consistent with your message. Do not try to be all things to everyone. Select an area or areas that you deem worthy of your brand, and then make sure you relate that message to existing patients and potential new patients.

For those physicians who take branding seriously, the payoff can be huge. The difference between good and great practice is in the details. Please pay attention to every aspect of yourself, your staff, and your practice to ensure it is consistent with your personality and the image you are trying to portray. Do not think of branding as taking patients from your colleagues or competitors. Think of branding as the opportunity to have your existing patients and potential new patients have your name and the name of your practice come to mind whenever a medical problem you treat or have as an area of expertise comes up in any conversation.

To start the branding process, you will need to gather your staff and conduct a brainstorming session. You should begin by writing down what you want to achieve and identify your target market. For example, if you are an orthopedist and wish to specialize in sports medicine, write down the ages of patients you want to treat, the nature of injuries you want to treat, and the ability of this patient population to pay for your services. Be as specific as possible to define the medical condition(s) and the demographics of the patients, payer mix, and what you can reasonably deliver

consistently. This latter situation or consistency is vital to the success of your branding process.

Your branding must sync with your skills, staff, facility, operating systems, and guiding principles. Set aside at least an hour for a branding brainstorming session with your team. Ask your staff to write down as many concise core messages they can think of that pertain to your practice in each of these categories:

- Courtesy (how you will treat patients, colleagues, and fellow providers).
- Punctuality or your level of commitment to being on time. We believe that this is one of the essential ingredients of branding: providing patients access to the practice and seeing patients on time. You can be the most outstanding expert in the area, but if patients have to wait four to 6 weeks to obtain an appointment and come to the office and wait 60 min to see the doctor, all of you will waste all of your branding efforts.
- Expertise in areas of your specialty. If you are an expert, this is where the rubber hits the road or how you differentiate yourself from others in the community.
- Referrals or how you will accept or forward communications and recommendations for care or services. You must place a priority on your communication with your referral sources. For the most part, this means sending a referral letter within 24 h after you have seen a patient referred by a colleague.

Next, consider the needs of your target market. Suppose you are an obstetrician specializing in infertility, and you need to establish a reproductive laboratory. In that case, you need to think about the technicians and other specialists who you will need to have in place. To have patients conduct all of their care at one facility and not have to go to multiple offices or laboratories is essential to make your practice user-friendly.

You have to identify your competitors. Do not think just of your local competitors. Consider those in the region and the rest of the nation, and depending upon areas of expertise, you may want to consider your global competitors. For example, practices that want to attract patients worldwide to come to their country for orthopedic procedures, significantly cheaper than the same procedure performed in America, organize the medical tourism industry in their countries. They are making it possible for patients to have visas, airline reservations, hotel reservations before and after their surgery, and even doctors who will participate in the postoperative care once they return to their home towns. This branding concept is to make it less expensive and hassle-free for patients who are willing to have surgery in such a setting. How are you different from the competitors? What makes you unique from those who offer the same services? For example, a urology practice in New Orleans is branding itself to provide urologic oncology care for patients from South America, a form of "reverse tourism." They have Spanish-speaking doctors and staff; they meet patients at the airport and provide transportation to the medical center. They essentially choreograph every aspect of the patient's care by providing outstanding customer service and the clinical skills of caring for the patient. To make this work, you want to list the unique benefits that patients might experience from being a patient in your practice. For another example, there is an academic practice in Boston specializing in treating urinary incontinence. This Boston practice has branded itself as a "one-stop-shop," which makes them attractive to the patients and the insurance companies, and the payors. They can evaluate the patient in one visit, conduct a complete history and physical exam, do all the diagnostic tests, discuss the treatment options, obtain consent, and do the pre-and post-op teaching on the first visit. This one-stop-shop concept contrasts the three or four trips that are typically needed by many other urogynecology practices because they cannot charge patients for diagnostic studies on the same day as the initial office visit when the E/M (evaluation and management) is generated.

During brainstorming sessions with your partners and staff, in order to get the best ideas, it is essential from the first session to avoid making any judgments on those who offer suggestions. You want to have as many unfiltered ideas and thoughts provided in this first brainstorming session. After this first brainstorming session, we suggest you publish your branding statement and share it with all of your staff before your next meeting. Your next meeting will allow you to refine your responses and answer the questions raised in your first meeting. At that second meeting, you will want to fine-tune your branding statement and then use it to create your strategy and tactics for implementing the branding message.

Displaying Your Brand

Look for opportunities to display your brand. If you have a website, take an objective look at it. Is there a way to add your updated brand message? What about your business cards? Perhaps you can have them redesigned to include your brand message. You might even create signage for your office to set the tone or display your brand. But more important than any of those tactics, find ways to share your message through your words, attitude, and behavior. No matter what you display externally, it is who you are internally that is your genuine brand.

Every successful business, including your medical practice, benefits from having a solid branding message. When creating your brand, make sure it is a proclamation and a promise and not a pitch. Because what you are delivering is a promise, and that is what the branding buzz is all about.

Back to the Case
Kaila's branding experience consisted of creating a website, with the permission of her multispecialty group, that focused on nutrition and the role of good nutrition in maintaining good health and using nutrition to improve many medical conditions. Kaila also began a monthly blog highlighting the importance of good nutrition. Kaila prepared a newsletter that she sent to exist-

ing patients and referring physicians. The newsletter was sent to her target market every quarter. Kaila created a slogan, "Kaila loves kale," which appeared on her website, stationery, and blogs. As a result, Kaila enhanced the number of patients she received from existing patients and other primary care physicians. Kaila soon found herself seeing patients with nutritional needs, using her skills as a nutritionist, and meeting the unmet nutritional needs within her community. She had a real sense that she saw the types of patients she wanted and felt that her practice was becoming a good fit for her skills and interests. Kaila was a real branding success story.

Bottom Line

Branding is not just for soft drink companies, bottled water, Amazon, and Nike shoes. Also, branding in healthcare is not just for the Mayo Clinic or the Cleveland Clinic. Nearly every practice and every hospital have the potential to create a brand or an area of expertise. The brand sets the practice or hospital apart from others in the community or the region. Be consistent and

use that brand to define the visual image, verbal communication, and the patient experience in all encounters. Einstein said, "If you can't explain it to a 6-year-old, you don't understand it yourself."

If you fall short in maintaining the promise to the patient of your brand at any stage, the relationship and implied trust will be at risk. Instead, create the best possible experience for your patients and establish a long-lasting brand that generates new patients and maintains the loyalty of existing patients.

Further Reading

Corbin CL, Kelley SW, Schwartz RW. Concepts in service marketing for healthcare professionals. Am J Surg. 2001;181(1):1–7.

Kemp E, Jillapalli R, Becerra E. Healthcare branding: developing emotionally based consumer brand relationships. J Serv Market. 2014;28(2):126–37. https://doi.org/10.1108/JSM-08-2012-0157.

Knowles H. Six things that make great healthcare branding strategies successful. January 10, 2018. https://medium.com/madison-ave-collective/six-things-that-make-great-healthcare-branding-strategies-successful-e2518cb0fa52.

Ries A, Ries L. The 22 immutable laws of branding. New York, NY: Harper Collins; 2002. p. 30.

Case Rochelle

Rochelle works with a small pediatric group practice and has recognized that she needs a medical assistant. Rochelle's partners agreed with her request and suggested she do the necessary screening and evaluation to find a suitable physician extender. Rochelle has never had to hire an employee. She realizes that she never learned about hiring or firing in any of her training. What should she look for? Where should she start?

Hiring the right employee that meets the requirements outlined in the job description is vital to the success of the practice. It is important to find the best employee available among the applicants for job openings in the practice. There will certainly be occasions when an employee must be terminated. This also requires tact, knowledge of the labor laws, and sensitivity to avoid further bruising egos and hurt feelings. This chapter will discuss the hiring process that has worked in the healthcare sector as well as other industries and professions and provide a guideline for the termination of an errant employee without running afoul of labor laws.

There has been a departure of healthcare workers from the healthcare profession following the pandemic of 2021–2022. This exodus has been referred to as "the Great Resignation" or the "Big Quit." It is not just nurses and allied health professionals who are leaving but also physicians who decide to leave their medical practices. As a result, record numbers of Americans in all professions leave their jobs. Many medical practices and hospitals are experiencing openings that are going unfilled. As a result, this places stress on the existing staff, which ultimately may impact patient care.

We will begin with the hiring process to find that match made in heaven and then conclude with the proper methods for terminating an employee. Hiring the right person to fill a staff position requires time and attention.

Finding the Match Made in Heaven

Like any other business, for the health and ultimate success of your practice, you must have high-quality, efficient, and dedicated staff. Someone not suited to your practice can create a negative impression among your patients and cause the morale of your staff to quickly decline. With today's tight healthcare labor market and competition from large hospitals and other industries that are offering higher salaries and more benefits, medical practices often have trouble competing with larger employers. The challenge of finding the right person for the job is made even more difficult. Does this mean that you should settle for a less-than-qualified employee? Certainly not! Despite other opportunities, job seekers still seem to find the idea of working at a medical practice attractive. A position with a private practice offers status as well as the gratification and enjoyment that come from helping others. By offering fair salaries and cooperative working conditions, you can build a top-notch staff. Hiring staff members is a delicate process and a skill that you will probably improve as you and your practice mature.

However, hiring is a process that requires time and patience. Being in a hurry to hire someone to fill a vacancy and making the wrong decision can lead to expensive turnover and a very uncomfortable work environment. Studies have shown that the average cost of employee turnover, whether you are correcting a hiring mistake or replacing a longtime employee, is two and a halftimes the salary of the worker you are losing. But turnover also brings hidden costs in addition to the tangible costs of salary and benefits. The time it takes to do interviews, the overtime you pay others to pick up the slack while you have a vacancy, and the impact on the morale of your existing staff can wreak havoc with your practice. One way to find your candidates is word of mouth using multimedia. You might consider taking advantage of job-listing services at local schools, universities, and professional organizations. Today there are websites where you can post job opportunities. One of the most popular job-listing sites is Craig's list (www.craigslist.org). This Internet site features job postings, classifieds, etc., and is favored as a networking tool for the younger generation of savvy job seekers. If you are looking for an associate, consider using Linkedin.com, which allows you to connect with potential physicians who are looking for positions.

Screening Your Applicants

Begin by requesting applicants to submit an electronic resume to your email address. You might ask your office manager to screen the resumes and then call the applicants to schedule an interview. Your office manager should speak to each applicant personally when they call your office the first time. This phone call is too important to be screened only by your receptionist. The office manager should specify the time of day when they can receive calls from applicants or set a time to return calls to the applicants. Another option to the telephone is to schedule a brief Zoom virtual visit. This allows the office manager to see the applicant and evaluate their communication skills, their dress, and their demeanor. After the office manager has screened applicants and narrowed down the choices, the doctor personally calls the finalists. Talking with an applicant personally allows you to evaluate:

- The applicant's telephone manners.
- The applicant's curiosity about you and your practice.

You want an active, vibrant individual who exudes enthusiasm. If you do not sense vitality and enthusiasm in a phone conversation with the applicant, your patients will not sense it either. Ask the applicant to send a handwritten letter along with their resume and application. Suggest a topic for the letter. For example, you might suggest that the applicant explain why they want the job, why the applicant is qualified for the job, or how the applicant could enhance your practice. You might also suggest that the letter address a nonmedical topic, such as the applicant's hobbies or last vacation. The letter can be scanned and emailed, faxed, snail-mailed, or hand-delivered to the office.

This letter will serve several functions:

- It allows you to see how quickly the applicant responds. In most medical practices, a speedy response can often be vital.
- It allows you to analyze the applicant's writing and spelling skills. (Obviously, you do not want to hire someone who cannot spell correctly or whose handwriting is more illegible than yours!) If the applicant is emailing the letter, this also allows you to evaluate their "email etiquette"—an important feature these days, when too many people fail to proofread or edit before they hit the send button!
- Finally, a written letter will frequently reveal something about the applicant that is not available in their resume.

The Interview Process

Encourage preparation. The interview will be more productive if you allow applicants to prepare. Before an interview, send the applicant a job description and information about you and your practice. If you have a primary care practice, you may want to send information on what you do, what kinds of patients you see, and what typical situations someone who works in your office might encounter. If you are a specialist, send the applicant information on the nature of your specialty or some educational material that you give to patients about the various diseases, illnesses, and conditions you treat. I am impressed when applicants demonstrate that they have read this information or have visited the practice's website and asked questions about anything they have not understood.

Make the most of each interviewing session. You can do this in several ways: the first few minutes of the interview can be used to break the ice. For example, you might tell the candidate about yourself, your practice, and the job description.

Next, consider providing the candidate at the time of their visit with a written list of questions (Fig. 15.1). Using a written list encourages candidates to do the talking. It is a good idea that you interview promising applicants more than once. First impressions are important, certainly, but most couples do not get engaged on their first dates! Many applicants will be eliminated after the phone call or first interview. Those still in the running need a second, third, or even fourth interview before the job offer is made.

Consider asking "curve ball" questions. At least one time during the interview process, ask the candidate a difficult question. In any medical practice, circumstances will often arise that require the staff to think creatively and respond quickly. Failure to react quickly can adversely affect the health of patients and might even lead to litigation. Suppose the candidate has worked in a medical office or has healthcare experience. In that case, you might ask a question such as, "What would you do if a patient called with a medical emergency and the physician could not be reached or located immediately?" Fig. 15.2

Fig. 15.1 List of questions to ask job applicants

Name

1. What are your strengths?

2. What are your weaknesses?

3. Why are you interested in changing jobs?

4. What was your best job? Your worst?

5. Tell me about your best boss.

6. Tell me about your worst boss.

7. What do you think your references will say when I call to inquire about your past employment?

8. What do you want to be doing one year for now? Five years from now?

1. If I did a procedure that did not have a CPT code, how would you attempt to obtain insurance coverage from a third-party payer?

2. How would you handle it if a patient began arguing with you in front of other patients about the cost of his visit?

3. If a patient called on the telephone and demanded that he be seen the same day as he called, and you knew that the problem was not an emergency, what would you tell him?

4. What would you say to a patient who requested that his records be sent to another physician? 5. If you saw a patient in a grocery store and you were with your spouse or significant other, how would you introduce them?

Fig. 15.2 List of "Curve Ball" questions to ask job applicants

contains additional examples of curveball questions you might consider asking.

Give a potential hire a "homework assignment." In addition to the curveball questions, which require immediate answers, we suggest that you present each applicant with a more complicated problem and allow them time to work on the response after the interview is over. For example, you may ask the applicant to propose a solution for a problem at the practice. How quickly the applicant responds to this "homework assignment" tells you about the applicant's creative problem-solving abilities as well as the strength of the applicant's desire to get the job.

Encourage the applicants to ask questions. This allows you to evaluate their level of interest in and curiosity about the job. If an applicant fails to ask any questions, this suggests that the applicant is intimidated by the interview process or is not very curious. If either is the case, you are learning something important. You want to hire people who are both curious and not easily intimidated. For instance, if an applicant's only question is about the salary or vacation pay that would be a clue to their priorities. If an applicant asked about furthering skills through seminars, night classes, or additional training, this might be an indication to put this applicant on the shortlist.

References

There is an unwritten rule regarding references: Do not give references out, but do not hire without them.

Many employers will make the mistake of calling the previous employer without any introduction and expect the previous employer to talk about the applicant and their employment history. Accept that the information you receive will likely not be complete and should not be the determining factor of whether you hire the individual. You can obtain information on an applicant through a background check (with proper authorization from the applicant). Still, you should not use criminal background information until after a conditional offer of employment has been made.

Many employers only give out a name, job title, and pay rate but will not provide specific information on performance and the applicant's termination because they are fearful of a lawsuit (Falcone, 2002). This situation can be avoided by asking the applicant to sign a release-of-information letter (see Fig. 15.3) and emailing or faxing it to their previous employers before your call. This avoids your cold calling a reference and not receiving any useful information.

Applicants will often not give you names of references unless they expect them to respond favorably. To get around this hurdle, ask applicants for additional references during later interviews. The length of time it takes them to respond will tell you something about the quality of the references.

Have your existing staff members interview each applicant. Your staff will tell you whether that person will be a team player and will make a good fit with the current staff.

Release Form

I am an applicant for employment with Dr. Baum. I am submitting a signed release form that provides you with permission to speak with Dr. Baum or one of his representatives regarding my previous employment and experience with you. I have read all the information in the attached request concerning your experiences with me as an employee. I agree with the content on the form and give you permission to release the information to Dr. Baum. I hold you harmless for any information you furnish regardless of the outcome of the application for employment.

Date:
Signature:
Notary Seal and Date

Fig. 15.3 Example of release of information letter

Pay attention to follow-up. Did the applicants return your phone calls promptly? Did they send you thank you notes after their interviews? Remember that the way they handle the business of looking for work today is how they will handle the business of working for you tomorrow. More important, the courtesies and manners they extend to you will be a barometer of how they will treat your patients.

Back to the Case

Rochelle got the word out in the medical community that she was looking for a medical assistant. She also posted a job description on Craig's List, but her best candidate came from one of her patients who had a daughter who was a trained medical assistant and looking to change jobs because of the great distance she had to travel from her home to her office. After thoroughly vetting Rochelle and a paid day to shadow her, Rochelle was hired, and both Rochelle and the medical assistant were happy with the decision.

Bottom Line on Hiring

Although the hiring process is time-consuming and stressful, it is essential for creating an excellent practice where outstanding service is provided by both the doctor and the staff. The costs of taking the time to hire the right employee are much less than the high costs of employee turnover.

Ready, Aim, Fire! Tactfully Terminating an Employee

The remainder of this chapter will discuss the legal process of terminating an employee and how to avoid running afoul of the labor laws and potentially risking a lawsuit if the termination is not done correctly.

Case of Terminating Theresa

Theresa was serving as office manager for a small group oncology practice. She had been with the practice for more than two decades when the practice merged with two other oncology groups in the community. Although Theresa was an excellent employee and was respected by the staff and the doctors, her skill level was not going to be adequate for managing a multi-million-dollar large group of oncologists. It became apparent that Theresa would have to be terminated. How does the practice terminate a good employee after so many years of service?

Termination of Employees: Dot Your i's and Cross Your t's

The overwhelming majority (95%) of private employers, which includes private medical practices, are nonunionized. Unionized employers, those that have contracts with unions covering wages, hours, and working conditions of their employees, are generally required by the contract to show that they had "just cause" to terminate an employee. This situation typically develops when an employee has been terminated and files a grievance with the union, which ultimately goes to arbitration. Arbitrators usually rule that the employer has the burden to prove just cause by a preponderance of the evidence, a high standard. Arbitrators often send terminated employees back to work even though the employer felt it had good reason to remove the person.

Why do we speak about unions in the context of this book, given that most private clinics and medical practices are not covered by union contracts? Since the enactment of the National Labor Relations Act of 1935, 29 USC §§ 151–169), and the Taft Hartley Act of 1947, 29 USC §§ 141–197, there have been significant changes in the laws affecting employment such that employees no longer need the help of a union to challenge their termination.

Those laws include:

- Title VII of the Civil Rights Act of 1964 (Title VII) (42 USC §§ 2000e-2000e-17) prohibits discrimination based on race, color, sex (including amendments by the Pregnancy Discrimination Act and the Civil Rights Act of 1991), national origin, and religion.
- Age Discrimination in Employment Act (ADEA) (29 USC §§ 621–634) prohibits discrimination based on age (40 and over).

- Title I and Title V of the Americans with Disabilities Act (ADA) (42 USC §§ 12,101–12,117) prohibit discrimination based on disability (including amendments by the Civil Rights Act of 1991 and the Americans with Disabilities Act Amendments Act (ADAAA)).
- Genetic Information Nondiscrimination Act (GINA) (24 USC §§ 2000ff-2000ff-11) prohibits discrimination based on genetic information.
- Uniformed Services Employment and Reemployment Rights Act (USERRA) (38 USC § 43) prohibits discrimination based on past, current, or prospective military service. Protects civilian job rights and benefits for veterans and members of reserve components.
- Section 1981 of the Civil Rights Act of 1866 (Section 1981) prohibits discrimination based on race, color, and ethnicity in the area of contracts.
- Most states and some municipalities have their own laws, which mirror many of the federal laws, and some provide protection beyond them, e.g., LGBT status.
- Family and Medical Leave Act (FMLA) (29 USC §§ 2601–2654) protects employees' rights to take up to 12 weeks of leave for medical and family care purposes.
- Workers' compensation laws prohibit retaliation against employees for making worker's compensation claims.
- National Labor Relations Act (NLRA) (29 USC §§ 151–169) prohibits termination because of an employee's protected and concerted activity on behalf of a group or for organizing or union activity.
- Fair Labor Standards Act (FLSA) 29 USC §§ 201–219) prohibits termination for exercising wage and hour rights.

How do these laws affect your decisions to terminate employees? Let's consider the "Bones Are Our Business Orthopedic Clinic," a clinic that has been in practice for 5 years and has five doctors and a support staff of 20. The clinic has experienced a decline in patients and the retirement of the head of the clinic. To meet these financial demands, as well as to deal with specific personnel issues, the clinic has taken the following actions:

1. Martha, an X-ray technician, is pregnant and has been restricted to lifting no more than 50 lbs.
2. Walter, a 61-year-old maintenance worker, had a heart attack and was restricted from lifting over 40 lbs. The clinic assigned Henry to help him when such lifting was needed. Martha heard about this and quit threatening to sue. The clinic advised her that she needed to go home, have the baby, and come back within 12 weeks.
3. Horace, an African-American male technician, had arrived late for work five times and had two unexcused absences within the past 3 months.
4. Sharon, a white female nurse, was late for work days on eight occasions and had three absences within the same time frame. The clinic terminates Horace but does not terminate Sharon because it deems her an essential employee.
5. William, a physician's assistant, went on active duty with his reserve unit 6 months ago and is now seeking to return to work. The clinic eliminated his position during his absence.
6. A patient complains that she does not want to be treated by Willie, a transgender male nurse, and she threatens to leave the clinic and take her large family, who are also patients, with her. The clinic terminates Willie to comply with the patient's request.
7. The clinic holds clinic-wide meetings for all employees and doctors every Friday morning. At one of the meetings, Jerry, an X-ray technician, complains that he and the rest of the staff are not fairly treated because they are not allowed to leave the clinic during their 45-min lunch break, for which they are not paid. Dr. Arthur, the head of the clinic, tells him that these are the rules, and if he does not like it, he can leave. Jerry responds that the clinic does not care about the employees, and he urges the rest of the staff to protest. Dr. Arthur terminates Jerry on the spot.

8. Nick, a Muslim physician's assistant, tells you he must pray five times a day. You tell him this would be too disruptive to the workplace and patient care, and he should look for other work.

What problems do you see with the above actions, and what laws do you think might apply? How can a doctor or a clinic avoid termination problems such as occurred at the Bones Are Our Business Orthopedic Clinic? The following steps are recommended:

1. Be familiar with the state and national laws that may apply to your employees.
2. Develop appropriate policies covering termination as a part of your employee handbook and/or personnel manual.
3. Educate the staff, especially the doctors and supervisors, as to the policies and legal ramifications covering employment termination.
4. Have the employees acknowledge in writing receipt of the policies and that they agree to comply with them.
5. Consistently apply policies and procedures to all employees without any exceptions.
6. Evaluations—be honest—do not sugarcoat the employee's deficiencies—this may come back to haunt you when you are considering termination. Make objective evaluations based on facts and not hearsay.
7. Consider placing a problem employee on an improvement plan, for example, 60 or 90 days, to achieve satisfactory performance. Review their performance every 30 days and document the improvement or lack of progress.
8. Document disciplinary actions as they occur and ensure that you have sufficient documentation to support a termination.
9. Ensure that the decision to terminate is based upon objective criteria and does not involve personal feelings.
10. Before deciding to terminate, conduct an impartial internal investigation and properly document the results of the investigation.
11. Determine if any employees have engaged in similar conduct and what disciplinary action was taken.
12. Analyze whether termination of the employee will have an adverse impact based on race, sex, age, or any protected category.
13. Where circumstances call for termination, act, do not delay.
14. Delivering the message to the employee:
    (a) Have a witness with you.
    (b) Arrange for the meeting with the employee to be private.
    (c) Collect and review the employees personnel file with particular attention to disciplinary write-ups.
    (d) Be prepared and rehearse for the meeting.
    (e) Discuss any employment agreements with the employee, including offer letters.
    (f) Present the termination decision to the employee and avoid arguing with the employee.
    (g) Have the employee's final pay and benefits prepared and have the check at the time of termination. You must decide if the employee is going to receive severance pay and have a waiver and release ready for their signature. For this action, you may need the advice of a labor or employment lawyer.
    (h) Be sensitive to the termination and recognize that this will be an emotional situation for the employee.
    (i) Allow the employee to speak, but do not argue with him or allow him to go on at length. If possible, do not interrupt the employee while they are talking.
    (j) Document the termination and have the witness also sign off on the document.
    (k) Obtain all clinic property from the employee, such as computer, parking pass, and keys to the office.
    (l) Disable electronic resources the employee had, including email, voice mail, passwords, and log-ins.

(m) Remind the employee of any continuing obligations, including non-competition and non-solicitation agreements and protection of confidential information and trade secrets.

(n) Escort the employee to his desk, allow him to gather belongings, and politely escort from the premises. If you anticipate resistance or violence, you may want to ask for a security officer from the hospital to accompany you and the employee.

(o) Advise the remaining employees of the termination either directly by the person who handled the termination or through other supervisors or managers.

(p) Consider how to inform patients of the action.

15. Determine what information will be provided to inquiries or references concerning the employee's employment and termination. You cannot go wrong if you give the dates and titles that the employee worked in the practice.

Following these guidelines will help you make the right decision and defend that decision if you are challenged by a discharged employee who is seeking damages for wrongful termination.

Back to the Case

Theresa had been a loyal employee and certainly did an excellent job when the practice was small and before the merger with the other two oncology groups. Theresa was given 4 months of pay and was told that her health insurance would be paid for 4 months after she left the practice. She was also informed that the practice would provide her with a favorable letter of recommendation, and she could use her previous employer as a reference. Theresa accepted the "goodbye gift" and left on good terms from the practice.

Bottom Line on Hiring and Firing

You may find the hiring process time-consuming and stressful, but that does not come close to comparing with the time and stress it will cost you if the candidate you hire is not a good "fit" with your practice. Follow the suggestions in this chapter, and you are likely to hire right the first time!

Circumstances surrounding hiring and firing are a source of angst among doctors, office managers, or human resources in the healthcare setting. The practice must develop skills and techniques to find the right person for various positions in the practice. Hiring takes time and energy, and mistakes can be very costly to the practice. Having the wrong employee in a position can significantly impact the efficiency and productivity of the practice. When the employee is not working out and fitting in with the practice, then comes the difficult process of terminating the employee. Termination can result in a deterioration of morale and can be very costly to find a replacement. Also of concern is the potential risk of liability for wrongful termination if the termination process is not followed, as we have shared with you in this chapter. This process of hiring and firing should not be minimized or delegated to a doctor or manager who does not have the skills to find the right person or the skills and knowledge to terminate an employee.

Further Reading

Da LH. How to manage problem employees: the big picture. J Med Pract Manag. 2021;36(4):205–12.

Falcone P. The hiring and firing question and answer book. New York: American Management Assoc; 2002.

Moriarty J. Business ethics: a contemporary introduction. London: Routledge; 2021.

Szalados JE. Employment and human resources law: an overview. In: Medical-Legal Aspects of Acute Care Medicine. Cham: Springer; 2021. p. 493–511.

Case Tomika and the Tail

Tomika is completing her training as an internist and plans to join a large group practice in the same community where she trained. She is married, her husband is finishing his training, and they plan to move closer to their families in 2 years. Tomika knows she will be employed in her current position for only 2 years. Her contract stipulates that she has a claims-made policy and that there is no tail coverage after she and her husband leave the community. What are Tomika's options?

One issue that every new physician must contend with is the subject of malpractice insurance. Medical malpractice insurance is one of the largest expenses a young physician will face in their career. The subject of malpractice is often shrouded in mystery and can be very time-consuming, especially if it is the first time confronted with this expensive decision. Young physicians who take the time to understand and buy malpractice insurance will save money and ensure they receive the right type and amount of coverage. This chapter will discuss the concept of malpractice insurance and what every young doctor needs to know about this issue.

Most malpractice policies cover the expenses incurred while defending and settling a malpractice suit. These include attorney fees, damages, arbitration, settlement costs, court costs, and punitive and compensatory damages.

Types of Malpractice Insurance

There are two categories of malpractice insurance: (1) claims made and (2) occurrence. A claims-made policy provides coverage only if the policy was in effect when the incident occurred and filed a lawsuit. Occurrence policies cover any claim for an event that takes place during the period the policy was in effect, even if the claim is filed after the policy lapses. Because a claim can be filed years after an event and after a claims-made policy expires, these policies often include a "tail" that extends coverage for a specified number of years beyond the expiration date of the malpractice policy. Tail coverage can be bought separately if it is not part of the original policy.

For example, suppose a physician has a malpractice claims-made policy and receives a malpractice lawsuit during their employment. In that case, the doctor will be covered under a claims-made policy. If the doctor has an occurrence policy and is sued *after* they leave the practice, but the policy was in effect while the doctor was

© The Author(s), under exclusive license to Springer Nature Switzerland AG 2023
N. Baum et al., *The Business of Building and Managing a Healthcare Practice*,
https://doi.org/10.1007/978-3-031-37623-8_16

practicing, the doctor will be covered and protected by the policy.

Tail coverage offers protection when a physician is changing jobs or retires. Sometimes the cost of tail coverage will be covered by a previous employer to protect itself or can be negotiated with a new employer. Occurrence policies generally do not require tail coverage but occurrence policies are only available in some states.

If you or your employer is buying a claims-made policy, be sure that the beginning date for coverage is accurate and matches the date on the prior policy to ensure no coverage gaps between policies.

The coverage can vary by state, specialty, and arrangements with hospitals or your employer. Some states require doctors to have minimum coverage, but you can request additional coverage depending on your specialty.

Generally, standard coverage limits are $1 million per claim and $3 million aggregate, which is the most the policy will pay in a year for all claims. However, certain states require different limits based on medical malpractice caps on damages. States with more litigious climates might require additional coverage.

Suppose a lawsuit is filed and found to be credible or legitimate. In that case, malpractice insurance will cover the injured patient's costs to a limit set by the state. Some states have patient compensation or catastrophe loss funds, which provide an additional layer of coverage over the primary policy limits. Doctors must pay into these state-run funds through a surcharge on medical malpractice insurance premiums. The rest is paid by the state's fund.

Finding a Malpractice Carrier

We emphasize that price certainly is one factor, but it should not be the only one in selecting a malpractice carrier. Most states have a few carriers licensed to sell insurance in the state. If you focus only on price, you might be hiring an unreliable or financially precarious carrier.

Make sure that the policy has a consent-to-settle clause. This clause prevents the insurer from settling a claim without the doctor's permission. Sometimes, insurance companies find it cheaper to settle a claim than to defend it. However, the doctor's reputation is at stake, and doctors are reticent to settle a claim if there is no evidence of malpractice.

The very best malpractice carriers will act as resources for their physician clients. They will offer advice on how to avoid claims and will hold the hand of the doctor during the process of any litigation.

A few suggestions for screening potential carriers include:

- Ask colleagues in the state where you plan to buy insurance about the malpractice carrier's reputation.
- You want to know their history of settling claims.
- Go to AM Best and check the carrier's financial position. AM Best provides the financial stability of the carriers and rates each carrier. Using this service, you can compare apples to apples (www.ambest.com).
- Check how long the carrier has been in business.
- Does the carrier specialize in specific medical fields such as obstetrics, neurosurgery, or anesthesia?
- Where is the carrier located? Do they have an office close to where you are going to practice?
- Do they want to have a relationship with you and meet you personally, or is it only through the Internet they communicate with their clients/doctors?

To Broker or Not to Broker

A broker has the depth of knowledge and the experience to know the coverage a doctor or practice needs and the best insurers to provide.

A broker helps keep us informed of what our needs are and what changes have to be made. For example, if a practice bought a general insurance policy 10 years ago, there was probably no provision for cyber insurance in case of a hack and loss of your data. A good broker will contact the doctor/practice and suggest that cyber insurance be added to the policy. Other insurance coverage risks include regulatory requirements such as compliance with the Health Insurance Portability and Accountability Act (HIPAA).

We suggest you contact your broker every 2–3 years and ensure you are up to date and adequately covered or if there have been new developments since the policy was purchased. Examples of a need for evaluation and changes in the policy include:

- Adding a provider
- Starting a new business, joint venture, or adding ancillary services
- Forming a new entity, i.e., sale of the practice to a hospital or merger with another practice
- Adding new services or equipment

Our take-home message is that if you can find a knowledgeable broker, it is much easier to hire them to do the heavy lifting, get the quotes, and inform you, the managing partner, or the office manager.

Back to the Case

Tomika approached her employer and asked about tail coverage. The large group practice said they could not make any exceptions regarding tail coverage for her. Tomika contacted a broker who found a tail-only policy at a reasonable premium that would be in effect for 5 years after she left the practice. Tomika purchased this policy and received additional compensation from the large group by offering her a "moving allowance" to help defray the extra cost of the tail insurance. Lesson learned: you can always get your own way if you have more ways than one!

Bottom Line

Malpractice insurance is required in every state. Most hospitals, ambulatory treatment centers, or outpatient surgery centers will require a malpractice policy to practice. For most employed physicians, medical liability coverage is usually provided as part of the employment contract by the hospital or the health system. It is essential to check your contract and make sure you have coverage if you leave the practice for any reason. The old CYA is now CYT or "cover your tail!"

Case Cassandra

Cassandra is a recent family medicine graduate who worked for 3 years in a primary care medical practice. She found that she was soon overwhelmed and was required to see more patients than she was comfortable with. As a result, she and the staff had to work overtime, increasing the practice's overhead. What are some solutions to her dilemma?

Healthcare has encountered a situation where the demand for our services exceeds the supply of physicians. Very shortly, the shortage of physicians will become even greater. When writing this book, primary care physicians are already in short supply. The American Academy of Family Physicians predicts a shortfall of 40,000 primary care physicians by 2020. Moreover, the US Bureau of Health Professions projects a shortage of 109,600 physicians in all specialties by 2020. One thing is sure—following the passage of the Affordable Care Act (Obama Care), 32 million additional Americans will have health insurance, and someone will need to take care of them. Who will provide medical care to millions of newly insured people? Upon passage of the Affordable Care Act, physician practices were overwhelmed by the increased demand. Many doctors stopped taking new patients; the concept of concierge medicine, also called direct primary care, has decreased the availability of primary care physicians. Physicians who continue to accept new patients have seen waiting times for appointments lengthen significantly. Visits to emergency rooms have increased by 7%, adding unanticipated costs to the program. To resolve this situation, physician practices and hospitals must proactively add capacity to treat many new patients. This chapter will identify mid-level providers and describe the role they can assume to increase the care we want to provide our patients.

Ideally, all Americans will have access to primary care physicians to help them maintain good health and prevent unnecessary emergency room visits. But primary care physicians are already in short supply.

One of the solutions to this dire situation is to use mid-level providers (MLP). This is an idea that is receiving recognition by the medical profession as well as patients. However, it is an area of controversy. However, mid-level providers are in our offices and hospitals, and the numbers are increasing rapidly. There is no going back, and we will not change that momentum.

© The Author(s), under exclusive license to Springer Nature Switzerland AG 2023
N. Baum et al., *The Business of Building and Managing a Healthcare Practice*,
https://doi.org/10.1007/978-3-031-37623-8_17

Who Are the Mid-Level Providers?

There is confusion in the medical profession about the names and titles associated with MLPs. Other terms that have been used for MLPs include limited-license providers, nonphysician providers, allied health providers, midwives, advanced practice providers, and even medical assistants.

Where Are MLPs Working?

Today, roughly 80,000 nurse practitioners (NPs) and 30,000 physician assistants (PAs) work in various settings around the country [1]. They have traditionally provided supervised care in rural and underserved settings, where they work under the supervision of a physician who may or may not be in the same office or community. In these settings, mid-level providers diagnose and treat a broad range of common medical conditions under supervision, referring the more complicated cases to the supervising physician. Many states have granted mid-level providers prescriptive authority, and in some states, NPs can practice independently of physicians. In our modern healthcare marketplace, clinics in pharmacies and other retail locations are often staffed with MLPs.

Over the last 30 years, the roles of MLPs have expanded well beyond the primary care environment. Today, mid-level providers work in hospitals, emergency departments, inpatient and outpatient surgical facilities, and specialty practices as part of the team that serves patients receiving ongoing treatment. It is often a mid-level provider who monitors diabetics, sees cancer patients between treatments, reduces bone fractures in the ED, or closes the surgical incision for the doctor at the end of surgery. As mentioned, many states now allow some MLPs to practice independently of supervising physicians.

MLPs include two distinct groups, physician assistants (PAs) and nurse practitioners (NPs). Their educational requirements and training are quite different. PAs receive three times more clinical hours in training than NPS. On the flip side,

NPs usually have more clinical work experience, which frequently balances out their lack of clinical training hours and perhaps levels the perceived training gap between the two groups.

The cultural, clinical training, and competencies of the two groups (PAs and NPs) are often nuanced, and the difference between NPs and PAs is subtle [2]. The big difference between PAs and NPs lies less in training and ability and more in a cultural difference or a difference in practice expectations. Depending on the state where MLPs practice, NPs increasingly are being delegated as independent practitioners free of physician supervision requirements. In contrast, PAs appear to have a career goal that takes them along a path to work dependently with practicing physicians.

It is important to understand that for lower-acuity patients, beyond the diagnostic work, 80% of the tasks (and time) to manage these patients do not require the skill sets of a physician. These tasks involve data gathering, reviewing past history, documenting the patient encounter, tracking and reviewing results, writing prescriptions, and other routine patient management tasks.

The physician's job is to engage in the critical portions of the patient encounter, that being the diagnostic decision-making, management, and treatment planning. By off-loading or delegating the perfunctory work, physicians gain leverage in productivity while simultaneously providing that critically important contribution to the quality of patient care. This is the direction we should be adopting regardless of whether the mid-level provider is a PA or an NP. Since the advice from physicians regarding medical care is often critical and time-sensitive, the MLP allows physicians to be more productive and more available to patients. This results in an improvement in the quality of care. From the patient's perspective, it improves the patient's experience and satisfaction with their care and will probably decrease healthcare costs. MLPs work throughout the entirety of healthcare, from health promotion and disease prevention to diagnosis that prevents and limits disability [3].

Clearly, it is important to understand the productivity and workflow advantages generated through the employment of MLPs. The average range of a mid-level provider in 2022 was $100,000–$140,000 per year. That is less than the cost of even the lowest-paid physicians. The average productivity of an MLP in the office setting is 1.6 patients per hour or about 80% of a physician's productivity. Adjusting the cost of an MLP for this variance in productivity generates a minimum of 50% improvement in the cost of care for this lower-acuity subset of patients. That is a significant improvement in financial margins. Theoretically, should we reinvest those margins—one could significantly increase the number of providers available to evaluate patients, thereby reducing wait times and improving both patient safety and patient satisfaction. This is where this workforce strategy begins to solve our demand management dilemma of balancing cost and service.

Compensation for MLPs

MLPs are nearly always paid a base salary based on years of experience, with extra compensation for overtime pay and additional payments for taking calls. MLPs participate in standard, all-employee benefit plans and receive additional continuing medical education benefits, including tuition reimbursement/repayment, paid time off for exams and certification, expenses for attending medical conferences, professional dues and subscriptions, and reimbursement for exams or licensure fees.

At the national level, PAs and NPs are paid similarly. According to the Bureau of Labor NPs earned a median salary of $120,680 and PAs earned a median salary of $121,530 in 2021. Outpatient care centers are the highest-paying workplaces for both NPs and PAs [4].

MLPs in surgical and other select medical subspecialties are paid 5–15% more than their primary care counterparts. Even so, salaries for MLPs are far lower than those of physicians. This suggests that mid-level providers may represent an option for increasing the capacity of physician specialty practices without significantly increasing payroll costs.

Some economists would argue with the ROI of MLPs by pointing to increased costs associated with their higher utilization of tests and labs. However, there is little data to support this argument. This does not mean that overutilization of resources is not an issue for many physicians and practices who decide to utilize MLPs. What is important is that oversight and appropriate supervision allows the physician to reduce this risk. The best advice is to have "rules of engagement" for the MLPs that flag complicated patients requiring complex workups and monitor high-cost procedures triggering physician engagement and oversight.

Outcomes and Liability of MLPs

Malpractice costs for mid-level providers are 10–20% of the cost of emergency physicians. There is no evidence in the literature supporting increased litigation or more significant malpractice claims related to independent MLPs in medical offices. In fact, the overall incidence of malpractice claims per provider is similar between MLPs and physicians, and payments for claims involving MLPs appear to be lower than claims against physicians. Also, the data suggest that patient outcomes for MLPs are comparable to or better than physicians [5].

Some states require physician oversight for all MLPs. While many MLPs have their own schedules and see patients autonomously, it is important to remember when physician oversight is necessary. State regulations dictate what degree of physician oversight is needed for MLPs, so it is essential to know these requirements.

Credentialing an MLP

Checking any professional medical credentials is essential, and MLPs are no different. Most states require that MLPs be certified to practice. State regulation requirements can vary, so it is important to verify what your individual state's regulations require for licensing. National certifications can be verified at:

- American Academy of Nurse Practitioners National Certification Board
- National Commission on Certification of Physician Assistants (NCCPA)

Where Do MLPs Come From?

Hospitals and medical practices can recruit MLPs directly from the medical schools and nursing schools that train them or can identify suitable candidates from their own staff and offer them the additional training they need to step into the role.

Several recruiting organizations can find MLPs for your practice. Examples include hiring mid-level practitioners (https://www.ihiremid-levelpractitioners.com/jobs/titles) and Staff Pointe (http://www.staffpointe.com/).

Soon, the medical community will be expected to serve more patients with fewer physicians. This reality will require a redesign in how medical care is delivered, and mid-level providers will likely play a more significant role than they do today. Every practice that is going to consider hiring an MLP should ask several questions:

- Does your practice have a backlog and inability to accommodate new patients? If a practice cannot see a new patient for four to 6 weeks, this may be ego-gratifying for the doctors. Still, this situation results in patients seeking their healthcare elsewhere.
- Is the practice paying costly over time to see patients at the end of the day?
- Are there signs of burnout in the physicians and the staff? (See Chap. 22).
- Are there delays seeing patients over 20 min? 20 min are considered by patients as the upper limit of a reasonable wait time. Longer wait times to see the doctor result in deterioration in patient satisfaction and poor online reviews.
- Where will your practice find MLPs to see an influx of new patients?
- Will MLPs be part of the solution to physician shortages in your practice?
- What strategies will you adopt to recruit and retain the needed MLPs?

- How will your organization compensate physicians for supervising mid-level providers?
- How your hospital or practice answers these questions will determine your need for an MLP.

Benefits of Hiring MLPs

Physician assistants have become increasingly popular over the last two decades, quickly becoming a valued member of many medical hospitals and medical practices.

Patient satisfaction is one of the greatest benefits of MLPs. Patients frequently report high satisfaction levels when visiting with an MLP. Many patients report that MLPs are more empathetic, and MLPs seem to have more time for them during the visit when compared to physicians [6]. These benefits of MLPs may be because they can spend more time per patient on health education and answering questions than other medical providers.

A significant advantage of hiring MLPs is that they can boost the practice's revenue [7]. If you compare an MLPs salary versus their revenue, they can produce three to four times their salary. Hiring MLPs can also have the benefit of freeing up physician time. This free time allows physicians to provide more focused and often higher grossing procedures and services.

There are a variety of scheduling options available to help boost your revenue. Having another healthcare practitioner helps if you are looking to increase your practice's productivity. Hiring an MLP can allow for patient care in tandem with physicians on a different schedule or in a satellite clinic.

"MLP-Lite" or Using a Scribe to Improve Efficiency and Productivity

One of the challenges impacting nearly every physician is the need to improve the efficiency of their practices. In the past, we had the luxury of low patient volumes and fat, juicy profit margins.

Today, it is the reverse: large patient volumes and razor-thin profit margins. As a result, to maintain incomes, physicians are motivated to improve the efficiency of their practices. One of the most effective methods to enhance the efficiency of any practice is to consider bringing an MLP into the practice.

A frequent complaint by physicians pertains to the increased amount of nonclinical administrative tasks they are asked to perform. Forty-six percent of physicians think that EMR use distracts them from patient care [8]. By utilizing scribes, physicians can concentrate on patient care and relieve the administrative burden. Employing scribes has also been shown to improve physician satisfaction and productivity [9].

How Does the Scribe Work?

The scribe interacts with a new patient after the doctor introduces themselves to the patient. The scribe then takes the history of the present illness (HOPI) and records the past medical history, and the review of systems. The scribe then presents the HOPI to the physician and accompanies the physician into the room. At this point, the doctor may ask a few additional questions or probe any aspects of the HOPI that are unclear or need a more in-depth questioning. The doctor conducts the physical exam, and the scribe then records the positive findings in the chart or the EMR. At this juncture, the doctor can discuss with the patient the diagnosis and the plan of management with the patient, and the scribe records the doctor's plan of action. The doctor can then answer any questions the patient may have. The scribe can give the chart or the computer to the nurse who will make the necessary arrangements for any lab tests, studies, or surgeries, provide the patient with sample medications and written instructions for the use of medicines, provide pertinent educational materials, and make the follow-up appointments. While the nurse is taking care of one patient, the scribe has moved to the next patient, staying one patient ahead of the physician.

Advantages of the Scribe

Most of all, the scribe improves the efficiency of the practice. With a scribe, doctors can be eyeball-to-eyeball with the patient and focus on communicating with the patient instead of writing or using the computer. As a result of using the scribe, physicians can see five to six additional patients each full day in the office. Also, coding may increase from a previous Level 2–3 to Level 4–5 as the scribe is more thorough in reviewing systems and past medical history and recording the fine nuances of the physical exam that are often neglected.

How Does a Physician Find a Scribe?

Good scribes who aspire to be physicians can be found in students taking a gap year between undergraduate school and medical school. It is our opinion that the scribe does not need to have a medical background. You are looking for someone with people skills and the ability to communicate with patients in a sensitive fashion. A scribe costs roughly $15–$20 an hour. We recommend starting at the lower end and moving up as the scribe becomes trained and comfortable in the scribe position.

The disadvantages of having a scribe are cost, time to train, and the fact that the physician has to change habits from writing in the chart or working the computers to allowing someone else to do the transcription.

In the beginning, this can be frustrating. Still, when you see how efficient you become, you will enjoy the luxury of having a scribe. As a matter of fact, when the scribe is absent or on vacation, you will realize how invaluable the scribe is and how effective the technique is in enhancing your practice.

Getting Started Using a Scribe

First, decide if you need a scribe. If most of your codes are Level 3 or less, you can improve your productivity by having a scribe. If patients need to wait more than 4–6 weeks to make an appointment for a routine visit, then you have a backlog of patients, and a scribe will help you reduce that backlog. If your last patient is scheduled at 4 or 4:30 and you are not finished with patients until 5:30 or 6:00, and your staff is working overtime, then a scribe will help improve the practice's efficiency. Finally, if you are considering moving to an EMR but are techno-phobic, then a scribe might be a natural segue to implementing the EMR.

Take-home message on scribes: Few of us can increase reimbursements or make cuts in overhead without impacting the quality of care and patient satisfaction. However, we all find ways to improve our efficiency and productivity. A scribe may be just what the doctor ordered.

The Economics of a Scribe

It is easy to calculate the return on investment of a scribe [10]. First, multiply the hours by the scribe's salary. For example, if the scribe's salary is $15/h and the scribe works 8 h, the cost of the scribe would be $90/day. Next, add the cost of benefits: insurance, parking, taxes, uniform, or about 25% of the salary. In this case, it would be $22.50 or $112.50/day.

Next, calculate the incremental increase in revenue by having a scribe.

Using a scribe requires determining how many more patients the provider can see in each period. In most circumstances, the scribe makes it possible to see an additional ten more established office patients a day and an additional four new patients/day. With an average reimbursement for a typical office follow-up patient of $75 and average reimbursement of $125 for a new patient, the daily incremental revenue is $750 for established patients plus $500 for new patients, or a total of $1250/day. Subtract the cost of the scribe $112.50, and that is an ROI of $1137.50/day.

This is perhaps the best investment you can make.

A scribe's economic benefit is usually seen after one to two additional patients a day, as that

is the breakeven for a scribe. If the scribe can increase productivity beyond two patients a day, then the added income will go right to the practice's bottom line.

Take-home message on using a scribe: There are advantages and disadvantages to using a scribe. There is no correct answer, and we encourage you to explore your options to maximize your practice efficiency. Your adoption will depend on your comfort after weighing the pros and cons.

Back to the Case
Cassandra investigated bringing on an MLP. She ran the numbers and showed the office manager that it was in the economic interest of the practice to hire an MLP. The scribe could see at least four additional patients each day, and any patients beyond the breakeven rate of two extra patients a day would make more money for the practice. This would increase access for patients in practice, reduce overhead costs, put less stress on Cassandra and the staff, and ultimately be a win-win-win for patients, staff, and Cassandra.

Bottom Line
Despite the issues and controversies surrounding the use of mid-level providers or scribes, this option will continue to grow. There is no question that hospitals and physician practices will need to change the way they deliver care as the healthcare environment continues to evolve. Changes that will affect our practices include the aging of our population, looming shortages of physicians and nurses, and increasing access to health insurance. These issues point to needing to care for more patients with fewer providers. Physician practices and hospitals will need to redesign work processes and introduce new technologies to increase efficiency, effectiveness, and employee satisfaction; retain employees and avoid turnovers; and attract a new generation of

employees, which will include MLPs. There is an anticipated shortfall of 40,000 primary care physicians by 2020. Moreover, the US Bureau of Health Professions projects a shortage of 109,600 physicians in all specialties by 2020 [11]. Given the long timeframe required to educate new physicians, it seems inevitable that MLP will be needed to fill the gap.

References

1. Agency for Healthcare Research and Quality. The number of nurse practitioners and physician assistants practicing primary care in the United States. Agency for Healthcare Research and Quality. https://www.ahrq.gov/research/findings/factsheets/primary/pcwork2/index.html.

2. NursingLicense. What is the difference between a Nurse Practitioner and a Physician Assistant? NursingLicensure.org. https://www.nursinglicensure.org/articles/np-vs-pa.html.

3. Institute of Medicine. The future of nursing: leading change, advancing health. Washington, DC: Academic; 2011.

4. Bureau of Labor Statistics. Occupational employment and wage statistics for nurse practitioners. BLS. 2022. https://www.bls.gov/oes/current/oes291171.htm.

5. Stanik-Hutt J, Newhouse RP, White KM, Johantgen M, Bass EB, Zangaro G, Weiner JP. The quality and effectiveness of care provided by nurse practitioners. J Nurse Pract. 2013;9(8):492–513.

6. Creech C, Filter M, Bowman S et al. Comparing patient satisfaction with nurse practitioner and physician delivered care. Poster presented at: 26th annual American Academy of nurse practitioners conference. 2011. Las Vegas, Nevada.

7. American Society of Clinical Oncology. Elements of successfully integrating a mid-level provider into practice. J Oncol Pract. 2005;1(3):93–4. (no author cited)

8. Alkureishi MA, Lee WW, Lyons M, et al. Impact of electronic medical record use on the patient-doctor relationship and communication. J Gen Intern Med. 2016;31(5):548–60.

9. Blank AJ, Gage RM. Annual impact of scribes on physician productivity and revenue in a cardiology clinic. Clinicoecon Outcomes Res. 2015;7:489–95.

10. Roberts LW. The ROI of medical scribes. Physicians practice. 2014. https://www.physicianspractice.com/ehr/roi-medical-scribes.

11. BHW. Physician supply and demand: projections to 2020. U.S. Department of Health and Human Services and Services Administration Bureau of Health Professions. 2006. https://bhw.hrsa.gov/sites/default/files/bhw/nchwa/projections/physician-2020projections.pdf.

Case Dr. Smith

Regarding upgrading her legacy EHR, Dr. Smith has been undecided. She is aware of several other providers in the community who are unhappy with their EHRs and worries she may end up just as dissatisfied. Moreover, the hospital has recently adopted an EHR that has so far not been successful. Her confidence is shaken and there are concerns over affordability as well as the mounting pressure from CMS to adopt a certified EHR or risk having reimbursements reduced. Despite recognizing the need for this to be done, the process of navigating this decision is extremely difficult and risky. This is not something she wants to get wrong as it could be one of the biggest decisions of her career.

Abstract: Adopting modern technology is no longer an option as first-generation EHRs are slowly approaching end-of-life and may not be eligible for incentives. This is even true for practices that do not intend to participate in Medicare or Medicaid. The payors and the government have imposed penalties for those who do not conform to IT standards and who do not adopt certified platforms.

According to the Office of the National Coordinator (ONC), the term "health information technology" (health IT) refers to the electronic systems that healthcare professionals and—increasingly, patients— use to store, share, and analyze health information. The most common platform for this is what is commonly referred to as an electronic medical record (EMR) system or an electronic health record (EHR) system. While EMRs can incorporate scanned images, computerized dictation, and/or any other method of electronically storing medical information, EHRs are certified platforms that are more comprehensive [1]. An EHR will typically be eligible for incentives and participation in an advance payment model that pays higher fees. For these reasons, it will be helpful first to understand the current state of the healthcare IT (HCIT) market and how it applies beyond our use of EHRs today.

The most notable state of our current HCIT market has to do with the incentives and penalties for the use and adoption of certified EHRs. As noted above, only EHRs have incentives and they must be a certified EHR. Products that are *not* certified are generally considered EMRs. Later in this chapter, this topic will be discussed in greater detail. However, to provide a quick background, the initial EHR incentive program was established in 2009 under the Obama administration with the passage of the *American Recovery and Reinvestment Act* [2]. We urgently needed incentives to stimulate the economy since it was on the verge of a second Great Depression. The healthcare IT industry was one of this bill's biggest beneficiaries. A total of $20 billion in incentives were allocated to promote the use of certified EHRs. We saw the fastest adoption rate for EHRs during this time.

Prior to this period, the Stark Law was relaxed under the Bush administration during his second term, which enabled hospitals to subsidize the cost of EHRs for their medical staff. These coordinated, concurrent initiatives sped up the adoption of EHRs and provided hospitals and clinics with numerous incentives to do so. Both programs are still in use to this day and they can be combined, though providers who are employed by hospitals generally get to keep the incentives. For private practices, hospitals may subsidize up to 85% of the cost of an EHR that meets certain conditions. In most cases, the hospitals have already selected the community EHR and therefore do not expect many vendor options.

The Affordable Care Act's program was primarily built around choosing and adopting a vendor with certified features and capabilities. To be eligible, doctors and hospitals only had to pick a certified vendor and attest to using the basic features of the EHR. There were no significant limitations or efforts to verify such. It goes without saying that this led to a massive explosion of new vendors trying to claim a piece of these funds. At the apex, there were over 600 certified EHRs on the market. Most are no longer existent and/or have since merged with other vendors to remain viable.

Today, incentive programs are more comprehensive and require some demonstrated outcomes. Fig. 18.1 provides a quick side-by-side comparison of the initiatives (Figs. 18.2 and 18.3).

In 2020, Meaningful Use has been superseded by MIPS and MACRA, and suppliers and providers who benefited from the previous incentive programs are now subject to enhance scrutiny and audits. The misleading assertion was supported by the absence of system capabilities required to maintain certification. When it came time to verify capabilities, the government found

that many of the vendors it had initially allowed to attest were not in compliance. The Department of Justice notably charged three significant suppliers with serious false claim breaches, which led to a multimillion-dollar settlement with the government. Key takeaway: It is the buyers responsibility to confirm that these systems have certification and that the version being sold is approved by CMS.

Although the attestation procedure is not new, the funding for the EHR incentive program has come under scrutiny. Providers and hospitals are required to give proof that they met all the requirements they pledged to uphold during the attestation process.[1] Those who are unable to provide the required documentation must return the incentive funds. And upon return, CMS will deduct the money from subsequent reimbursements and/or may levy further penalties for noncompliance. The security risk analysis (SRA) is one of the prerequisites that is most commonly overlooked.[2] Due to the pass/fail nature of this SRA, HHS can easily audit this requirement. Practices are typically requested to repay the incentive money if they cannot provide proof that they perform an annual SRA. To pass an SRA, a practice must have up-to-date HIPAA privacy and security policies, as well as documentation of staff training and knowledge assessments. Figure 18.4 outlines instructions to help you conduct a risk analysis that is appropriate for your organization. For further information, an excellent reference is the U.S. Department of Health & Human Services' HIPAA Security Rule page for professionals.

The first requirement of the HIPAA Security Rule is a risk analysis (updated in 2013 by the

---

[1]Attestation is a process of making a claim/statement without the requirement of submitting supporting documentation to validate these claims/statements. The government accepts these statements without verification but reserves the right to audit at any time to ensure the statements are accurate.

[2]Measure: Conduct or review a security risk analysis in accordance with the requirements under 45 CFR 164.308(a)(1), including addressing the security (including encryption) of data created or maintained by CEHRT in accordance with requirements under 45 CFR 164.312(a)(2)(iv) and 45.

Original EHR Incentives	Current EHR Incentives
•The Vendor must be certified by the Certification Commission for Healthcare Information Technology (CCHIT).	•CCHIT (Certification Commission for Healthcare Information Technology). The Certification Commission for Healthcare Information Technology (CCHIT)
•Meet Meaningful Use (MU) Standards MU was based on five main objectives, according to the Centers for Disease Control and Prevention. They were: (1) Improve quality (2) safety (3) efficiency (4) reduce health disparities, and (5) increase patient engagement	•Meaningful Use +++ MU has now shifted to a Merit-based Incentive Payment System and is combined with the Medicare Access and CHIP Reauthorization Act (MACRA), the Medicare EHR Incentive Program, commonly referred to as meaningful use, was transitioned to become one of the four components of the new Merit-Based Incentive Payment System (MIPS), which itself is part of MACRA. MIPS harmonizes existing CMS quality programs (including meaningful use), the Physician Quality Reporting System, and Value-Based Payment Modifiers. MIPS consolidates multiple quality programs into a single program to improve quality care.

•Compensation
The payout was over five (5) stages with phase one starting with 15 core requirements and 10 menu requirements. All core requirements are mandatory. Additional core requirements were added each year by CMS. There were two payout tracks.
    1.Medicare Track: Eligible providers could receive up to $44,000 if all stages for all years were met. (See Figure18.2.)
    2.Medicaid Track: Eligible providers could receive up to $63,750. The only requirement for phase one was a signed contract with a certified vendor. The requirements for Medicaid were lower because Medicaid practices have less access to capital. To qualify for the Medicaid track, the provider would have to have a minimum of 30% Medicaid patients. (See Figure 18.3.)
	•Compensation as an up or down adjustment to the provider's Medicare payments.
	The first year started at a plus or minus of 4%, and it is set to go up to plus or minus 9% by 2021. Additional incentives can be gained through alternative payment models, but the risk is higher.

Fig. 18.1 Original and current incentives compared

Omnibus Rule). Per 164.308(a)(1)(ii)(A), a CE or BA must "conduct an accurate and thorough assessment of the potential risks and vulnerabilities to the confidentiality, integrity, and availability of electronic protected health information (ePHI) held by the covered entity or business associate" [3].

While there is no preferred approach, most risk analysis and risk management processes have steps in common. According to CMS, these include the following:

- Define the scope of the risk analysis and collect data regarding the ePHI pertinent to the defined scope.

- Identify potential threats and vulnerabilities to patient privacy and to the security of your practice's ePHI.

- Assess the effectiveness of implemented security measures in protecting against the identified threats and vulnerabilities.

- Determine the likelihood a particular threat will occur and the impact such an occurrence would have on the confidentiality, integrity, and availability of ePHI.

- Determine and assign risk levels based on the likelihood and impact of a threat occurrence.

- Prioritize the remediation or mitigation of identified risks based on the severity of their impact on your patients and practice.

- First Calendar Year (CY) for which the EP Receives an Incentive Payment

	CY 2011	CY 2012	CY 2013	CY2014	CY 2015 and later
CY 2011	$18,000				
CY 2012	$12,000	$18,000			
CY 2013	$8,000	$12,000	$15,000		
CY 2014	$4,000	$8,000	$12,000	$12,000	
CY 2015	$2,000	$4,000	$8,000	$8,000	$0
CY 2016		$2,000	$4,000	$4,000	$0
TOTAL	$44,000	$44,000	$39,000	$24,000	$0

Fig. 18.2 Original MU payout—Medicare. (Source: CMS)

Maximum Incentive Payments for Medicaid EPs Who Are Meaningful Users in the First Payment Year

	Medicaid EPs who begin MU of certified EHR technology in					
	2011	2012	2013	2014	2015	2016
2011	$21,250					
2012	$8,500	$21,250				
2013	$8,500	$8,500	$21,250			
2014	$8,500	$8,500	$8,500	$21,250		
2015	$8,500	$8,500	$8,500	$8,500	$21,250	
2016	$8,500	$8,500	$8,500	$8,500	$8,500	$21,250
2017		$8,500	$8,500	$8,500	$8,500	$8,500
2018			$8,500	$8,500	$8,500	$8,500
2019				$8,500	$8,500	$8,500
2020					$8,500	$8,500
2021						$8,500
Total	$63,750	$63,750	$63,750	$63,750	$63,750	$63,750

Calendar Year (row label, left axis)

Fig. 18.3 Original MU Medicaid payout. (Source: CMS)

The first requirement of the HIPAA Security Rule is a risk analysis (updated in 2013 by the Omnibus Rule). Per 164.308(a)(1)(ii)(A), a CE or BA must "conduct an accurate and thorough assessment of the potential risks and vulnerabilities to the confidentiality, integrity, and availability of electronic protected health information (ePHI) held by the covered entity or business associate" [3].

While there is no preferred approach, most risk analysis and risk management processes have steps in common. According to CMS, these include the following:

- Define the scope of the risk analysis and collect data regarding the ePHI pertinent to the defined scope.

- Identify potential threats and vulnerabilities to patient privacy and to the security of your practice's ePHI.

- Assess the effectiveness of implemented security measures in protecting against the identified threats and vulnerabilities.

- Determine the likelihood a particular threat will occur and the impact such an occurrence would have on the confidentiality, integrity, and availability of ePHI.

- Determine and assign risk levels based on the likelihood and impact of a threat occurrence.

- Prioritize the remediation or mitigation of identified risks based on the severity of their impact on your patients and practice.

- Document your risk analysis including information from the steps above as well as the risk analysis results.

- Review and update your risk analysis on a periodic basis.

---

[1] Attestation is a process of making a claim/statement without the requirement of submitting supporting documentation to validate these claims/statements. The government accepts these statements without verification but reserves the right to audit at any time to ensure the statements are accurate.

[2] Measure: Conduct or review a security risk analysis in accordance with the requirements under 45 CFR 164.308(a)(1), including addressing the security (including encryption) of data created or maintained by CEHRT in accordance with requirements under 45 CFR 164.312(a)(2)(iv) and 45.

Fig. 18.4 Conducting a HIPAA security rule risk analysis

- Document your risk analysis including information from the steps above as well as the risk analysis results.
- Review and update your risk analysis on a periodic basis.

An SRA tip sheet is available at https://www.cms.gov/Regulations-and-Guidance/Legislation/EHRIncentivePrograms/Downloads/2016_SecurityRiskAnalysis.pdf.

Source: https://www.hhs.gov/hipaa/for-professionals/security/index.html

Moving beyond the trends of incentives and auditing, we are now seeing emerging new markets of innovation enabling caregivers to go beyond their internal EHRs. The push for interoperability has moved the market toward an application programming interface (API) model.[3] The best example of an API strategy can be seen within companies such as Apple, Amazon, Google, and other organizations.

For instance, Apple offers its platform (Operating System) as the framework and has made its application programming interface (API) available to anyone who seeks to develop software that would operate within it. Amazon now has a worldwide network of distributors, giving retailers from all over the world a platform to promote their products and services. In order to allow developers full access to the Amazon

---

[3] An application programming interface is an interface or communication protocol between a client and a server intended to simplify the building of client-side software.

data center and to enable interoperability, Amazon has also released Amazon Web Services (AWS) and its API.[4] Most of the major vendors that had previously offered their EHRs installed on on-premises servers located on-site at the practice are now operating on the Amazon (or similar) cloud platforms. These tech giants are disrupting the old model of isolated systems running as on-premises silos. They also have provisions in their agreements that allow for data mining, which some claim is becoming the new currency. In short, the trend is toward having a vast ecosystem of applications that are all connected to a single, globally accessible platform. As a result, millions of private innovators are building and developing applications across a myriad of markets and verticals, including the healthcare industry.

Another major trend is the concept of an open application programming interface (API), which is when software development allows the open market to have integration with its platform/operating system.[5] The best example of this concept is the App Store provided by some of the largest cell phone device manufacturers such as Apple and Android. Millions of applications are built to run on these devices. As a result, the consumer becomes dependent on the device because they are necessary to run the applications. Creating this ecosystem drives consumers to the devices supporting their favorite apps. It also makes it particularly challenging to change a device because it often means giving up many of the applications designed for these devices. Major vendors such as EPIC, CERNER, Allscripts, Athena, and others have taken notice and recently started publishing their API to encourage the private market to develop solutions to enhance their platforms

and the end-user's experience. This action not only creates an ecosystem of solutions, but it also speeds up development and lowers costs by allowing third-party companies to do innovation as a complement to the core EHR platform. It is also an excellent strategy to tie the consumer to a product the provider depends on, thus creating a complete ecosystem. Notwithstanding, unlike Apple and Amazon, EHR vendors can still be very proprietary and selective with who they permit access to their API.

The EHR vendor may even attempt to block access if the application competes with any of the inherent features and functions already provided by the EHR vendors and/or an existing partner. Some EHR vendors will create a "developer approved" marketplace and only allow innovators who agree to share in revenue to get their endorsements as a preferred partner/application. While it is understandable for an EHR vendor to align exclusively with innovators who best support their objectives, there may be instances where the practice and/or hospitals require interoperability outside of the core EHR vendor's ecosystem of application. The quick answer might result in more costs, but we will cover how to handle this in the vendor contracting process later. To create an interface that does not already exist, the EHR vendor will probably charge between $10,000 and $20,000, or, worse yet, it may completely reject the request altogether.

With the recent development of the twenty-first Century Cures Act, there has been a significant shift toward an open API model. Vendors are now required to publish these APIs, allowing practice and innovators to develop their own patient-facing platforms on top of their EHRs. This is akin to the iPhone app store. The iPhone has its own operating system (iOS), but Apple has published its APIs so innovators can create compatible apps. As a result, there is an entire ecosystem of consumer-facing platforms compatible with the iPhone. The same is starting to happen with EHRs. The industry has seen remarkable innovation since EHRs were introduced 20 years ago. The improvements in internet speed and access, cloud computing, and web-enabled solutions have been major accelera-

---

[4] Amazon Web Services is a subsidiary of Amazon that provides on-demand cloud computing platforms to individuals, companies, and governments, on a metered pay-as-you-go basis.

[5] An application program interface (API) is a set of routines, protocols, and tools for building software applications. Basically, an API specifies how software components should interact. Additionally, APIs are used when programming graphical user interface (GUI) components.

tors in this growth. Many thought spending and investing in EHRs was a one-time commitment, but the market continues to expand and evolve. The next section will provide some insights into this anticipated growth.

Projected Growth

As the world changes and technology progresses, hospitals and other medical professionals must do the same. As the technology in the world has expanded, the Healthcare IT market has skyrocketed, and with it, the reach of hospitals and other medical practices. Projections are that the market worth will climb sharply to $324.9 billion by 2026, an astronomical growth from $187.9 billion in 2019 [4]. The figure below (Fig. 18.5) charts the projected increase in the marketplace.

With the growing healthcare technology market, hospitals and medical practices have had to make, and will continue to make, a number of

critical decisions to ensure that they continue to stay current and modern. One of the most significant decisions hospitals and other medical professionals must make is selecting the next phase of IT investing. For some, it will be starting over and replacing their old, commercially discontinued EHR. These practices/hospitals will have to grapple with data migration options and costs. Some may turn to third-party options such as data archiving solutions to retire their legacy systems. For others, it will be building and expanding off of their existing platforms and exploring options for innovation. Some examples include the following:

- Artificial intelligence
- Process robotics
- Telemedicine
- Telemedicine with clinical chatbot support
- Advanced electronic patient communication
- Predictive analytics
- Listening devices in the exam room

Fig. 18.5 Latest 12-month public company multiples. Source: Projected Growth - Beyond EHR: Using Technology to Meet Growing Demands and Deliver Better Patient Care (ebrary.net)

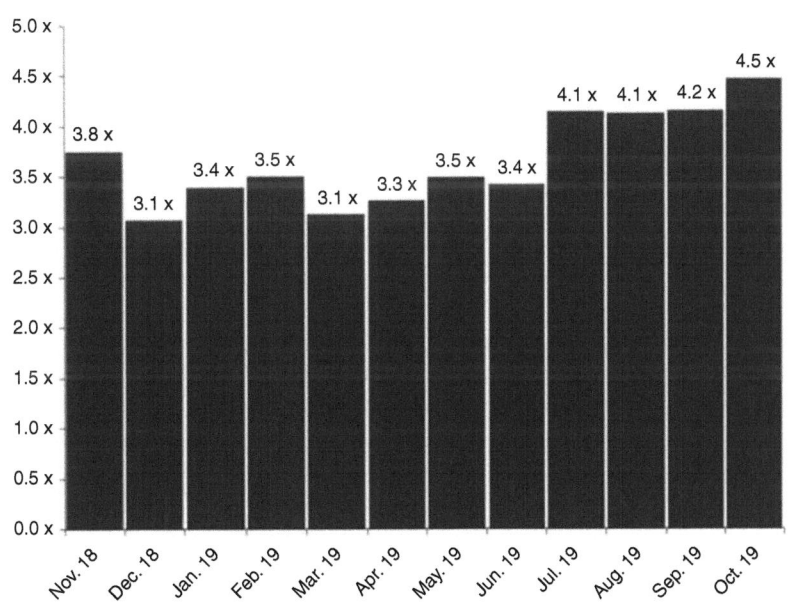

Latest Twelve Month ("LTM") Public Co. Multiples:

Average Enterprise Value ("EV") / LTM Revenue by Month |

Patients today have a greater willingness to take an active role in their own health and make lifestyle changes to improve it as technology and medicine have advanced. Basic fitness apps for their phones and fitness trackers like Fitbits, Apple Devices, or other smart watches are some of the tools these patients are incorporating into their regular lifestyle. By tracking their activities and workouts with apps such as the Health app or MyFitnessPal, users can determine whether they are consuming enough calories to maintain a healthy lifestyle. Some behavior health organizations have apps that can track the movements of their patients. When activity is low, they send a social worker to check on the patient. There are other apps that enable users to input data about the food they consume, allowing them to monitor their eating patterns and determine if they are meeting, exceeding, or falling short of their caloric needs. These fitness trackers monitor all movement, not just exercise, and provide users with an accurate estimation of their daily activity and calorie expenditure. This enables them to observe a typical day and identify which foods to eat and which to avoid. These tools assist doctors with patients because they now have an accurate measure of the patient's activity, which allows them to find faults in their daily lifestyle and prescribe changes that fit the patient's shortcomings. By having a detailed record of the patient's lifestyle, the doctor can prescribe specific changes, whether it is to diet or exercise, before prescribing a medication. Even if the doctor must prescribe medicine, they can give one that works best for the patient that suits their lifestyle. About 90% of patients, according to research conducted in the emergency department, would be interested in using these technologies, yet they are seldom used. What would be the reason for this?

Issues concerning these tools include reservations about their effectiveness as well as concerns about privacy and security. Consumers are wary of entering more personal information into technology in light of recent security breaches at companies such as Facebook. Although this concern is legitimate, it should not discourage consumers completely as technology continues to grow and develop. In addition, many of the creators of the apps have installed robust security protocols that make hacking and stealing information extremely difficult. The concern about effectiveness is an argument often presented by those who oppose the change to a more technology-based world. However, technology will progress; those who resist will have the option to go along with the changes or fall behind. As medicine progresses and the market grows, all medical professionals must incorporate these technologies into their practices so that they can accurately diagnose patients. By incorporating these tools into their daily lives, patients can take charge of their health and at the same time, doctors can expect a greater patient base by incorporating patient engagement technologies into daily practice.

The expanded application and importance of artificial intelligence (AI) is a further component of the expanding Healthcare IT market. Medical experts need a system to keep track of the molecular changes that occur as diseases and illnesses develop and evolve. AI comes into play in this situation since it can swiftly evaluate data and assist doctors in finding patterns. Medical experts and researchers can see where, how, and why a disease is changing attributable to this pattern recognition. By recognizing these characteristics, medical professionals can treat illnesses with the appropriate prescriptions and researchers can find a cure more rapidly [5].

Scientists can enter information into a database for quick analysis rather than manually processing it, which could take days. This analysis aids in the search for treatments for diseases including cancer and certain neurological conditions. One of the pioneer AI systems in operation is called IBM Watson, named after its founder, Thomas J. Watson. Watson is an IBM supercomputer that combines AI and sophisticated analytical software for optimal performance as a "question answering" machine. It can process data within seconds and help scientists find trends and patterns in data instantly. By incorporating these systems into medical practices, medical professionals are better able to analyze patient data and find patient patterns quickly. AI systems significantly speed up data analysis for scientists that can help them find cures more rapidly, which then helps medical professionals treat more patients. Additionally, medical procedures are accelerated by AI, which makes doctor labor more productive. Due to its higher efficiency, the rising usage of AI has substantially influenced the present trend in the healthcare IT market.

Most people lead busy schedules, and many of them choose not to see physicians because they lack the time or resources to do so. Instead, they believe that they can self-diagnose by consulting resources such as Google and WebMD. However, the industry is experiencing a growth in the use of telemedicine. Telemedicine is the communication between medical professionals and their patients through a two-way device, enabling doctors to treat and interact with their patients remotely. With the growing Healthcare IT market, telemedicine is becoming increasingly popular because it is a convenient alternative for patients to seek treatment; they can receive care from the comfort of their own home [6].

Telemedicine and telestroke are increasingly available in ambulances. For instance, paramedics can use Bluetooth stethoscopes when a patient is being transferred to the hospital during an emergency. Doctors can hear the heartbeat from the hospital, find the most effective treatment before the ill or injured person arrives, and administer rapid treatment The future growth of the Healthcare IT market will be aided by telemedicine and virtual care as a result of the impending Generation Z's reliance on technology. As a result, they will engage in telemedicine more frequently than earlier generations. Telemedicine, which many members of the younger generations would use, will account for the majority of the market value doubling. Doctors and other medical professionals will need to incorporate more telemedicine into their practices if they want to keep up with the trends and advance with the market. The market has also been driven by COVID-19 to reconsider engagement strategies, including the idea of virtual visits and a remote workforce. We are also witnessing a rapid growth of what is referred to as the "digital front door" as a result of COVID-19. This is the notion of complete self-service from check-in to check-out. Some experts predict the front desk at doctors' offices will soon be a thing of the past much like cashiers at grocery stores. As more practices and hospitals adopt advanced automation, it will contribute to their growth, increase access, and make the practice more appealing to the high-tech consumer (patients).

As the Healthcare IT market shifts and develops, medical professionals must recognize what is changing the market so that they can incorporate these tools into their practices. Along with selecting an appropriate EHR system, they must include a variety of other resources that are currently contributing to the growth of the market. Integrating patient engagement tools, artificial intelligence, and telemedicine into their practices will enable them to grow along with the Healthcare IT market. As the market begins to increase and double, it is up to hospitals to incorporate these resources to keep up with the demand [7].

Predictions

Growing up in the 1970s, I remember watching the Jetsons cartoon and seeing flat screens, flying robots, robotic vacuums, smart watches, tablet computers, and moving sidewalks. Even though all of this was made up and a work of fiction at the time, in 2022 we already have the same technology. To that end, here are some practical as well as peculiar predictions due consideration:

A Hospital at Home: The hospital of the future may be in the comfort of your own home. This concept is currently being developed and tested by the Johns Hopkins School of Medicine and the Public Health Departments in some markets. This innovative care model is expected to lower costs by nearly one-third and reduce complications. So far, patients and caregivers alike have provided favorable feedback.

Ambulance ride services are similar to assistance such as Uber and Lyft. The high cost of an ambulance service is not in the transportation. The ambulance comes with a fully-trained emergency medical team and expensive lifesaving equipment, when, in many cases, the patient just needs a ride to the Emergency Room. Both Uber and Lyft are looking into the possibility of offering a ride-sharing service where the driver is a licensed caregiver for non-trauma-type situations.

The chatbot will see you now. This was alluded to previously, but several companies are currently developing chat-bots that treat patients based on algorithms and responses to Q&A. Technology is also being developed that may detect signs of stress, pain, or both in a patient's voice and assess whether the level of care has to be escalated.

Self-treating pathways for consumers: Consider a child who has a chronic ear infection; the mom knows it is an ear infection based on the previous ten ear infections. The parent typically understands what is required to treat it or could follow a prior procedure. There might be an at-home diagnostic tool for straightforward issues that would validate what the parent already knows and then open secure access to treatment delivered directly to the home.

Digital phenotyping: *Phenotypes* are physical traits such as eye or hair color, height, voice, shoe size, and the like, influenced by *genotypes*. *Phenotyping* is when these traits are used in clinical research for the discovery of diseases. In the age of digital technology, researchers have partnered with technology companies to track how users interact with the web in order to better understand peoples emotions, thoughts, and behavior. Major technology corporations such as Google, Amazon, Facebook, and Netflix, are already collecting and storing enormous amounts of data on each click we make online, including monitoring our movement and private messages. Consider the scenario that someone with a highly social digital phenotype 1 day becomes reclusive and isolated. Perhaps they are now exploring a website that deals with depression or suicide or watching videos that promote violence or school shootings. Could this be used to help with early intervention before someone gets hurt, or is this an invasion of privacy? You may have already noticed that your phone can track your online activity down to the specific apps you used most frequently, thus the data are being collected. How will it be used, and can we strike a balance between the good and the requirement to uphold individual privacy rights?

Wearables: Devices we wear on our bodies already exist, but they will become increasingly advanced and include more interoperability with our caregivers.

A spoon full or microchip: A digital pill that looks like any other capsule on the market today, but it also has an edible sensor within. After consumption, the sensor starts reporting medical information. The technology that makes up the pill, as well as the data transmitted by the pill's sensor, is part of digital medicine. The FDA has recently approved such a device but has not yet researched the best approach to return it when it exits the digestive system.

Back to the Case

Dr. Smith spoke with colleagues and identified an EMR that would meet all of her needs including documentation, billing, and quality reporting.

Bottom Line

One of the best ways to produce content that will make people cringe 10 years from now is to write a chapter about technology market trends. Although it is impossible to predict where current and emerging technology will lead us, change will be profound and disruptive. We are aware that the expense of healthcare is still rising, and access is poor, despite all of the finest efforts made thus far. While healthcare IT will not solve all the present challenges, it will play a major role and is expected to become even more prolific within our healthcare delivery system and personal lives. The opportunities and possibilities are endless, given the difficulties we face today.

References

1. Polaris Market Research. Global healthcare IT market share will reach to US $324.9 billion by 2026. Digital Journal. 2022. https://www.digitaljournal.com/pr/global-healthcare-it-market-share-will-reach-to-us-324-9-billion-by-2026-polaris-market-research.

2. American Recovery and Reinvestment Act of 2009, H.R.1, 11th Cong., 2009.

3. U.S. Department of Health and Human Services. The security rule. HHS. 2022. https://www.hhs.gov/hipaa/for-professionals/security/index.html.

4. Markets and Markets. Press release: Healthcare IT market worth $390.7 billion by 2024. Markets and Markets. https://www.marketsandmarkets.com/Press-Releases/healthcare-it-market.asp.

5. Jiang F, Jiang Y, Zhi H, Dong Y, Li H, Ma S, Dong Q, Shen H, Wang Y. Artificial intelligence in healthcare: past, present and future. Stroke Vasc Neurol. 2017;2(4):230–43; https://svn.bmj.com/content/2/4/230.abstract.

6. Bazolli, Fred. 12 trends that will dominate healthcare IT in 2019. Health Data Management. 2019. https://www.healthdatamanagement.com/list/12-trends-that-will-dominate-healthcare-it-in-2019.

7. Birnbaum F, Lewis DM, Rosen R, Ranney ML. Patient engagement and the design of digital health. Acad Emerg Med. 2015;22(6):754–6. https://doi.org/10.1111/acem.12692; https://www.ncbi.nlm.nih.gov/pmc/articles/PMC4674428/.

Team Building for Healthcare Practices

Case Victor

As the coronavirus disease 2019 (COVID-19) pandemic began to wane, Victor, and endocrinologist in a multi-specialty group began to feel burned out. His practice had experienced some attrition and he was becoming increasingly frustrated with the administration of his hospital. Victor wondered what he could do?

There has been a deterioration of morale in most medical offices and in hospitals. A contributing factor is the Great Resignation which refers to large numbers of employees, including physicians leaving the healthcare profession.

Many medical practices and hospitals are experiencing openings that are going unfilled. As a result, this places stress on the existing staff, which ultimately may impact patient care. In the following blog, I will discuss practical suggestions to stem the exodus of good healthcare employees from leaving the healthcare arena. This blog will cover the reasons employees are leaving the profession.

About 1 in 5 healthcare workers have left medicine since the pandemic began. (Masson G. About 1 in 5 healthcare workers have left medicine since the pandemic started. Becker's Hospital, Review, November 2021) Employee turnover is one of the costliest challenges faced in healthcare today and only threatens to become more problematic as the demand for care exceeds the available supply of healthcare workers. When healthcare workers quit, it is estimated that replacing them averages the cost of an entire year's salary for that position. The obvious conclusion is that a hospital or practice that doesn't work on employee retention will result in understaffing, financial insolvency, and deterioration in patient care.

The US healthcare sector has lost nearly half a million workers since February 2020, according to estimates from the Bureau of Labor Statistics. Eighteen percent of healthcare staff have quit since the pandemic began, while 12% have been laid off, according to survey research company Morning Consult. Of the remaining workers, 31% have thought about leaving their employer, according to Morning Consult. (Yong E. The Atlantic, November 2021.) why healthcare workers are quitting in droves.

In 2022, nearly 1.7 million people have quit their healthcare jobs—equivalent to almost 3% of the healthcare workforce each month, according to the U.S. Bureau of Labor Statistics.

It is not just nurses and allied health professionals who are leaving but also physicians who decide to leave their medical practices.

With the Great Resignation comes increased workload on existing employees. Just imagine it is Monday morning and there's a message left with the answering service that the receptionist and one of your medical assistants have called in to say that they won't be coming to work. Do you call a temp organization and they send you a person who has never worked in a medical office and is unfamiliar with the scheduling process? Or will you try to make do with your existing staff and wreak havoc with your schedule? Do you call patients and reschedule several patients and only see those that are deemed necessary and urgent? None of these options are very attractive and likely to cause stress for the existing staff and will probably cause problems with patient care. The best answer is to anticipate in advance that this situation of a suddenly absent employee(s) may occur. Then cross-train your staff so that employees can work in other positions. This allows the full schedule of patients to be seen without delays or disruptions and that patients are not aware that there is a shortage of employees.

All practices but especially small practices benefit from cross training. When staff members are prepared to work in multiple positions, owners and managers can ensure that all employees have enough work to keep them busy while keeping staffing needs to a minimum.

Staffing shortages are not just a result of COVID-19. When there are not enough employees that could mean that fewer workers will be required to take care of more patients. Shortages and the extra work burden may lead to burnout and personal illness.

When there is not enough staff, sometimes mandatory overtime will be necessary for some working employees. Working extra hours can affect sleep quality and work performance, leading many employees to change to a different type of employment.

The other major issue that impacts staff morale is burnout. Before the pandemic, between 35 and 54% of US nurses and physicians experience one or more symptoms of burnout. Now, burnout has increased in frequency, and more physicians, nurses, and healthcare employees are leaving the profession because burnout has resulted in mental and physical issues. A recent survey of 1000 healthcare professionals showed that 28% had quit a job because of burnout.

The pandemic has created additional responsibilities, new workflows and the daily reality of potential viral exposure for doctors and staff and have all increased the stress and exhaustion already felt by so many providers. Burnout, in turn, can lead to lower quality care and medical errors, negative health outcomes, and patient dissatisfaction.

Medicine can be a physically and emotionally demanding job. Often there is not enough staff for the number of patients, and the demand placed on providers has only increased in recent years. The patient volume and acuity of illnesses have increased, and there is not enough staff to meet that demand. Many healthcare staff is burnt out and leave the profession to regain their physical and mental health.

A few suggestions for enhancing moral and team building include:

Effective Staff Meetings

There are three types of staff meetings. There are formal or standard meetings, which are often held monthly. Less formal meetings are held during lunch and may be sponsored by a pharmaceutical company or one of the vendors that call on the practice. These meetings do not have an agenda. They provide an opportunity to have open discussions about the practice. The third meeting type of staff meeting is very informal and usually without any structure but just for the staff to share issues that may affect patient care or even non-medical and non-clinical discussions. Staff meetings are held more often if there are any problems or new programs being introduced into the practice.

When organizing staff meetings, keep the following points in mind:

1. Avoid meetings on Monday and Friday.
2. Meeting in the morning when everyone is rested.
3. Limit the meeting to 30–40 min.
4. Avoid interruptions-turn off cell phones and have answering service pick up call.
5. Serve refreshments.

Starting on a Positive Note

Many positive events and circumstances happen to the staff. We think it is important to share those positive comments with all the staff. At the beginning of a staff meeting ask that everyone related compliments some positive incident that has happened since the last meeting. Such incidents might include successfully dealing with a difficult patient, getting a new uniform, or an employee receiving an accolade or award. We suggest starting the meeting with these comments, which creates a positive atmosphere and avoids having the staff meeting as a gripe session.

Another suggestion is to ask everyone to contribute one idea that will help improve the practice. Each suggestion is recorded in the notes kept during the meeting. Ideas which are implemented are rewarded wither verbally or monetarily, especially if the cost savings are significant. Remember to avoid criticizing any of the staff's suggestions. If you do, you will stifle future creativity if you indicate that some of the ideas are ridiculous or useless. Creating a positive atmosphere is a prerequisite for creativity. If your team isn't happy, engaged, and feeling good about their work, then your practice won't be having the best results regarding care for the patients. This also impacts patient satisfaction as well as your online reputation.

Stimulating Staff Involvement

Have you thought about what your patients feel and what they experience when they interact with your practice? Did you ever wonder how it feels like to grow old? What is it like when you have difficulty lifting your hand above your head? How does it feel when you've recovering from a heart attack? Perhaps looking through the lens of a patient can be very helpful in identifying the doctor-patient encounter from the patient's point of view.

Role-playing is another technique for enhancing morale within the practice. For example, one staff member can assume the role of an irate patient calling to complain about a bill and another staff member can attempt to calm the patient and solve their problem. The rest of the staff can critique the dialogue.

Another example is a senior citizen simulation for your younger staff members to understand the limitations and problems that older patients have navigating a medical practice. This is accomplished in the following fashion:

A middle-aged "team" member is converted to a senior citizen by (1) making her hard of hearing by placing a cotton ball in each ear, (2) impair her vision by giving her glasses that distort the reading material, (3) making her arthritic by having her wear gloves and immobilizing one leg with a splint (see Fig. 19.1). Prior to the staff meeting, she is asked to go to the bank in the building and make a transaction, enter the office, and sign in at the reception desk, and take a seat and try reading some of our material on patient education.

The team member then changes back to the reality of a middle-aged lady. We then started the staff meeting and she explained that she had trouble reading materials at the bank and in our reception area. She also had difficulty getting into and out of the chairs in the reception area. She also had problems using the doorknobs to open doors in the restroom and the exam room. Finally, she had trouble hearing the receptionist in the office and the teller at the bank.

What did we learn? We learned that the font size on our print material in the reception area was

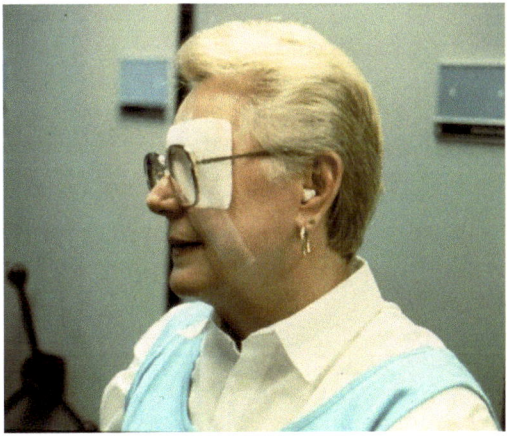

Fig. 19.1 Example of senior citizen simulation by using ear plugs and impairing her vision

too small. We learned that most of the chairs in our reception area and the exam rooms were not senior-friendly. We learned that one of the staff members may need to help seniors with their paperwork because of difficulty with fine motor skills like writing. We also added door handles to facilitate seniors' ability to open doors. But, most of all we increased the sensitivity of the entire staff about the unique concerns of the elderly and how we might provide better care of them.

Every staff meeting should end with a summary of what has been accomplished and the creation of a "to do" list for the next meeting. This list should be distributed to all the staff members and to staff that were unable to attend the meeting.

For a staff meeting to be effective, doctors and office managers must be good listeners and accept constructive criticism. Listening is probably one of the most difficult things for a doctor to do at a staff meeting. If good ideas are suggested, implement them. Show your employees that the time spent during staff meetings is well spent.

The take-home message on staff meetings is important to make the staff meetings fun, enjoyable, and positive. By adding a little sparkle, you can make those meetings a team building experience that will generate positive results for your practice.

Back to the Case

Victor decided to enlist the help of some of his colleagues who ran team building exercises for businesses. Victor used the information to improve his staff meetings, and minimized meetings when they were not necessary. Victor noticed improved morale and improved patient satisfaction with his practice.

Bottom Line

Team building by dressing-up for Halloween or doling out employee of the month certificates will not be effective in today's healthcare environment.

Today, it is possible to simulate learning and especially the concept of empathy using virtual reality. The University of New England put this theory to the test by incorporating simulations via VR in the medical school curriculum. The participating students were found to better understand such conditions and saw an increase in their empathy for the elderly [1].

Another university that explored the potential of VR in medical education is the University of Michigan. Students used the MPathic-VR app to train their communication skills with a virtual human, which proved to be very helpful when delivering difficult news [2].

This technology has become more affordable and accessible. VR headsets are now less than $5 with the Google Cardboard [3]. I think that the next generation of doctors is very comfortable with VR and is open to technology as a teaching device especially in the area of enhancing communication and developing patient empathy.

Bottom Line: Perhaps it is time for us to try and understand what our patients are experiencing in our practices. Simulations are one way to accomplish this goal. Another more modern approach is the use of virtual reality which is readily available and also affordable.

References

1. Dyer E. Virtual humans help aspiring doctors learn empathy." Science Daily. 2017.; https://www.sciencedaily.com/releases/2017/04/170427091749.htm.

2. Kron FW, et al. Using a computer simulation for teaching communication skills: a blinded multisite mixed methods randomized controlled trial. Patient Educ Couns. 2017;100(4):748.

3. Google VR. Get your cardboard. Google. https://arvr.google.com/cardboard/get-cardboard/.

Case Valda

Valda is a dermatologist with fellowship training in MOHs surgery. She has been in practice for 18 months and wants to do more MOHs surgery than general dermatology. Valda believes she doesn't have to depend on referrals from primary care physicians or internists. However, she can reach out to the public and inform them of her areas of interest and expertise. How should she proceed?

The new physician can carve and sculpt their practice using ethical marketing techniques. This chapter will focus on the new physician and how they can grow and use marketing techniques to create an ideal practice.

Everyone who went to medical school has learned how to diagnose and treat medical conditions. However, few doctors received training on how to market and promote their skills in an ethical yet effective fashion. The reality is everyone will be required to use ethical marketing techniques to succeed.

There are four ingredients of a successful marketing program to generate new patients: internal marketing, external marketing, the internet and social media (see Chap. 21), and the ability to attract referrals from colleagues and other referral sources. This chapter will focus briefly on internal and more in-depth external marketing.

Internal Marketing

Internal marketing is considered the low-hanging fruit, readily available to every physician before considering the more expensive marketing opportunities. It is much easier to start in one's backyard by ensuring that current patients have a positive experience. If they have a positive experience, those patients will share it with others who may become patients in practice.

Most physicians are probably very familiar and comfortable with internal marketing because they may never have considered it marketing. The tactics associated with this sphere of marketing include informing and educating patients about available services and actively asking them to refer family and friends. For example, suppose the doctor performs a new office procedure, and the patient has a good experience. In that case, providing the patient with educational materials to share with friends who might be interested in the procedure is easy. You can expect that one of

© The Author(s), under exclusive license to Springer Nature Switzerland AG 2023

N. Baum et al., *The Business of Building and Managing a Healthcare Practice*,

https://doi.org/10.1007/978-3-031-37623-8_20

every three patients will pass the material to family, friends, and others. This process will result in new patients who call to schedule an office visit and inquire about the procedure.

Another aspect of internal marketing is treating patients respectfully and improving patient satisfaction. So, too, is upgrading the décor of the reception area, and changing from a phone tree answering system, so that every patient can quickly speak to a human in practice, not a computer. Employees are part of the internal marketing program as your employees will tell their friends, family members, and others about the physicians in practice and their areas of interest and expertise. It is therefore essential to educate, train, and engage staff so they are knowledgeable and enthusiastic about the practice and can pass that enthusiasm onto the patients.

Internal marketing can be relatively inexpensive. However, it is a slow process that requires regular attention to the numerous details that help patients recognize that their physician is highly skilled and that the medical practice is friendly, accessible, caring, and compassionate.

External Marketing

External marketing is more than making potential patients aware of practice services and areas of expertise. The public doesn't mind marketing if they believe the information is honest, straightforward, and provides educational value. However, external marketing or getting the word out to the public is the component of any marketing program that makes some physicians uncomfortable. It is not uncommon for physicians to often think that marketing is synonymous with advertising. It is possible to inform the public about a physician's areas of interest and expertise without spending large amounts of money—and doing it ethically and professionally and does not violate the Hippocratic Oath.

There are inexpensive techniques to increase a physician's visibility within the community, the region, or the nation. These techniques do not require additional staff or assistance from the hospital's public relations and marketing departments. The essence of external marketing is writing and speaking. The rest of this chapter will focus on these two components of external marketing.

Examples of External Marketing

The physician can offer public seminars on popular wellness, nutrition, and cancer prevention topics. The practice may sponsor support groups that match the physician's interests and expertise. Support groups can target audiences according to specific diseases, diagnoses, treatments, and even specific demographic groups such as senior citizens, certain ethnic groups, or millennials.

Suppose you are conducting a seminar on a disease or condition. In that case, it is a good idea to have a patient with a specific diagnosis or condition attend the meeting or the support group. The patient describes how the problem affected their quality of life, details about the procedure they care to share, and their experience following the procedure. Support group meetings or lectures can occur in the hospital, ambulatory treatment center lobby, or the practice's reception area. Potential patients will get to know the physicians that sponsor the support group and their areas of expertise, and they'll know where to go when a medical issue arises.

Charity auctions and similar community events are another low-cost marketing opportunity. The physician may offer their services as part of an auction for a school or local charity. For example, one can consider a donation of a no-scalpel, no needle vasectomy to a local school's annual auction. The title in the auction book could be "School Tuition Getting You Down? A No-Scalpel, No-Needle Vasectomy Is a Solution." Even if those attending the auction don't respond on the day, a few men will probably call the office to make an appointment for the procedure weeks, months, or even a year later. The cost of this kind of external marketing to the practice is negligible.

Targeted Marketing

Serving the healthcare needs of various ethnic populations presents a unique marketing opportunity for culturally competent physicians. It is best to begin by identifying the ethnic community to target. That may depend on area demographics, one's ethnic background, and the languages you or your staff speak. There are ethnic community websites and directories that offer the physician the opportunity to be included. For example, the Vietnamese Yellow Pages can be easily reached through http://www.yellowpages.vn

Most cultural groups also have a word-of-mouth network. Suppose a physician treats a few members of an ethnic group in the community. In that case, word will travel fast, and they will become lifelong healthcare providers to their community. Another benefit to marketing to various ethnic communities is that grateful patients will often refer family members from their native countries who come to the United States for their medical needs. If the physician can communicate with their relatives, these relatives will likely use that practice for their medical care. An advantage of attracting patients outside of the United States is that there are no insurance issues to contend with, and the doctor receives a full fee-for-service basis without the necessity for discounts.

Writing for Recognition or Deciding to Start Writing

Writing articles for the lay press will increase the physician's visibility, credibility, and profitability. It is not likely that a physician will receive many referrals from an article that appeared in the *JAMA* or *The New England Journal of Medicine*. However, writing articles for local newspapers and magazines can effectively promote the practice and one's areas of interest and expertise—and bring in new patients. For example, the physician can create compelling and interesting articles about new procedures, new treatments, a unique case with an excellent result, or new technologies, such as stem cell transplants to treat certain leukemias, multiple myeloma, and some lymphomas. An advantage of writing articles is that they have a long shelf-life compared to radio and T.V. appearances, which only reach those who are listening to or watching the program.

Why Write?

Anyone published in professional journals knows that an article may require hundreds of hours of time and energy. Writing an article for a local magazine or newspaper takes only a fraction of the time needed for a peer-reviewed paper and can generate dozens of new patients. For example, an article called "The Prostate—A Gland of Pain and Pleasure" that appeared in a senior citizen bulletin generated nearly 50 office visits, five minimally invasive procedures, one radical prostatectomy, and one penile prosthesis surgery. Although these efforts may add to your prestige within the medical community, the return on your investment, i.e., money-wise and marketing-wise, is meager.

Our take-home message: You can effectively promote your practice and area of interest and expertise by writing articles for local newspapers and magazines.

Published bylined articles in the lay press increase your visibility, credibility, and, ultimately, your profitability. People are more likely to believe what you say if you have written it down first and had it published.

You can become a media resource by writing articles for the local press. Reporters and editors will notice your pieces. Often, they will contact you for articles or ask you for quotations to be included in articles they are writing. And, if you are responsive, they will keep you in their databases as a contact person to call on whenever your specialty is in the news. For example, the regional newspaper contacted a local urologist when Lance Armstrong developed testicular cancer. Information was provided to the health and science reporter on testis tumors which focused on the importance of testicle self-examination and how early detection of testicular cancer can cure this disease. When Senator John McCain developed a brain tumor, the newspaper called the urologist who wrote the article on testicular cancer for information for a story on the treatment of brain cancer. This condition was not his area of medical expertise. The urologist contacted a neurosurgeon who was delighted to be interviewed as the local expert on the subject.

Selecting a Topic

Topics of interest to lay readers in your community undoubtedly include wellness, nutrition, cancer prevention, sexually transmitted diseases, such as AIDS, and sports medicine. You can create an interesting article about new procedures, treatments, or new technologies, such as lasers, to correct vision problems.

Do some research before you select your topic. Note what medical stories receive local and national attention on television. When a public figure, such as an athlete, entertainer, or politician, has a medical problem, you might contact the local print media and offer to serve as a local expert on the subject. In most instances, newspapers prefer to print an article with a local twist rather than use wire service articles. Give some thought to the demographics of your surrounding area. Suppose there is a substantial population of baby boomers in your area. In that case, you can be sure that topics related to menopause, bone health, heart disease, and joint preservation will interest them. If, on the other hand, there are lots of young families in your community, any topic related to pediatric medicine or parenting will get their attention.

Study the health news section of your local newspaper. Read national women's magazines, such as *Redbook, Family Circle, Allure, Self, and Vogue*, which often have excellent coverage of health issues. The print media is interested in the personality profiles of healthcare professionals and exceptional people coping with disability, illness, or the unique circumstances surrounding an illness.

Ideally, you should try to select a topic that is familiar to you. Then either find a new angle that will excite the readers in your community or tie the subject matter to a current event. The purpose of any article is to inform, entertain, or persuade the readers; the best articles will do all three. Characteristically, physicians are capable of writing to inform the reader. Your challenge will be to arrive at a style and content that elevate the information above a simple explanation. If your article contains appropriate anecdotes and humorous stories, it will be more likely to attract and hold the reader's attention.

One caution in selecting a topic: Avoid controversial subjects, such as abortion and euthanasia, unless you are willing to take the heat.

Titles Are Terrific

A title should be like a billboard on the highway. With a billboard, you have 3 s to capture the driver's attention. The same applies to the title of your article.

In this age of information overload, you have just a few seconds to entice the reader to look at the headline and decide if they deem your article worthy of further reading.

Chris Garrett (www.chrisg.com) provides ideas and suggestions on creating titles that can attract viewers and keep them viewing your online material.

The advertising genius David Ogilvy said, "It has been found that the less an advertisement looks like an advertisement, and the more it looks like an editorial, the more readers stop, look and read." We need to make our material feel and look editorial, not a sales pitch for our areas of interest or expertise.

Think about Station WIIFM, or "What's in It for Me?"

Without a compelling headline, you will not attract attention, and your article will not be read. If you write a killer headline, you will get more readers, and readers will share it with friends and contacts.

Your title should grab the attention of the reader. The title might use a statistic, claim, fact, jingle, rhyme, or indicate a benefit.

It is essential to be as specific as possible. Highly specific approaches work much better to draw attention and create belief than generic and vague statements that can come across as untrustworthy. Rather than say, "Get great results," try "New treatment reduces the risk of cancer recurrence by seventy-five percent."

Try to create curiosity. "Are you having a problem in the bedroom? If so, below are suggestions to put energy into your love life." It is well known in the media that the topic of sex has an allure and will almost guarantee viewers want to know more information. One of the best examples is the title, "More Sex Is Safer Sex," by Steven Landsburg. Who could resist picking up this book about "unconventional wisdom of economics"!

Another suggestion is to provide powerful benefits. Does the headline offer a solution to their problem? If so, your title will take the viewer to the next level. The next level means picking up the phone and making an appointment (or, if you have a well-constructed Web site, they can make an online appointment from your Web site).

Discoveries in healthcare or stories about celebrities and politicians with certain medical conditions are always hot topics for articles for local publications. For example, there was an announcement that fish oil could be a promoter of prostate cancer. The article "Something Fishy About Fish Oil and Prostate Cancer" interested many men taking fish oil to protect against heart disease. This article received dozens of comments and patients calling for more information because it was so current.

"How-to" articles share a technique to achieve something practical and beneficial. A healthcare example of a how-to would be "10 Steps for Preventing Urinary Tract Infections," which is far better than the "Diagnosis and Treatment of Urinary Tract Infections."

The take-home message is that titles that work create a trigger and an emotional reaction. Remember, we do not just want interest; we want the reader to take any action—which means becoming a patient in your practice. You can do this by writing terrific titles.

Pitching to Publish

If you have met the health editor of a newspaper or magazine, you can contact them with your suggestion for a story. Otherwise, the standard approach is to send a query letter (Fig. 20.1 is an example of a query letter). This letter describes the subject of your article, indicates the angle you will take, and includes some information about yourself. The query letter is the equivalent of a sales pitch. You will need to study the publication to which you submit your query. Is your article appropriate? Are you targeting the right audience for your article? Once you have written a query letter, you must ensure it gets to the appropriate editor. If necessary, you can call the editorial desk and ask for the name and title of the editor for the section for your article or where you have seen other related articles appear. Take that one extra minute to ask for the correct spelling of that editor's name and title—nothing is more indicative of amateurism than misspelled words, names, or titles. Keep in mind that the editor is a very busy person. Hopefully, your letter creates an impression on the editor.

Your query letter should be a condensed version of your proposed article, with a beginning (or lead), a middle, and an end. The editor will look for a "hook" or unique opening to attract the reader. After all, if your query letter is dry and uninteresting, how can the editor expect the story to be any different? Start the letter with the most interesting aspect of what you want to write. Start with an eye-opening statistic, such as the number of people in the community affected by the health problem you will discuss. The following paragraph might describe the benefits of the article to the reader. The third paragraph mentions your qualifications to write the article. (In most cases, having the initials M.D. after your name will qualify you as a reliable and credible resource.) The last paragraph offers additional information, including how and when to reach you. Limit the query letter to one page.

One of the best hooks for an article was in a query letter by an executive from Chemwaste Corporation. This recycling company was concerned with environmental issues. The letter

January 25, 2017
Mr. Michael Lafavore
Executive Editor
Men's Health
Box 114
Emmaus, PA 18099-0114

Dear Mr. Lafavore,

Did you know that even after introducing the "miracle drug" Viagra, some men still suffer the tragedy of the bedroom?

I am a urologist in private practice in New Orleans, Louisiana. One of my areas of interest is diagnosing and treating Impotence. I have written articles on this subject in professional and lay publications. I have co-authored a book for men entitled ECNETOPMI: (Impotence) It's Reversible. I see these men by the scores every week.

I would like to suggest an 800- to 1,000-word article for your publication, *Men's Health*. We are proposing a positive an article that reassures men that help is available for nearly all men who suffer from this problem. Our message is that "no one needs to suffer the tragedy of the bedroom."

I am enclosing my curriculum vitae, several articles that I have written on this subject, and a copy of the book on Impotence.

I look forward to hearing from you.

Sincerely,
Neil Baum, MD

Fig. 20.1 Sample query letter

began: "It takes 75,000 trees to provide the paper for a single edition of the Sunday *New York Times*. Better yet, we can preserve the trees if we recycle, and our children can climb one." 1 That hook captured the reader's attention and motivated them to read the rest of the query letter.

Once you have sent the query letter, you must be prepared to track it. Unless you have a scientifically proven cure for cancer or a better drug than Viagra to treat erectile dysfunction, a follow-up call is a necessary part of the getting-published game. Some writers send a self-addressed, stamped envelope or request a reply to an email submission with the query letter to make it easier for the editor to respond. An excellent suggestion is to include with her query a stamped, self-addressed postcard with boxes next to the following statements:

- Received your query and will reply in __ weeks.
- Received your query, but we are not interested at this time.
- Received your query and want to talk to you right away.

If the editor is "still thinking about it," offer to provide additional information. Make the call short and call back in a few weeks. If you do not get an answer within 2 months, politely let the editor know that you intend to submit your idea to another publication. Then do it.

The etiquette regarding email is still evolving when it comes to contacting an editor whom you do not know personally. If the editorial desk will give you the editor's email address, use it, but do not abuse it. Common sense should prevail in an email conversation, as with phone conversations. Do not bug the person with frequent messages sent too soon after your query. Suppose you have established a personal connection with a local editor. In that case, sending your query letter as a Word document attachment to an email is perfectly fine. Make sure you proofread all emails and attachments before hitting the send button! It pays to take the extra time to make a good impression.

Remember, there are other places to publish besides the local newspaper. If you are targeting Baby Boomers, contact the local branch of the AARP (American Association of Retired Persons, the national magazine of AARP (www.aarp.org;

601 E Street NW, Washington, DC 20049) and offer to write an article for their newsletter. Start with a query letter to AARP, the national magazine of AARP. If pediatric parents are your target audience, contact parenting and children's magazines. There are also many city and regional magazines that accept articles written on healthcare issues. *The Writer's Market*, edited by Robert Brewer and published every year by Writer's Digest Books, is an excellent resource for possible outlets for your writing. It is available at bookstores, at your local library's reference desk, or through the Internet at Amazon.com and other booksellers.

Personally deliver the article to the editor to establish a face-to-face relationship. This latter advice certainly applies if the publication is a local one. If you do not hear from the editor within a few weeks, follow up with a telephone call. Always ensure you deliver your article on time and in the format requested (hard copy, CD, or digital file via email). That is the most valuable commodity to a busy editor. Suppose an editor has agreed to publish your masterpiece and has to badger you for the final copy. In that case, you will never write again for that editor or publication.

Capitalizing on Your Clips

You can get additional marketing mileage from your articles long after publication. For example, the articles can be framed and hung in your reception area or examination rooms. Your patients would rather read your articles than see your diplomas on the wall. Copies of the articles can be sent to your referring physicians and patients as bill stuffers along with their monthly statements. Add the articles to your website and have your staff mention to patients when they call for an appointment that information on their condition is on the website.

One of the advantages of writing articles is that they have a long shelf-life compared to radio and T.V. appearances. If you have negotiated to keep all reprint rights, you can submit the articles to other publications for a second printing—and

usually, get paid a small fee for giving them the right to reprint your article. Add the articles to your CV. Add these articles to a book in your reception area. Have copies available for patients asking for copies. Finally, you can send copies to the local radio and T.V. stations and suggest an interview for a story on the subject.

Rejection Is Not a Four-Letter Word

Do not expect to publish every article you write or to get a positive response to every query. Never forget that John Grisham, the lawyer turned bestselling novelist, was rejected dozens of times before finding a publisher. Also, J.K Rowling, the author of the blockbuster Harry Potter books, has a rags-to-riches story from a welfare recipient to a billionaire in less than 5 years and is one of the wealthiest women in Britain.

Everyone hates rejection. Physicians are programmed to get people well and expect quick results from our patient interactions. Consequently, many of us are reluctant to attempt to use print media for marketing our practices. However, you will find that getting published is not especially difficult once you learn to accept the rejections that come with the territory.

Our take-home message: Writing skills can be learned and polished like medical skills. The more you do, the better you get. The better you get, the more patients you will attract to your practice.

Public Speaking

Most doctors are out of their comfort zone regarding public speaking. We are very comfortable one-on-one with patients, but when we stand in front of strangers, our palms become wet, our voices tighten, and we grip the podium as if hanging on a cliff. Jerry Seinfeld humorously described the fear of public speaking this way, "People's number one fear is public speaking. Number two is death. Thus, if you go to a funeral, you're better off in the casket than doing the eulogy."

Most doctors and healthcare professionals pride themselves as good communicators. After all, that is how we take a history, discuss our findings with our patients, and then provide them with advice for restoring or maintaining their health. Except for bedside presentations to faculty or a presentation at grand rounds, we have received little training on public speaking. Few of us are able or comfortable in front of the T.V. camera. For the most part, public speaking is a learned skill. With just a little practice and preparation, all of us can become good or even excellent public speakers. As a result, we can learn how to make a presentation in front of peers, before lay audiences, and not be uncomfortable in front of the T.V. camera. The audience can learn more about a specific medical topic and how it applies to their health through public lectures. Few doctors are natural-born public speakers. But after acquiring effective public speaking skills, there will be an increased demand for our speaking services and a commensurable increase in the number of new patients filling our appointment books.

One can start researching lecture opportunities by contacting meeting planners at various church groups, service organizations such as Rotary, Kiwanis, Lions Club, Knights of Columbus, and AARP, as well as patient advocacy organizations such as the American Cancer Society, American Diabetes Association, American Heart Association, and Us Too.

Next, send the meeting planner a brief biography outlining credentials, a list of previous groups where you have presented, and a few testimonials from meeting planners or audience members. It is also helpful to attach a fact sheet (Fig. 20.3) and relevant articles, especially those you have authored.

Collect the email addresses of everyone who attends the program and keep in touch by sending out a quarterly newsletter. It is also necessary to have business cards to give to potential patients and a handout that includes a few essential facts from the presentation and all of the speaker's contact information. Distribute handouts or practice brochures *after* the program so that the audience focuses on the speaker instead of reading during the presentation.

There are three essential areas of concern for public speakers:

1. Preparation for the program.
2. The actual program, and finally.
3. After the program is over.

Before the Program

You need to know and review your slide material thoroughly. Be comfortable with the material on every slide. We have found that the best speakers can discuss any slide without having to look at the slide. Avoid reading from the slides. Reading from the slides results in boredom and loss of interest on the part of the audience. If you are looking at the slides, you are not looking at the audience, and you will lose your ability to connect with the audience. You need to know how long the program lasts and how long you are allowed to speak. We suggest you practice with a timer and ensure you do not exceed the allotted time.

Audiovisual Requirements

Before the program, communicate with the meeting planner and determine who will be responsible for the audiovisual equipment. Find out if the venue will provide the computer, the projector, and the screen. If not, let them know what you will bring and what kind of computer you have and make sure it is compatible with their projector. You can learn this the hard way. For example, if you bring a MAC computer that doesn't have the appropriate cable to connect to the LCD projector, which is only P.C. compatible. Also, you will probably not require a microphone for a small group. A microphone may be helpful if you are speaking in a loud restaurant.

We recommend that you are the first to arrive at the program. This way, you can be sure that the computers, LCD projector, screen placement, and seating area are all in order before the program. Nothing can sidetrack a speaker if they find a computer or equipment problem. Your thumb drive with a USB port does not load onto the facility's computer, or your PowerPoint program from a MAC computer does not work on their P.C.

It is a good idea to look at the agenda from the meeting planner before the program. Are you speaking before a meal, which I believe is the least favorable time, as you are almost holding the audience hostage to hear the program before they eat?

We think preparing a handout for the program is a good idea. We suggest you don't distribute the handout before the program as you want your audience to focus on you and your slides and not on the handout. Tell the audience that you will be providing a summary of your presentation so that it will not be necessary for the audience to take notes during your presentation.

Prepare an Introduction

You need to prepare an introduction. We suggest you write your introduction and send a copy by email to the person introducing you. Tell the introducer that you are providing them with the introduction as a "suggestion" and that they are welcome to modify it if they wish. Most introducers or meeting planners are delighted to have your introduction. They will use it just as you have written it. It is a good idea to bring a hard copy as many introducers will download a copy and remember to bring it. Fig. 20.2 is an example of an introduction you can easily modify for one of your programs.

The Opening

It is the first and last 30 s of any speech that has the most impact. Therefore, give the opening and closing of your talk a little extra thought, time, and effort. Avoid opening with this humdrum line: "Ladies and Gentlemen, it is a pleasure to be here tonight." It's wasting too much of those precious 30 s.

Opening a speech with a joke or funny story is conventional wisdom. Before you do, ask yourself these questions:

- Is it appropriate to the occasion for the audience?
- Is it in good taste?
- Does it relate to me (my practice) or the event or the group? Does it support your topic or its key points?

A humorous story, and an inspirational vignette, which relates to your topic or audience, will capture an audience's attention. However, it may take more presentation skills than you possess initially.

You know the questions you hear most at a cocktail reception or professional society meeting. Well, put the answers to those questions in your speech. An excellent way to open your speech is to give the audience the information they most want to hear. For example, a scientist prepared a speech for a woman's group. Since most of the audience didn't know what scientists are like or what they do, he told them what it was like to be a scientist. "Being a scientist is like doing a jigsaw puzzle in a snowstorm at night…you don't have all the pieces…and you don't have the picture to work from." You can say more with less.

Dr. Neil Baum is a urologist in private practice in New Orleans, Louisiana.

He is a Professor of Clinical Urology at Tulane. He has written ten books, and one of his books, *Impotence It's Reversible,* has sold thousands of copies, including in Latin America. His presentations are famous for providing helpful information on common medical conditions such as prostate cancer, urinary incontinence, and Impotence.

Dr. Baum is also an amateur magician and usually includes at least one special effect in his presentations.

Today's talk is also the title of his new book, *What's Going On Down There-the Complete Guide to Women's Pelvic Health.* Please help me welcome Dr. Neil Baum.

Fig. 20.2 Neil Baum bio and introduction

The Closing

The closing should be one of the highlights of your speech. Summarize the key elements of your presentation, i.e., an overview of the medical problem you discussed, preventive measures used, and what are effective treatments. If you're going to take questions, say, "Before my closing remarks, are there any questions?" Finish with something inspirational that ties into your theme.

The scientist told of the frustrations of being a scientist, and he closed by saying, "People often ask, 'why should anyone want to be a scientist?'" His closing story told of a particularly information-intensive medical conference he attended. The day's final speaker opened with, "I am a 32-year-old wife and mother of two. I have AIDS. Please work fast!" The scientist got a standing ovation for the speech.

After your talk, hang around and don't be in a hurry to leave. Be available to answer questions and have plenty of business cards, brochures, and articles about the topic you have presented. You want every audience member to leave with a piece of paper with your contact information. Fig. 20.3 is an example of the FAQ handout on overactive bladder.

Overactive Bladder: You Don't Have to Depend on DependsTM!

Overactive bladder is a common disorder that affects millions of American men and women. Most people with this condition suffer in silence and do not seek help from a healthcare professional. Fortunately, most sufferers can be helped.

- Affects 33 million American men and women.
- Can result in reclusive behavior.
- Source of tremendous embarrassment.
- Cause of recurrent urinary tract infections.
- Hinders workplace interactions.
- Limits personal mobility.
- Causes skin infections.
- Leads to falls and fractures.
- May lead to nursing home institutionalization.
- Expensive—economic cost exceeded $35 billion in 2015.
- Help is available. No one needs to depend on DependsTM!

If you would like additional information on this topic, or you are interested in having Dr. Baum speak to your group, please call (504)

Overactive Bladder: You Don't Have to Depend on DependsTM!

Overactive bladder is a common disorder that affects millions of American men and women. Most people with this condition suffer in silence and do not seek help from a health care professional. Fortunately, most sufferers can be helped.
- Affects 33 million American men and women
- Can result in reclusive behavior
- Source of tremendous embarrassment
- Cause of recurrent urinary tract infections
- Hinders workplace interactions
- Limits personal mobility
- Causes skin infections
- Leads to falls and fractures
- May lead to nursing home institutionalization
- Expensive—economic cost exceeded $35 billion in 2015
- Help is available. No one needs to depend on DependsTM!

If you would like additional information on this topic, or you are interested in having Dr. Baum speak to your group, please call (504) 891-8454 or write to Dr. Baum at neilbaum@hotmail.com.

Fig. 20.3 Example of a fact sheet on possible meeting topic for women

891–8454 or write to Dr. Baum at neilbaum@hotmail.com.

Use of Social Media and Websites

Website development and social media use are beyond the scope of this publication. Using a website and other social media tools is an excellent method of demonstrating your areas of expertise and connecting with potential new patients. A properly constructed website can target potential patients and be used as a magnet to attract new patients to your practice.

Your website is a filtering device that reaches out to potential patient's multiple times. When the time arrives that they might need your medical services, they can reach out and contact your office for an appointment.

You must have a method of collecting the email address of every person who lands on your webpage. The easiest way to do this is with a signup form.

Back to the Case
Valda contacted her hospital's public relations department and offered to speak at any local service organization, club, church, or school. She started with speaking engagements at the local Junior League (www.ajli.org) and an independent living facility where dozens of residents would likely need her services for MOHs surgery. She wrote several articles in local publications on the importance of sunscreens and seeing a dermatologist for the early warning signs of melanoma. Within 6 months, she doubled the number of MOHs cases that she did in her office with minimal expense and no paid advertising.

Bottom Line
Public speaking and writing for local publications are the best ways to achieve local recognition. It is an ethical way of communicating with your peers and the public and an opportunity to showcase your areas of interest or expertise. It all begins with reaching out to local editors and meeting planners, sending a compelling query letter, and then writing or preparing a program that has a call to action such as give us a call if you have any questions or would like additional information.

Resources

1. Ailes R, Kraushar J. You are the message-secrets of the master communicators. Homewood, IL: Dow Jones-Irwin; 1988.
2. Brewer R. 2008 Writer's Market. Writers Digest Books; 2008; http://www.amazon.com/2008-Writers-Market-Robert-Brewer/dp/1582974969.
3. Slutsky J, Baum NH. Public speaking for the healthcare professional. Street Fighter Press; 2017; Amazon.com.

Case Sammy

Sammy had an undergraduate degree in business with extensive knowledge in computer science, as he spent his younger years as an avid video game player and developer. Sammy joined a five-person orthopedic practice following residency. The practice hired a high school student to convert the three-colored practice brochure into an electronic format. The student cut and pasted the document into the free WordPress.com website builder in less than one hour. Despite trying to have a presence on social media, the site has remained idle for more than a year. What is Sammy's next action step regarding social media?

Just a few decades ago, placing a shingle or a sign on a doctor's office door was all that was permitted for a doctor to identify their practice. In 1847, when the American Medical Association (AMA) was established, it included a ban on physician advertising as part of its original code of ethics. In the years since then, great disapprobation was shown toward physicians who attempted to promote their services to the public. Some physicians—particularly young ones—became concerned when their advertising attempts met with censure from local, state, and national medical societies. In 1906, the Missouri Medical Society rebuked a local newspaper for publishing an ad by a physician: "… not one line of this obscene advertising would be possible without the publishers also being liable to prosecution. The publisher is as culpable as the physician who prostitutes his profession."

Little progress in physician marketing was made until the 1970s and 1980s, as doctors were limited to inserting a small ad in the local newspapers as an acceptable method of announcing their practices. Doctors learned ethical marketing methods in the late 1980s and early 1990s and started promoting their practices. This began with patient brochures, newsletters, and local presentations to service organizations. In the late 1990s, doctors developed web pages. These were static web pages, and there was no interaction between patients and their doctors. The first medical web pages were brochure-ware when the threefold, colored brochure was transferred electronically to the web page.

Then, in the 2000s, large group practices like Cleveland Clinic, Mayo Clinic, and the Lahey Clinic developed a presence on Facebook, YouTube, Twitter, and other social media sites. This launched a new era of practice promotion. This new era is referred to as Web 2.0. This allowed a two-way interaction between the viewers and the medical practice. Dialogue and communication enable patients to become more involved and true participants in their health care with their physicians. The exciting part of Web 2.0 is that small medical practices with a few doctors or only one doctor can compete with large groups. Social media is now very affordable, which levels the playing field and allows solo practices to market just like the large group practices and medical centers. The days of the Yellow Pages are now caput, i.e., over!

Today, every medical practice will need to participate in social media. This chapter will discuss the advantages of social media and the role of online reputation management, which is so critical to the success of any physician and medical practice.

This chapter is written with small practices in mind. We will teach you how to start your own blog site and generate fans and followers on Facebook and Twitter. We will share how to develop a YouTube presence for under $200, which includes the camera and editing software. We do not want to mislead you, as you will not have a Steven-Spielberg-quality video. Still, you will have a video showcasing your areas of interest and expertise and direct patients to your website and your practice. After reading this chapter, you will be able to have a social media presence, and you can anticipate generating several new patients every day. This very exciting technology is not as daunting as implementing an electronic medical record (EMR) into your practice. This is like adding new clinical technology, like ultrasound, into your practice. However, the return on the investment for social media is far greater than any clinical technology that is currently available.

We think that this is an exciting time for young physicians. With reimbursements decreasing and overhead costs rising, it is imperative to find new methods to improve practice visibility using ethical marketing methods and to promote the doctors and the practice. Social media is that opportunity, and it is available to everyone. We want you to consider this new technology as the shingle for ethically marketing and promoting your practice.

Why Use Social Media?

When Wayne Gretzky was asked about his excellent hockey skills, he said, "I skate to where the puck is going to be, not where it has been." If you ask a successful medical practice that makes good use of social media where they place their marketing materials, they will tell you they create and post where the patients and potential patients are hanging out, i.e., on the Internet through social media. Practices need to be where the patients are. Having a presence on a social media site is like locating your office in a prime location with easy access to highways or mass transit. With a presence on Facebook, LinkedIn, and other sites, you create more opportunities for more people to learn about you and your medical practice.

Social media allows you and your practice to stay in touch with existing patients and offers a way to provide value to your current patients. You can reach potential patients with a social media presence, including your website. These potential patients can search for you on social media sites and review the recommendations of friends and family. You can even use social media to enhance your professional relationships and partnerships by networking with colleagues focused on medical issues. Ultimately, social media allows you to raise your stature in the profession.

By using social media, you generate more traffic to your website by providing links to it. Also, your social media pages create more traffic to your website and your practice. You can expect that social media will increase your ranking in search engines which results in higher rankings in search engines, such as Google.

One of the best applications of social media is the opportunity for interaction with patients, such as answering questions, providing advice, and giving existing and potential patients a sense of what kind of physician you are. And it does not hurt to convey an appearance of being tech savvy, especially if you are reaching out to a millennial audience. Finally, ratings from patients on social media sites are essential to supporting the all-important word of mouth that builds a medical practice. This is particularly important for young physicians who want to establish themselves in the community with a positive reputation.

Social media will increase your ranking in search engines which translates to more links and enhance your rankings in search engines, such as Google.

One of the best applications of social media is the opportunity for interaction with patients, such as answering questions, providing advice, and giving existing and potential patients a sense of what kind of physician you are. And it does not hurt to convey an appearance of being tech savvy, especially if you are reaching out to a millennial audience. Finally, ratings from patients on social media sites can be an important way of supporting the all-important word of mouth that builds a medical practice. This is particularly important for young physicians who want to establish themselves in the community with a positive reputation.

Social Media Examples for Healthcare Practices

LinkedIn

LinkedIn is considered the most prominent social media site devoted to the needs of educated professionals, including physicians. LinkedIn was launched in 2003 and has more than 135 million members in over 200 countries.

More than two million companies, organizations, and practices have LinkedIn pages, and more than one million LinkedIn Groups are devoted to specific topics or professions.

LinkedIn is a way to promote yourself, especially if you are searching for a job. But LinkedIn is used in dozens of other ways: to communicate and share insights with like-minded colleagues, to do market research on new ideas, and to form business partnerships.

It is easy to get started on LinkedIn: simply set up your profile and invite other people in the LinkedIn network to connect with you. Dozens of medical practices have LinkedIn accounts. Prospective patients can search for you on LinkedIn, or they may seek you out because you

share a mutual connection with another LinkedIn member. You can join a group of like-minded physicians on LinkedIn or form a group to share ideas and insights.

You can set up a free LinkedIn profile. The free version is a great way to get started. However, if you become an active LinkedIn user and regularly exchange communications and links with other members and leading groups, you may want to consider one of the paid plans.

Because it is designed for educated professionals, LinkedIn is the social media site that most closely meets the needs of physicians. But LinkedIn does not have the mass of users that will make it truly valuable as a form of patient outreach. For that, you need to look at Facebook.

Facebook

With more than 2.27 billion and 1.15 billion users daily, Facebook is almost synonymous with social media [1]. After becoming popular among college students, Facebook entered the mainstream and is now the primary way many people keep up with family and friends: providing updates, posting photos, arranging meetings, and the like.

With so many Facebook users spending hours on it every week, it was inevitable that medical practices would use Facebook to promote their products and services, provide customer support, test ideas, and let existing patients and potential patients know what is happening in their practices. Facebook accepts advertising, but more importantly, when users declare that they "like" a product, they advertise that fact to all their friends and followers. For the medical profession, especially for the new physician, who has always relied primarily on word of mouth, this is a critical way that Facebook can help build a practice.

Overall, doctors have not been leaders when it comes to using Facebook. But that is likely to change. Various surveys have shown that over half of all doctors graduating from medical school have both a diploma and a profile on Facebook. Organizations like the Mayo Clinic have given it their seal of approval. The American

Medical Association and many medical specialty organizations all have Facebook pages.

Facebook offers numerous benefits to a healthcare practitioner. A well-designed Facebook page becomes almost like another website. You can have all the key information about your practice on Facebook: address, phone, office hours, services provided, etc. The hundreds of millions of users and the hours they spend every month is a significant market for your practice. Many people now do their web searching on Facebook on either the site itself or by asking friends and family for referrals.

Posting new information on Facebook makes it easy to educate patients by providing engaging, accurate health information and advice. And then, there is the potential for interactivity, including the ability to answer questions, have patients set up appointments, and refill their prescriptions.

We caution against "friending" patients. The American Medical Association has taken a strong position on this, advising medical staff and students to reject any approaches by current and former patients to avoid the risk of blurring the boundaries of the doctor-patient relationship.

Because of these issues, the right approach to Facebook is to keep a business or practice page separate from your personal page and monitor it closely. Another option is to look at a social media vehicle where you are in more complete control, such as Twitter.

Twitter

Every day, more than 500 million "tweets" (messages of up to 140 characters) are sent by more than 326 million active Twitter users. Twitter was initially popular with politicians, celebrities, and sports figures, who used it to stay in touch with thousands of fans.

But for easy and fast mass communication, Twitter is excellent. As a result, it is another example of a social media tool that can be used in your practice.

What you do with Twitter is limited only by your imagination. You can tweet messages about newsworthy issues and provide links to interest-

ing content. You can inform people of your involvement in events and activities such as attending national meetings and tweeting what new information is being presented. One of the beauties of Twitter is that it is possible to tweet while the meeting is taking place in real-time.

Getting started is easy. Go to Twitter.com and sign up. Choose a short, descriptive name and put a good description of yourself under the "bio" section, so people will know your background and followers can differentiate you from spammers. Registering as "skin doctor," your Twitter name becomes @skindoctor.

Begin by "follow" some people on Twitter. There are lots of places that give you lists of current Twitter users, including lists of physicians. (Try twellow.com or twibes.com.) Also, once you start with Twitter, it is easy for it to get out of control. A program like TweetDeck or Hootsuite, which is available for free, can help organize your tweets.

All the same issues with patient privacy and the patient-doctor relationship that are generated by Facebook apply to Twitter as well. It is imperative to pay attention to professional, ethical, and patient privacy concerns, which should preclude all other considerations in using any social media platform.

Blogging

A blog (the word is a blend of the terms "web" and "log") is a type of website where new content is posted regularly. In many ways, blogs are the most personal social media outlets. There are easy-to-use blogging templates, and when you write your blog postings, you are not limited to a specific word count as in the 140 characters of Twitter.

Before blogging became popular, interactive discussions online typically occurred (and still do) in online forums where participants created running conversations devoted to specific topics.

The evolution of easy-to-use blogging software such as WordPress, Movable Type, and Typepad's is easy to produce and manage. The first blogs often took the form of an online diary or journal. It is estimated that over 164 million active public blogs exist today, with over one million posts each day being added.

Typically, blogs are interactive. You write a blog post and allow visitors to your blog to leave comments. A typical blog combines text, images, and links to other blogs, web pages, and other social media related to its topic.

Of all the social media vehicles, blogs give you the greatest opportunity to establish your own voice and expertise. The ideal scenario is that your blog posts are seen as valuable, so people send a link to your blog to others. This increases your rankings in search engines, attracting more patients, thus making the investment of time worthwhile.

The best blogs are short and to the point. We suggest about 10–300 words as this is all most people have the time to read. Over time, short blogs will build credibility with your viewers.

You want to use content that differentiates yourself and your practice from your competitors. Try to use actionable content such as "how to" and FAQs. This gives your readers action steps that they can use to enhance their health.

Your blogs should allow comments. Allow readers to post comments on your blogs. You can post a question to initiate additional comments. Note that visitors interacting and writing comments about your blog will attract search engine algorithms that will move you to the first page of Google.

Getting Started

Before launching your social media presence, spend a few minutes every day reading, listening to, and watching what others are writing and doing. Start by paying attention to what others notice (blog, posts, comments, and retweets) and what appeals to you, and identify your comfort zone. We recommend you participate in other people's conversations before starting your social medial presence.

When you are ready to take the social media plunge, start slowly, build a foundation, and add more media to the mix. Start by connecting with people you know in real life and then broaden your set of connections.

Let us share a bit of advice: take private conversations offline. Never mention a patient's name or even allude to a patient so that the patient could possibly be identified in the content.

Taking advantage of social media tools costs nothing or relatively little. But social media is far from free. Allocating the time to manage and keep them up to date is your highest cost.

Plan on allocating several hours a week on social media, including research and writing, providing the content for tweets, Facebook, and blogs. If you cannot spend time cultivating your social media strategy, consider hiring a freelancer or agency to assist you with creating compelling content.

You cannot maintain a social media presence by being absent on your social media sites. If you are going to be involved in social media, plan on contributing regularly. We suggest publishing content to your blog, Facebook page, or LinkedIn group weekly.

Just as you cannot disappear, you cannot be wildly inconsistent in the kind and quality of information you provide. Your goal is for your audience to view you as a consistent, reliable source of medical information.

One unique aspect of social media is that it is a conversation, not a monologue. You need to hold up your end of the conversation. Try not to dominate it or expect that you can maintain the dialogue with material that is interesting to you but not to your audience.

Keep the needs of your target audience in mind. What do they want to know, and what do you want to know about you and your practice? Develop a unique perspective with core messages that you communicate regularly. Remember, content is king. Your content must attract and hold the viewer. The word technophiles use is "sticky," and your goal is to attract and inform viewers, have them stick on your site, and eventually call your office for an appointment.

YouTube for Medical Practices

An excellent opportunity to showcase you and your practice is by making videos and uploading those videos onto the YouTube site. There are nearly 150 million viewers on YouTube each month. Every 60 s, more than 300 h of HD quality video uploaded to YouTube contribute to a massive collection of 1.3 billion videos [2].

YouTube is a medium where people can upload and share their videos for free. YouTube is not always a platform considered social media. Still, it qualifies because you can interact with your viewers through videos, comments, and even video responses.

Video is an increasingly important aspect of any Internet marketing campaign. Video attracts people to your website, engages them, and keeps them on it longer. Many people use YouTube as a search engine, preferring to have their answers in video and audio rather than reading text.

Why Is Video Important?

Video is an essential medium for representing your practice on the Internet. Along with your website, blog, and various forms of social media, your mission is to provide your patients, both potential and existing, the best and most comprehensive information in the best format for them. Video has a high perceived value in this arena.

Just as people are inclined to understand and believe what they see on television, video on the Internet has the same effect. Allowing a potential patient to find a basic answer to a medical question in a form where you as the physician can talk to them is a compelling opportunity.

One of social media goals is to be on the first page of a Google search, and search engines love video. At the time of writing this book, search engines are only able to catalog that a video exists on your website. However, in the future, search engines can scan the audio of your video file for keywords. This will provide even better results from your videos. Adding your videos to video sites, such as YouTube, will further increase your visibility on the Internet.

Getting Started on YouTube

Video is not difficult or expensive. Excellent results in creating videos are achieved without investing in expensive equipment or hiring professional video services.

Creating Your Own Videos

A video camera does not have to be expensive. In fact, many portable video cameras now record in high definition. Smartphones, such as the iPhone, have a video camera that incorporates those records in high definition. iPhones even feature the ability to upload directly to YouTube without moving the file to a computer.

We also suggest purchasing a universal or flexible iPhone holder which contains a Bluetooth remote shutter. The cost is $5.00–10.00 [3].

Self-produced videos require you to control your own sound and lighting. If there is a well-lit area of your home or office, then that could double as your video studio. You also can record your videos outside to have natural light.

Invest in a lavalier microphone if your camera can use an external microphone. This will allow for the superior sound quality of your video.

Editing a video that you shoot yourself should not be difficult. Most computers come with software to simplify the editing process. This software allows you to add a title frame, text subtitle, images, and anything else you wish to add to your clip.

Once your video is edited, you are ready to upload to YouTube. Visit www.YouTube.com to sign in. If you have not yet used YouTube, click "Create Account" to proceed.

It is also essential to make sure your channel and videos are public. This way, they are cataloged by search engines and viewable by prospective patients.

Once your account is created, you are ready to begin adding content to YouTube.

Start by uploading your first edited video by clicking "Upload and Share Your Video."

By clicking "Upload Video," you will navigate to the video file on your computer.

Aside from having your videos on YouTube, placing them on your website, in a blog post, or on Facebook for additional availability to your patients and potential patients is helpful.

You can link your video to an e-newsletter, on your website, referenced in an article, or in a blog post with a similar topic. We suggest that the video also be loaded onto your EMR to show patients while they are in the exam room preparing for the doctor-patient encounter. Finally, we encourage your front office or receptionist to guide patients to the YouTube site to watch videos before coming to the office on various medical topics that interest patients.

Like anything in medicine, there is a learning curve, and you will find the first foray into video production will be time-consuming and may take several hours. If you stick with it, you'll see how easy it is to create a five to 7 min video that can drive new patients to your office.

Online Reputation Management

A patient with a computer and access to social media can now quickly and effortlessly comment on your practice and services. Although social media is a powerful marketing and practice promotion opportunity, this tool is also a double-edged sword. Most comments about physicians are positive. However, a negative one may be posted by a disgruntled patient. The remainder of this chapter will focus on protecting your online reputation.

Patients rely on referrals and word of mouth to make decisions about their health and choice of doctor. This process can now be done online. From social networking and Google searches to online review sites like Healthgrades, Yelp, RateMDs, and ZocDoc, patients can research and find information about their physician almost instantly.

Individual consumers also rely on their personal networks and peer recommendations. Overall, one study found that 72% of patients ranked the healthcare provider's reputation and personal experience as the top driver for choosing a provider [4].

We live and die by our reputations, our most precious possession. Our reputations are created the minute we receive our medical diploma. They take years to build but are so fragile that they can crumble in seconds or a few mouse clicks. Look at what happens to athletes and movie stars who use a phrase that is politically incorrect or get caught driving while intoxicated. They tumble from their pedestal in a nanosecond.

In today's digital age, where news is instant, thanks to social media, blogs, and search engines, your practice reputation can instantly turn for the worse. The Internet has dramatically altered the way people gather information. Social media has impacted governments, nations, and societies.

With the ease of using social media and online reviews, it is likely that a patient, or even a fellow physician, can target your practice and wreak havoc on your reputation. We will provide you with methods that you can use to protect yourself.

First, most online reviews of physicians are positive 70–90% of the time [5]. However, most physicians have five or fewer reviews on any site [6].

At a minimum, a physician should monitor their practice reputation by "Googling" their name to identify what information about their practice is already visible online. If you are like most of our colleagues, these reviews will be positive. However, do not be surprised if one or two are negative. Let's face it; even the most well-known and experienced physician cannot possibly satisfy every patient that walks through the door. The easiest way to see what others say about you is to sign up for the free Google Alerts (www.google.com/alerts).

The advantage of these alerts is that you see if it is essential or something you need to investigate further or respond to. You can also set up alerts on Facebook, LinkedIn, YouTube, and Twitter to notify you when messages are posted.

The Topic of Online Reviews

One common patient complaint is the wait time to get an appointment. Another frequent complaint is spending too much time waiting in the reception area and exam room to see the doctor. Both issues can be resolved by careful attention to your scheduling process. Patients will even judge their medical experience by how the phone is answered, how long they were left on hold, and if there is ample parking near the office.

Suppose you hear a complaint on more than one occasion. In that case, you can be sure that multiple patients have that same negative experience. Still, they are not vocalizing or writing about that negative experience. Therefore, it is imperative to take notice of these negative responses and correct them.

Ethically Creating Positive Reviews

The facts remain that most patients are delighted with their medical care from physicians. However, 40% of negative reviews are related to poor telephone technique and etiquette, failure to obtain access to the practice, and general patient service issues not involving the doctor [7].

Whether we like it or not, online reviews are here to stay. They can significantly impact the perception of your practice from both new and existing patients.

In the past, one of us (NB) tried encouraging patients to provide an online review. The patients received a card requesting they go to the review sites and provide us a favorable review (Fig. 21.1). This approach was an abysmal failure with a response rate of only 1%. This was hardly worth my staff's time to give out the cards.

Most physicians are appreciated by their patients. There isn't a day that goes by that most of us receive glowing compliments from our patients. (It is one of the best reasons to become a doctor as no other profession enjoys receiving many compliments from their customers or clients!) When a patient compliments the doctor or one of the staff members, we ask them if they wouldn't mind posting this on a review site, such as healthgrades.com. Most patients who offer a

Thank you for helping us to serve you better!
Was it easy for you to get an appointment in this office? Yes No
Is your general impression of this office favorable?
Yes No
Was the office staff friendly and concerned?
Yes No
Did the doctor adequately answer your questions?
Yes No
Would you recommend this office to someone else?
Yes No
Do you have any additional comments?

Fig. 21.1 Card given to patients to rate their experience with the practice

flattering remark will agree to provide the comment to the online review site. To capture the compliment at the point of service (POS), we use a free kiosk in our office provided by outcomeshealth.com and direct them to leave a review while they are in the exam room.

Finally, to make these reviews impactful, we ask the patient to add their name to the review. A review by Kate Smith, San Antonio, is better and much more credible and believable than "KS."

When patients compliment the staff or the physicians, ask the patient to make their comment public by submitting their positive comments to one of the many review sites. You will be amazed that a patient pleased with your staff's service will be happy to take 5 min to review your practice. You might consider posting a sign in a prominent place within the office that you appreciate an online review.

Just imagine that if you have 20–30 positive reviews for every negative review, what impact that will have on the potential new patient? If the scale swings to the predominance of positive comments, the few negative ones will be drowned out in a sea of compliments that reflect the true nature of your practice.

Managing a Negative Review

A bad online review is inevitable, just like a lawsuit is part and parcel of the medical profession today. Our advice: do not panic and do not overreact. The reality is you cannot make everyone happy.

If your ratings are mostly positive, there is often little reason for concern. Most favorable ratings with a smattering of bad ratings are likely perceived as more credible than 100% five-star ratings. It is likely that a couple of negative ratings balanced by mostly positive ratings may have the unintended consequence of increasing the positive perception of you and your practice.

If the review is off the wall or inappropriate, you should check to see if the comment violates the website's terms of use. Many sites have formulated rules constraining how reviewers should behave. For example, the use of inflammatory language is prohibited. If you identify that the comment violates the terms of use, you can submit a letter to the review site of a violation. The site is not obligated to take down the post but might consider honoring the terms of use policy.

Suppose you believe the post of the negative comment is inaccurate, and you can identify the post's author, what should you do? We suggest sending a letter or calling to the writer's attention that their post was incorrect. Then politely request that the writer amend or review the negative post. Often a polite request will remedy and correct a negative review. Some sites, like Yelp, allow doctors to privately respond to patient reviews without publicizing their comments.

We suggest you respond to negative reviews, especially if the complaint is non-clinical. You can explain how your practice works but refrain from publicly talking about the specifics of any one patient's experience. You are permitted to do this without violating HIPAA privacy laws.

To be perfectly safe, you should ask patients for their permission to reply publicly to their reviews or, if appropriate, post an apology. Once you have received written consent from the patient, an apology shows that you are listening to patients and taking steps to address their concerns. Going public with your apology potentially turns the adverse situation of a bad review into a more constructive experience [8].

Patients are seeking and leaving reviews about you and your practice online. It's time to embrace this digital age and actively manage your online reputation. Do not let one disgruntled patient ruin your reputation. Our advice is to take an active role and generate positive reviews to drown out any negative remarks made by an occasional disgruntled patient. Remember, your reputation is elastic and can be changed.

TikTok

TikTok is the fastest-growing social media platform ever created. It has created over a billion users in a virtual nanosecond. The concept is primarily embraced by users 16–29 years of age. TikTok reached over two billion downloads

worldwide as of April 2021. Over 850 million users a month log in to the video platform. It currently has more than 30 million users in the United States and was the most downloaded social-media app in 2021.

Tik Tok is a popular app that delivers interesting and unique special effects to create short-duration, attention-grabbing videos that have the potential to go viral. Tik Tok is the potential to create 15 s of videos that give users recognition and popularity. This free app provides opportunities to create creative short videos for countless worldwide viewers.

The major advantage of TikTok is that it provides an excellent opportunity to entertain your patients. Your only limit is your creativity. The program is especially suitable for people aged 12 and older. This app allows every doctor to make interesting videos and gain instant publicity.

In addition to being free, one unique feature is that beginners don't require specialized equipment to create videos. Everything can be accomplished with a mobile device with a video recorder.

A major proportion of users post their humorous videos with the purpose of entertaining others. For the healthcare professional, the purpose could be patient and community education. The beauty of TikTok is its simplicity. You don't need skills in editing videos and adding background music while using this app. This app brings you the most straightforward interface by featuring audio and video editing options for ease of use.

At the time of this publication, few medical practices and physicians have embraced TikTok as a social medium to communicate with existing and potential new patients. It can be mindless fun and a source of entertainment. Still, it's also a social media option to pay attention to the potential to educate a younger population segment.

Back to the Case

Sammy quickly recognized that he did not have the time, energy, or skills to develop a website and a social media presence. He contacted a marketing company with extensive experience in medical websites and social media. He divided the responsibility of creating content for the website and social media with two other younger doctors in his practice. He committed his practice to create one YouTube video a month. Within a few months, his practice was on the first page of Google. More importantly, he received two to three calls or responses daily from the website and from viewers on the Internet requesting appointments.

Bottom Line

The days of Dr. Marcus Welby have disappeared. Today's physicians have more in common with Mark Zuckerberg and Bill Gates than with Marcus Welby. The advent of technology differentiates the doctors of today from the doctors of decades ago. We have grown comfortable with computers in diagnosing and treating diseases; now, we must get comfortable using computers and social media to help communicate with patients.

Currently, there is one primary care physician for every 1500 patients. It is estimated that, by the end of this decade, there will be one primary care physician for every 5000–6000 patients. The challenge is to see and care for additional patients, educate them, and preserve the quality of care that patients are accustomed to while avoiding the ever-present threat of litigation. That is where the Internet and social media come in as a solution to some of the problems impacting physicians today.

There is good news. Statistics suggest that the doctor-patient relationship is changing, and patients will not receive the kind of care offered by Dr. Welby, doctors must embrace the digital age, which includes social media. They will have to think creatively about how to communicate with patients, educate them, and teach them about wellness instead of being available to treat only illness. Doctors will have to utilize the new digital solutions to lead to a complementary relationship between the doctor and the patient.

References

1. Noyes D. The top 20 valuable facebook statistics. Zephoria Digital Marketing. 2018. https://zephoria.com/top-15-valuable-facebook-statistics/.
2. Iqbal M. YouTube revenue and usage statistics. 2018. Business of Apps. http://www.businessofapps.com/data/youtube-statistics/#2.
3. https://www.walmart.com/ip/Acuvar-6-5-Flexible-Tripod-Universal-Mount-iPhones-Samsung-phones-Many-Smartphones-Bluetooth-   Remote-Shutter-eCostConnection-Microfiber-Cloth/253466155?athcpid=253466155&athpgid=athenaItemPage&athcgid=null&athznid=PWVUB&athieid=v0&athstid=CS020&athguid=30c0f326-914-16825b93f1e24d&athena=true.
4. PwC Health Research institute. Customer experience in healthcare: the moment of truth. PwC. 2012. www.pwc.com/es_MX/mx/publicaciones/archivo/2012-09-customer-experience-healthcare.pdf.
5. Lagu T, Hannon NS, Rothberg MB, Lindenauer PK. Patients' evaluations of health care providers in the era of social networking: an analysis of physician rating websites. J Gen Intern Med. 2010;25(9):942–6.
6. Gunter J. For better or maybe, worse, patients are judging your care online. Obg Manag. 2011;23(3):47–51.7.
7. Tehrani AB, Feldman SR, Camacho FT, Balkrishnan R. Patient satisfaction with outpatient medical care in the United States. Health Out Res Red. 2011;2(4):e197–202.
8. Ventola CL. Social media and health care professionals: benefits, risks, and best practices. Pharm Ther. 2014;39(7):491–9.

Case Ben and Hurricane Katrina
Ben had been the dean at a southern medical school for two years when a Category 4 hurricane struck his city. The storm led to massive destruction of his city's infrastructure, and the resulting flooding damaged many of the facilities on his campus. Ben evacuated to a city 350 miles from home and was trying to plan for the future of his school. Unfortunately, the storm had disrupted major communication systems, including cell phone service and email. The easiest course of action might be to suspend his school for a semester, an idea favored by the president of his university. Still, Ben was concerned that this course of action might have dire consequences as faculty and students may choose to go elsewhere, costing the school a loss of tuition, grants, and clinical dollars. How should Ben proceed?

Every institution and medical practice experience a crisis. These crises include financial, personnel, public relations, and even natural disasters. Although some crises can be predicted, such as a downturn in the economy or the implementation of new federal regulations that alter Medicare payments, many crises like natural disasters are unexpected. Surviving a crisis involves a management style that is quite different from that of managing typical business operations. Successful crisis management often results in a stronger institution following the resolution of the crisis [1].

The first step in managing a crisis is to identify your leadership team. In his book, *Good to Great*, James Collins describes this process as "getting the right people on the bus" [2]. Identifying specific job descriptions for the leadership team at the beginning of a crisis is often less important because the right team will usually effectively solve problems. Recovery from a crisis is not achieved through the micromanagement of a single leader but through creating an empowered team that can make decisions, solve problems, and thinks out of the box.

When Tulane University School of Medicine was recovering from the devastation of Hurricane Katrina, a group of leaders was assembled in Houston, Texas, to plan to reopen the medical school. The small group worked closely, and each was empowered to make decisions consistent with the overall goal of reopening the school. Although the dean had the final say on decisions, the success of the recovery was closely linked to teamwork and cooperation [1].

Once your team is identified, the next step is quickly establishing a recovery plan with clear objectives. This involves setting a single thematic goal that is clear, concise, and consistent throughout the organization. The public, your employees, and your patients want to feel that the situation is controlled and managed adeptly.

Although crisis management is complex, raising the tendency to have multiple goals, a thematic goal should identify the single top priority. If everything is important, then nothing is important.

A thematic goal requires a definable action and a time frame for results. The thematic goal should dictate the organization's steps during the recovery and the time frame in which milestones are expected to be reached. Suppose the thematic goal is to open a new clinic to recover market share by a particular date. In that case, the business strategy should center around this goal. The thematic goal becomes the defining rationale for strategic planning.

Any change in operation that is inconsistent with or irrelevant to the goal should be questioned and dismissed. In crises, management needs to be coordinated, iterative, and precise. Since time is of the essence, efficiency and agility are essential in the planning process.

A crisis requires quick action. After establishing a thematic goal, the team needs to set measurable objectives. Having measurable outcomes ensures accountability for all management decisions at all levels.

Establishing an effective and comprehensive communication plan is almost as important as selecting the crisis team and identifying a plan with goals. In any crisis, stakeholders must know that the leadership team has everyone's best interests. To properly communicate during a crisis, identify a spokesperson, preferably someone with training in communicating with the media, and communicate often. In medical practice, your stakeholders include your patients, your employees, the hospitals where you work, other referring physicians, your community, and the public. Think broadly. Are there other stakeholders who may feel left out if not directly contacted?

In 2017, Adidas sent an email to all finishers of the Boston Marathon stating, "Congrats, you survived the Boston Marathon!" [3]. This email was sent four years after three people were killed

and several hundred injured by an explosion near the finish line. Adidas recognized its mistake and quickly apologized for its perceived lack of sensitivity. Their quick response and apology prevented a worse public relations disaster. In the aftermath of Hurricane Katrina, leaders at Tulane University School of Medicine created a "war room" where the team would meet to discuss each objective (obtaining housing for the students, bringing faculty to Houston, providing financial resources for students in need) and where they were in the process of accomplishing this objective. Frequent communication kept the team on task and helped them feel accountable for the overall thematic goal of getting the school back into operation [3]. During the time of crisis, frequent status updates are imperative.

Nothing is better at breaking down silos than a crisis. Silos are bad in business because they lead to distrust, conflicting goals, and turf wars where people on the same team can work against each other. Nearly every silo can be attributed to leaders who have not fostered interdependence between different units of an organization. The silver lining of a crisis is that it brings people together toward a common goal. When a country goes to war, a president's popularity typically increases due to a sense of loyalty. To break down silos, identify key objectives, gather consensus, and involve as many constituents as possible.

During a crisis, honesty is essential. Successful recovery depends on the ability of leaders to communicate recovery plans and to have people trust their decisions. During the first Iraq war in 2003, Iraqi Information Minister Mohammed Saeed al-Sahaf, nicknamed "Baghdad Bob" appeared on TV daily to predict an Iraqi victory and deny the American Baghdad invasion even when US tanks were seen on the screen behind him. Sahaf did not waiver from his story until Baghdad fell [4]. American forces captured and interrogated him and ended up in Abu Dhabi, where he dropped into obscurity. The term "Baghdad Bob" is now used colloquially to refer to a leader who confidently attests to something everyone else sees as false.

If you are a leader in a time of crisis, set an example. Be honest, show integrity, and take charge. The mayhem imparted by a crisis requires people to act quickly and follow through with plans. You need to be the first to volunteer and the last to go home. It is also important to show emotion and empathy when appropriate. No one wants a leader who appears detached from their organization. Some crises are emotion-driven by their very nature. For example, physician suicide is an unfortunate reality that confronts practices, medical staff, and medical schools. Suicide produces feelings of guilt, sadness, and anger among survivors. A good leader in this type of crisis does not appear detached but one who is warm, consoling, and emotionally involved in such a time of sorrow.

An example of not showing leadership and understanding occurred in May 2010 when the British Petroleum Deep Water Horizon rig exploded in the Gulf of Mexico, killing several roustabouts on the rig. During the crisis, the CEO of British Petroleum, Tony Hayward, opted to take time off to sail with his son instead of dealing with the Gulf of Mexico oil spill. This was an example of a leader MIA just when his company, the families of the men who were killed, and those who were injured in the explosion needed to see a leader demonstrate ethical principles of responsibility, accountability, and humanistic care. The case of the BP oil spill in 2010 provides an example for understanding how these principles are valued by public opinion in a crisis and how the communication actions by a corporation in this type of circumstance might have a long-term effect on the image of the organization [5].

This is a textbook example of how not to conduct a crisis management resolution. (By the way, Tony Hayward was relieved of his CEO position a few months later).

Finally, with any crisis, plan for next time. What will you do the next time your competitor opens an office down the street from you? What will you do with the next market crash? The next product recall? The next drug shortage? In his book, *The Black Swan*, Nassim Taleb describes a black swan as an unpredictable event with significant impact [6] After the event, the facts are interpreted such that the event appears less random. The term black swan comes from the assumption that they represent a rare species mutation, yet they are reasonably common. The danger of black swans is that the human brain uses black swans to create the illusion that we know more than we do. The human brain is programmed to focus on specifics rather than generalities. For example, following 9/11, every airport has instituted a rigorous screening process assuming that airplanes would be used as weapons in future attacks on America.

The next terrorist attack is probably less likely to be via a weaponized airplane than a mass poisoning of our water supply. Preventing such an attack using airplanes remains the goal of airport security. But we do not focus on the generalities of making our world safer for everyone.

Do not assume it to be a black swan when planning for the next crisis. In New Orleans, the next hurricane is not likely to be complicated by levee breaches. A narrow focus will not make the next crisis easier.

In healthcare, the next epidemic will not be AIDS, so to assume that efforts to reduce the spread of HIV will be effective for a future epidemic is foolhardy. We suggest planning with a general approach. This includes planning for personnel changes, financial stresses, and changes in hospital management through mergers and acquisitions. Do not plan for specifics such as planning for the subsequent merger with a for-profit or planning for a medication shortage.

Back to the Case
Ben decided that he would not suspend school operations for the semester. Realizing that his city would not be ready for a medical school for at least 6–12 months, Ben moved the medical school to a city 350 miles away. Ben gathered a management team including his associate deans, key chains, key faculty, and key students. His management team communicated with students, faculty, and staff, assembled a curriculum, organized housing, and created an alliance with other medical schools in the new location to train

clinical students and residents. The school remained in the new city for the entire academic year and even recruited a new medical school class from their new location. Finally, after moving back home after 10 months, the team marveled at what they had accomplished with little resources [7].

Bottom Line

1. Crises happen and, by their very nature, are unexpected.
2. Crisis management involves deliberative steps, including identifying your leadership team, articulating a recovery plan, communicating effectively and often, breaking down silos, being honest, leading by example, and plan ahead for the next crisis.
3. In planning ahead, do not be deceived by black swans; the next crisis will never be identical to the last one.

References

1. Kahn MJ, Sachs BP. Crises and turnaround management: lessons learned from recovery of New Orleans and Tulane University following Hurricane Katrina. Rambam Maimonides Med J. 2018;9(4):e0031.
2. Collins J. Good to great: why some companies make the leap…and others don't. Harper Business; 2011.
3. Calfas J. Adidas apologizes after sending "you survived" email to Boston Marathon finishers. 2017. http://time.com/4745066/adidas-boston-marathon-email/. Accessed 14 Jul 2022.
4. Posetti J, Matthews A. A short guide to the history of 'fake news' and disinformation. ICFJ. 2018;7(2018):2018–07.
5. Valvi AC, Fragkos KC. Crisis communication strategies: a case of British petroleum. Ind Commer Train. 2013;45(7):383–91.
6. Taleb NN. The black swan: the impact of the highly improbable, vol. 2. Random house; 2007.
7. Krane NK, Kahn MJ, Markert RJ, Whelton PK, Traber PG, Taylor IL. Surviving hurricane 8. Katrina: reconstructing the educational enterprise of Tulane University School of Medicine. Acad Med. 2007;82(8):757–62.

Case Lancelot

Lancelot is the youngest member of a five-person neurologic practice. One of the senior members appears to be detached from the practice and his patients. The senior doctor is consistently late to start his clinic. He is receiving negative comments on his lack of compassion and caring on online review sites. The older doctor is involved in a lawsuit involving a patient who contends he missed diagnosing a brain tumor. In summary, the more senior doctor is depressed. What is Lancelot, the young doctor in practice, to do?

This chapter will discuss the prevalence of burnout in the healthcare profession, review the causes of burnout, provide the most common signs and symptoms of burnout, and finally, offer active solutions for burnout.

Physician burnout is reaching epidemic proportions. That's the bad news. The good news is that burnout is easily recognized, and solutions to this common problem exist.

Most articles report a prevalence of burnout in approximately 50% of all physicians. Our profession is witnessing a trend of young doctors deciding to take alternate career paths in technology,

consulting, and healthcare policy instead of pursuing a career in clinical medicine.

Also, we are seeing a rise in online communities of dissatisfied and disaffected doctors looking to change careers and even have their own "club," the Drop Out Club and Physicians Nonclinical Career Hunters (www.docjobs.com and www.nonclinicaldoctors.com) [1].

Another issue of great concern to our profession is that burnout is more common among physicians than other US workers and non-medical professionals [1]. There are increasing numbers of disillusioned physicians, with increasing depression seen in physicians and the highest rate of suicide in our profession. The burnout rate is emblematic of the problems facing our profession. We want to emphasize that burnout isn't just impacting older or near retiring physicians. More than 50% of medical students, residents, fellows, and early-career physicians are already experiencing burnout [2].

Definition of Burnout

Burnout is characterized by a state of emotional, mental, and physical exhaustion caused by excessive and prolonged stress. Although burnout can occur in any profession, burnout occurs most frequently among people in the caring professions of medicine, nursing, social work, counseling, and teaching.

© The Author(s), under exclusive license to Springer Nature Switzerland AG 2023
N. Baum et al., *The Business of Building and Managing a Healthcare Practice*,
https://doi.org/10.1007/978-3-031-37623-8_23

Causes of Burnout

The most common cause of burnout include:

- Workloads over seventy hours a week.
- Loss of autonomy.
- Electronic medical record (EMR)
- Increased paperwork.
- Night and weekend call
- Risk of litigation
- Demanding patients
- Loss of work-life balance.
- Onerous regulations
- Managing the business of medicine
- COVID-19

For the most part, physicians can manage difficult situations, especially in the clinical arena. However, there are now external factors that increase the stress that physicians must face regularly [3].

In the past, medical education emphasized the concept of high touch. Today that concept has been replaced by high tech. New physicians today are being micromanaged by many outside forces that make all physicians, young and older, feel a loss of control and feel less valued.

For the most part, physicians can manage difficult situations, especially in the clinical arena.

In the past, it was common in medical education to emphasize the concept of high touch to physicians in training. Today that concept has been replaced by high tech. New physicians are being micromanaged by many outside forces that make all physicians, young and older, feel a loss of control and feel less valued.

Autonomy is the ability of physicians to exercise their judgment of how to spend their time, attention, and resources. In the recent past, the doctor controlled the decision when to see the patient, time spent with each patient, tests to perform, medications to prescribe, and recommended treatments. The autonomous doctor did all these activities without asking for permission or obtaining authorization. Today, control and autonomy no longer exist. The current methods in medical reimbursement force physicians to spend less time with each patient, more time

looking at a computer than the patient, adhere to guidelines and complete large amounts of paperwork. Doctors become discouraged when caring for patients requires focusing on the monitor rather than the patient. Most physicians complain of the tsunami of electronic paperwork. Filling out paperwork is not why anyone decided to become a doctor. Most physicians remain altruistic and have a mission to treat patients and change the world—not to check boxes on paper or an electronic record. Doctors often feel they are treating a computer rather than a patient.

When young physicians transition from training to private practice, adjusting to a new environment, following rules from the government, insurance companies, and hospitals all limit the time physicians can spend with a patient. Those rules also require that each doctor-patient encounter complies with the Health Information Portability and Accountability Act (HIPAA), Accountable Care Organizations (ACOs), quality indicators, MIPS, and MACRA (see Chap. 12 for more information on MIPS and MACRA)

In the past, medical education emphasized the concept of high touch. Today that concept has been replaced by high tech. New physicians today are being micromanaged by many outside forces that make all physicians, young and older feel a loss of control and feel less valued.

Autonomy is the ability of physicians to exercise their judgment on how to spend their time, attention, and resources. Doctors were in control of the decision when to see each patient, how much time to spend with each patient, what questions to ask them, when to see them next, what kinds of tests to perform, what medications to prescribe, and what treatments to recommend without asking for permission or obtaining authorization. Today, physician control and autonomy no longer exist. The current methods in medical reimbursement mandate that physicians spend less time with each patient, more time entering data on a computer, and completing large amounts of paperwork. Doctors become discouraged when caring for patients requires focusing on the monitor rather than the patient. Most physicians complain of the tsunami of electronic paperwork. Filling out paperwork is not why anyone decided to become a doctor. Most physicians remain altruistic and have a mission to treat patients and change the world—not to check boxes on paper or an electronic record. Doctors often feel they are treating a computer rather than a patient.

Physician training teaches the young doctor to focus on the patient. Then there is a transition to the real world of private practice, which requires adjusting to a new environment that limits the time physicians can spend with patients. Those rules also require that the doctor-patient encounter complies with the Health Information Portability and Accountability Act (HIPAA), Accountable Care Organizations (ACOs), quality indicators, MIPS, and MACRA (see Chap. 12 for more information on MIPS and MACRA).

If we had to select one of the major causes of burnout, it would be the electronic medical record. Physicians who must transition from paper charts to electronic records describe the computer as shackles or handcuffs and that every "additional click of the mouse inflicts a nick on physicians' morale"[4].

For many physicians, the EHR has become the final straw. Although intended to overcome the inherent flaws in a paper-based system, the EHR has produced its own problems. The most significant impact is a loss of eye contact with the patient. A previous article in JAMA tells it all. It's a drawing by a pediatric patient of her experience with her doctor. (Drawing available at https:// t w i t t e r . c o m / T h e L a n c e t / s t a-tus/1170306723019743233/photo/1) You can clearly see that the patient recognizes that the doctor is paying more attention to the computer than to her or her mother.

Another complaint of young doctors is the time involved in completing the electronic record and additional paperwork long after the encounter with the patient is completed. They spend one to 2 h of uncompensated time working at home each evening to keep up. One study involved ambulatory care in four specialties (family medicine, internal medicine, cardiology, and orthopedics) in four states (Illinois, New Hampshire, Virginia, and Washington) [5].

What a sad commentary to our profession that prides itself on high touch in addition to high tech with loss of interaction with our greatest commodity, our patients. The electronic record requires the doctor to be a data collector rather than focus on the outcome. This is compounded by the fact that most electronic medical records are built and created with the primary purpose of billing and not caring for patients. The technology intended to improve healthcare, i.e., the EMR, is generating burnout and one of the most common reasons for doctors deciding to leave the practice of medicine.

Symptoms of Burnout

Burnout is reasonably easy to recognize. Usually, it is not possible to see it in yourself. Still, others can quickly identify doctors experiencing burnout and can lead them to help.

In the early stages of burnout, the doctor will appear anxious and will be worried and sad. Uncontrolled anxiety may become so serious that it interferes with the doctor's ability to work productively and may cause problems in his\her personal life.

The burned-out doctor has a short fuse and unexplained outbursts. Partners and colleagues of the burnout doctor may notice irritability between the doctor and the staff and the doctor and his\her patients. If anger reaches the point where it turns to thoughts or acts of violence toward family or coworkers, this is a sign that professional help is needed.

Burnout doctors will often complain of chronic fatigue. The doctor may note a lack of energy and feel tired and lethargic on most days. If burnout goes untreated, the doctor may feel a sense of fear and anxiety and be unable to function in the office or hospital setting.

Another symptom of burnout is insomnia. The doctor often reports trouble falling and staying asleep. As a result, the doctor is exhausted upon awakening in the morning.

It has been the observation of one of us (NB) that burned out physicians, including both men and women, experience a decrease in libido and male physicians report erectile dysfunction.

The burned-out doctor will complain of loss of concentration and forgetfulness. It is common for doctors experiencing burnout to forget to attend meetings, are chronically late for the clinic, have delays reporting for surgery, and miss significant events in their personal lives.

When burnout is untreated, the doctor may experience physical symptoms such as chest pain, palpitations, shortness of breath, vague abdominal pain, and headaches. These symptoms cannot be allocated to burnout and must be medically evaluated.

Even in its earliest stages, burnout is often accompanied by a loss of appetite. As a result, unexplained weight loss occurs.

The depressed doctor needs to obtain professional help as soon as possible. In the early stages, the burned-out doctor may feel mildly sad, occasionally hopeless, and may experience feelings of guilt and worthlessness. In later stages, the doctor may experience depression and hopelessness, which put those who suffer from depression at risk for suicide.

The colleagues and partners of a burned-out doctor will notice an erosion of the doctor's productivity.

The burned-out doctor does not complete projects on time. They are the ones that have incomplete medical records in the office and at the hospital.

The burned-out doctor doesn't complete charge sheets, resulting in compensation delays. The doctor will have a litany of excuses but never seems to "climb out from under the pile" of work or responsibilities.

Solutions for Burnout

In Patrick Lencioni's book, *The Three Signs of a Miserable Job* [6], job satisfaction is discussed from a management perspective. Lencioni identifies three characteristics that make a job untenable: anonymity, irrelevance, and a term he coined, "immeasurement." Anonymity among employees leads to feelings of frustration and isolation. Irrelevance leads to a loss of sense of meaning with work. Immeasurement, defined as the lack of accountability standards and metrics, leads to a lack of sense of how one is doing their job, and they lack a sense of fulfillment. All three of these, anonymity, irrelevance, and immeasurement, lead directly to physician burnout.

When looking for physician solutions to burnout, the three signs of a miserable job need to be addressed. To protect against anonymity, we suggest getting involved in organizied medicine. This can be done on the local, regional, or national level. We recommend starting by becoming engaged in the hospital committee. Become the "go-to" person for quality medical care, credentialing, or pharmaceutical approval. At the regional or national level, become involved with your special day or subspecialty societies. Develop a reputation in your area of interest and expertise.

Become Relevant

Create a situation where you have decision-making capacity, either as someone who is part of a committee that writes guidelines for medical conditions for your hospital or helps decide strategy for allocating funds for projects. Many hospitals in healthcare systems now employ a chief wellness officer. Perhaps aspiring to be this person or at least being on a wellness team can increase your sense of value. Teaching medical students, residents, fellows, or mid-level providers can provide a sense of job satisfaction. This helps you stay up to date with your specialty. Additionally, psychosocial theory suggests that we all seek mastery over internal and external forces to establish a sense of wellness. Teaching allows us to feel competent, confirming our sense of worth.

We also recommend that you insist on measurement. Ask your supervisor or your group,

"What is expected of me in the upcoming year?" Develop a 1- to 5-and 10-year plan with milestones and stay on schedule. Demand feedback. Work on improving those things you are deficient in and even better at those things you do well.

As for other solutions to the burnout crisis, there is evidence of debt exposure to arts and humanities decreases burnout among medical students [7]. The authors of this study speculate that the humanities stimulate a part of the brain associated with pleasure, improving the quality of life. Interestingly, in this study, there was no difference between active participation in the heart (playing an instrument, writing a play, meaning a picture) and passive participation (listening to music, seeing a play, going to an art museum). We do not suggest that the entire problem of burnout can be solved with a single rock concert. Still, personal wellness is undoubtedly part of the solution.

Finally, create safe places for physicians to talk. The hospital workplace or a medical office can be demoralizing and difficult to control. Narratives are powerful communication tools; people feel good about talking about themselves. Feeling part of a team or connected can relieve feelings of isolation in talking with others experiencing the same problems and provide support. Sometimes confiding in a friend or colleague offers a sense of control.

Of course, the best solutions to burnout are to create systems, including the process of making entry into the electronic health record, that are efficient with respect to time and effort. Limiting work hours, providing time off, and allowing for work-life equilibrium are also important strategies. Sharing decision-making among hospital liters and physicians also helps create a sense of control. The burnout issue among physicians is complex, and there is not a one-size fits all solution. All physicians, hospitals, and health systems need to address the issue of physician burnout to provide the best care for our patients.

Back to the Case

It was clear to Lancelot that he was dealing with a burned-out doctor. Since Lancelot was the youngest doctor in the practice, he was uncomfortable confronting the older doctor about the recognition of burnout. Lancelot approached two other older physicians in the practice and made sure they were aware of Lancelot's observations. The more senior doctors appreciated Lancelot's observation, met with the depressed doctor, and strongly recommended he receive professional help. The older doctor saw a psychiatrist specializing in substance abuse and burnout. The doctor received treatment and took two months of recommended leave of absence. His partners were very supportive, and he successfully returned to practice and remained very appreciative of Lancelot recognizing the reality of the situation.

Physicians may be reluctant to volunteer that they are suffering from burnout, as in the case of Lancelot's senior partner. There are online burnout self-assessment programs. These are free and allow the physician anonymity. These tools help screen for burnout. It helps physicians look at how they feel about their job and experiences at work, so they can get a feel for whether they are at risk of burnout. One of these free online tools is available at https://www.mindtools.com/pages/article/newTCS_08.htm.

The self-assessment tool consists of 15 questions (see Fig. 23.1) that, upon completion, provide a score interpretation ranging from "no sign of burnout" to the extreme "You are at a very severe risk of burnout-do something about this urgently."

Bottom Line

Burnout is not a condition we can ignore. Nearly 50% of doctors, including medical students, residents, fellows, and young doctors, are experienc-

Fig. 23.1 Self-assessment tool of burnout

1.I feel run down and drained of physical or emotional energy.
2 I have negative thoughts about my job.
3 I am harder and less sympathetic with people than perhaps they deserve.
4 I am easily irritated by small problems, or by my co-workers and team.
5I feel misunderstood or unappreciated by my co-workers.
6 I feel that I have no one to talk to.
7 I feel that I am achieving less than I should.
8 I feel under an unpleasant level of pressure to succeed.
9. I feel that I am not getting what I want out of my job.
10 I feel that I am in the wrong organization or the wrong profession.
11 I am frustrated with parts of my job.
12 I feel that organizational politics or bureaucracy frustrate my ability to do a good job.
13 I feel that there is more work to do than I practically have the ability to do.
14 I feel that I do not have time to do many of the things that are important to doing a good quality job.
15 I find that I do not have time to plan as much as I would like to.

ing the signs and symptoms of burnout. The causes are a feeling of powerlessness, loss of autonomy, and the intrusion of technology intended to improve healthcare but detracts from the care we provide our patients. The signs and symptoms are easily recognized, and effective treatment is available for the impaired physician.

References

1. Shanafelt TD, Boone S, Tan L, et al. Burnout and satisfaction with work-life balance among US physicians relative to the general US population. Arch Intern Med. 2012;172(18):1377–85.
2. Dyrbye LN, West CP, Satele D, Boone S, Tan L, Sloan J, Shanafelt TD. Burnout among US medical students, residents, and early career physicians relative to the general US population. Acad Med. 2014;89(3):443–51.
3. Fred HL, Scheid MS. Physician burnout: causes, consequences, and cures. Tex Heart Inst J. 2018;45(4):198.
4. Zulman DM, Shah NH, Verghese A. Evolutionary pressures on the electronic health record: caring for complexity. JAMA. 2016;316(9):923–4.
5. Sinsky C, Colligan L, Li L, Prgomet M, Reynolds S, Goeders L, et al. Allocation of physician time in ambulatory practice: a time and motion study in 4 specialties. Ann Intern Med. 2016;165(11):753–60.
6. Lencioni P. The three signs of a miserable job. San Francisco: Jossey-Bass; 2007.
7. Mangione S, Chakraborti C, Staltari G, et al. Medical students' exposure to the humanities correlates with positive personal qualities and reduced burn-out: a multi-institutional study. J Gen Intern Med. 2018;33(5):628–34.

Case Phillipe

Phillipe is a nephrologist who joined a small practice in a rural community in the Mid-West 3 years ago. He had an income guarantee for his first 2 years and was very productive, earning a bonus during his third year in practice. However, his wife, a social worker, was unhappy in the community and could only find part time work leaving her professionally unfulfilled. As a result, Phillipe considered terminating his relationship with the practice.

Physicians are under a tremendous amount of pressure in today's healthcare environment as costs escalate, reimbursement declines, and the threat of malpractice continues. Normal workplace stresses are exacerbated by longer hours, less pay and less tolerance for error, which can lead to disappointment and ultimately the decision to leave a practice.

Reasons for a medical divorce or termination of employment agreements are usually divided in two categories: "for cause" and "without cause." For-cause termination generally means that a party to the agreement can terminate the agreement, often immediately, if the other party breaches or violates the agreement in some way. The employment agreement should clearly spell out each of the causes for which the employment can be terminated. The causes for termination should be objective and reasonably within the employed physician's control but not so restrictive as to leave the employer without recourse if some unexpected behavioral or performance issue arises.

Common causes for termination with cause may include loss or suspension of a medical license, losing medical staff privileges at the hospital, failure to obtain or maintain insurance participation, failure to obtain or maintain board certification, conviction of a crime or felony, patient safety-related issues, or use of illegal drugs or abuse of controlled substances. For some types of cause, a physician may negotiate a provision requiring that the employer provide advance written notice of the complaint that, if uncorrected, will lead to termination, thus allowing the physician adequate time either to change the objectionable behavior or to find new employment.

Physician employment agreements can also be terminated without cause, which means that either party can terminate the agreement at any time. Without cause termination usually requires notice of a certain number of days without having to identify any specific reason for the termination. It is common for contracts to state that termination without cause may be invoked by either party following a specified period of advance written notification, which is usually 90 or 180 days.

This type of termination provision can offer protection for both parties since, in the absence of a without cause provision, each party is obligated to abide by the terms of the initial agreement for the entire term unless they are able to find a cause for termination or are willing to breach the contract. If a departing physician chooses the latter option, this may result in a lawsuit for breaching the contract.

If you are planning to terminate your relationship with your employer, we suggest that you follow these steps to make the medical divorce as painless as possible [1].

1. Prior to notifying your employer of your decision to depart, review all documents, especially the contract you have signed. It is best to do this with an attorney. Documents will most likely include an employment agreement, a shareholders' agreement (if the practice is a corporation) or an operating agreement (if the practice is a limited liability company), and, in some cases, a deferred compensation arrangement. During your review, pay careful attention to information about advance notice provisions, the details of retirement, and non-compete restrictive covenants. These are the key components of your contract.

   It is critical that you understand and adhere to what you have promised to do and what has been promised to you via these contractual agreements.

2. Next, review the practice's policies with your attorney. In addition to reviewing any documents you have signed, you should review any of the practice's policies applicable to employment and departures. Some employment agreements indicate that the practice's general policies and procedures may be applicable even if they are contrary to the physician's employment agreement.

3. One of the most important aspects of your departure is to develop a plan for notifying your patients of your departure. Many states have a requirement that all patients be notified when a physician is departing a practice. Some states even require or suggest 30 days

prior written notice before a departure so that patients will have sufficient time to transfer their record sand care if they desire to change physicians. If you are not familiar with your state's requirements, contact a healthcare attorney in your area for advice.

In addition to sending letters to your patients, think carefully about how you will address your departure when you speak with patients in person. For example, you would never want to be in a situation where you felt compelled to lie to a patient. Often practices and departing physicians will agree on what to tell patients who inquire about the tenure of the departing physician. Some practices display placards in the reception area informing patients of a physician's departure. Voice mail systems can also be modified to provide new contact information after the physician has departed.

Think about patients first. When scheduling your departure from the practice, take reasonable steps to ensure that you are not leaving any patients in a bind. For example, if you are an obstetrician, you would not want to plan your departure during a week in which you are anticipating five deliveries. The key is to prevent patients from falling through the cracks because of tensions between the departing physician and the practice. You and the practice have an obligation to provide proper care for your patients. The take-home message is to consider the patient first and do not do anything that puts the patient's health in jeopardy.

High-risk patients should be sent a letter by certified mail, with return receipt requested to confirm their receipt of the notification. High-risk patients are those who are more likely to experience adverse outcomes and feel that they have been abandoned if their departing physician is unavailable for ongoing care. Examples would include recent postop patients and those currently being followed for serious or chronic conditions. Keep a copy of the notification letter and certification material in the patient's record.

Active patients who are not high risk should be sent a letter by regular post. Examples of active patients include those seen within the last 12–18 months. Again, we suggest that you keep a copy of the notification letter in the patient's record.

Finally, notify other patients who will not be receiving a letter by placing a notice in the local newspaper with the largest local circulation. We also recommend placing a sign in the reception area about any changes in physician employment.

The practice should also provide a script for phone receptionists on what to say. This should include information on how to contact the departing physician.

If the departing physician will not be available for ongoing care if they are moving out of the area, the letter should provide this information but should also explain that care is available at the same location from other physicians in the practice. You should tell those patients who choose to seek care elsewhere that, upon their written authorization, a copy of their medical record will be forwarded to their new provider.

If the departing physician will be available for ongoing care, explain to patients that the physician is leaving the practice but is still available in the area. Tell patients that they have the choice of staying with the practice or continuing to see the same physician in his or her new location. Instruct patients who choose to follow the physician that, upon their written authorization, a copy of their medical record will be forwarded to the physician at his or her new location.

To expedite the transfer of records, you should consider including an authorization form with the letter of notification. If your practice is going to charge the patient for the photocopying costs, you should inform the patient what the fee will be. Any material that is related to patient care should be considered part of the medical record, should be considered confidential, and should be provided to the new physician. Both the practice and the

new physician should keep a copy of the medical records.

For patients who stay within the practice, the patient should be notified about the change in provider. The patient's preferences should be honored either to stay in the practice or continue with care with the departing physician.

If the care will be provided by another practitioner with the same scope of practice as the departing physician, simply inform the patient of the new provider's name. However, if the care will be provided by a practitioner with a different subspecialty, you should verify that the patient's clinical needs can be safely met by the new provider.

Fig. 24.1 is a sample of a letter you might consider sending to your patients announcing your departure.

4. Review advance notice provisions. Your contract may require that you give your practice advance written notice of your departure. If you fail to give notice, the practice could claim breach of contract, and you could be held legally responsible for the cost of hiring a *locum tenens* physician or the cost of recruiting a new physician to fulfill the remainder of your term. Further, many deferred-compensation arrangements are linked to the amount of notice given. Some require an extraordinarily long notice period (such as 1 year) before the physician can qualify for any deferred compensation payments.

5. Review your retirement plans. This will ensure that your departure date does not result in unnecessary forfeitures. For example, some retirement plans require an employee to work the entire year prior to becoming eligible. While it may be convenient to resign shortly before Christmas so that you can spend the holidays at home, it could be a monumental mistake if it results in losing nearly 1-year of retirement benefits. Further, many retirement plans have vesting schedules that depend on the number of years you have worked with the employer in order

Notice of Leaving Practice (Patient)

Dear (patient's name):

It is with mixed emotion that I am [announcing my retirement from active practice; relocating my practice; etc.] as of [date]. This decision has not been made lightly, as I have enjoyed working at _____.

As of [date], Dr. _____ will be taking over my practice. [Describe the new physician's background in 1-2 sentences]. Dr. _____ can be contacted at the address below:

[Name of Physician and/or Clinic] [Address]
[Telephone number]
[E-mail]

If you prefer, you may obtain the services of another physician. If you choose to do so, I would recommend proceeding as soon as possible to ensure a smooth transition for your health care. The local Health Region keeps a list of physicians who are accepting new patients.

Your medical records are confidential, and a copy can be sent to another physician or released to you or another person only through your consent. I will be pleased to provide a summary of my care while you have been my patient, and with your consent, will arrange to have a copy of your file transferred to your new physician's office. Please sign the enclosed authorization form and return it to our office as soon as possible before (date) so that we may make the appropriate arrangements concerning your file.

It has been my great pleasure to have provided you with health services in the past, and I am grateful to have had the opportunity to meet some wonderful people throughout my years in practice. Best wishes for a healthy future.

Sincerely,

Dr. _____ [title]

Fig. 24.1 Notice of leaving practice (Patient)

to receive your deserved retirement compensation. You and your attorney should review the details of your plan so that you do not unwittingly forfeit significant amounts of retirement money.

6. "CYT" or cover your tail! Many practices obtain "claims made" malpractice insurance policies that insure you for claims made during your term of employment. This means that if a malpractice event occurs while you were employed but the claim was not filed until after you have left the practice, the malpractice insurer will not cover that claim because it was not made during your employment. To prevent this, you need to procure a supplemental policy, commonly referred to as "tail coverage," which insures you for claims made after your employment terminates. While some employers will contractually agree to pay tail insurance, a thorough review of your employment agreement will determine who is responsible for procuring tail coverage.

Whether the practice pays for tail coverage often depends on the type of termination. For example, practices often agree to pay for tail coverage in the event that employment is terminated by the practice without cause, meaning there was no violation on your part. For example, if the practice was sold or merged with another group, the malpractice might not cover you in the event of a claim after the practice is sold or merged. Likewise, physicians often agree in their initial contract negotiation to pay for tail coverage if the physician terminates their employment without cause.

This tail coverage can be significant, especially if you are an obstetrician or in another high malpractice risk field. Thus, regardless of who is responsible for procuring tail coverage, that party should provide a certificate of insurance to the other party. Do not be seduced into foregoing the purchase of tail coverage. The cost of successfully defending a medical malpractice action is lifestyle altering and you do not want to do this on your nickel.

While you can purchase tail coverage that has no end date, many malpractice carriers offer 1-year, 3-year, 5-year, or 7-year tail coverage policies. These finite tail coverage policies as opposed to lifetime coverage are generally less expensive. If you live in a state with a limited statute of limitations on medical malpractice insurance claims, these finite tail coverage policies can save you money without leaving your tail exposed.

If you are responsible for tail coverage, you may be able to negotiate with your new practice to provide you with sufficient funds to purchase it. Or, in limited circumstances, the new practice may provide coverage through a new policy with a retroactive endorsement date. This is referred to as "nose" coverage. Our take-home message is to check out both your tail and your nose so that you are covered in the event of a malpractice suit after you leave a practice.

- There are several companies that will provide you with free quotes on tail coverage. (https://www.cunninghamgroupins.com/request-a-free-quote/ or 866–213–3035) or The Doctors Insurance Agency, http://www.doctorsagency.com/blog/entryid/1137/-the-cost-of-tail-the-doctors-company-, 800-553-9293).

7. Parting with the patients' charts. Be aware that patient lists, patient charts, and other patient demographic information are property of the practice, not the departing physician. Employment contracts usually reinforce this stipulation in the contract. Rarely do practices agree that patient charts are the property of the departing physician. These assets belong to the practice and cannot be taken by the physician without the practice's consent. You should note, however, that most states allow the patient to request that his or her chart be forwarded to a departing physician, in which case the physician can, at that time, receive the chart from the practice. Usually, the practice will charge the patient for copying the chart. Importantly, the departing physician cannot merely request a copy of the chart be sent to them in their new practice.

8. Taking employees with you is a no-no. Your contract may contain provisions against your soliciting the employment of existing employees of the practice. Even without these prohibitions, you should not actively solicit the employment of existing employees, especially prior to your departure. Some states would consider this behavior an egregious act and courts would find favor with the employer if a physician were to "raid" the practice for employees. It is, however, not uncommon for employees to solicit the departing physician prior to departure. This creates a quandary because although you may need new employees, you do not want to appear to be soliciting from the existing practice. Before you make any decisions, revisit your employment contract and your state's laws regarding the issue. This is another area where a healthcare attorney can be very helpful.

9. Review noncompetition covenants. A noncompete covenant may prohibit you from practicing within a certain geographic radius of your current practice for a designated period of time, often 2 years. The radius is usually determined by your practice's location and could range from 5 miles in a suburban area to 50 miles or more in a rural area. Many departing physicians are of the opinion that these covenants will not be enforced; however, the courts in most states will uphold them if they are reasonable. For this reason, you should review the covenant as though it will be enforceable in accordance. Litigating a covenant, either from the employer or departing physician's perspective, is expensive. Do not hesitate to contact an attorney if you have any questions.

10. Even when leaving a position under less-than-ideal circumstances, the departing physician should leave adequate forwarding information. Patients may need to contact the departing physician. Payors may need to contact them as well, especially where audits and adjustments that are the responsibility of the departing physician are concerned. If the practice has to respond it does not know where the departing physician is located, complaints to the medical board are a certainty. And a physician does not want a complaint when they are trying to obtain licensed in another state or obtain hospital privileges at another institution.

Dependent upon the provisions of contracts and state law, both the departing physician and the practice may need to notify various third parties:

- The malpractice insurance carrier that needs to know of any changes in order to ensure coverage of the care rendered in both the prior and future practice settings.
- Managed care companies with whom you have contracts.
- The medical staff committee of hospitals where the departing physician has privileges. If he or she is on-call at the hospital, notify the emergency department as well.
- The state board of medicine (if required by state law).
- Legal counsel for assistance as needed in contract provisions and employment law.

Fig. 24.2 is a letter you might consider using to notify colleagues of your departure from a practice.

We strongly advise securing the counsel of a healthcare attorney with any contract-related matter. Just as the words cure, remission, and no evidence of disease are pleasant words to the ears of the treating physician and their team, divorce is a pleasant word for healthcare attorneys.

Although physicians are transitioning from volume to value, attorneys are still reimbursed by the volume of cases they have and they will be just delighted to help you through a potentially expensive experience. That is why we suggest that you seek the counsel of an attorney with healthcare experience and an attorney who has experience managing medical termination on behalf of an employed doctor. We also recommend that you ask your attorney who you are considering hiring for an estimate of the charges for managing your case. You cannot hold their feet to the fire but they should provide you with a ballpark cost of managing your case. If the attorney comes back with a response that they just "log in their hours" and then give you an hourly fee, then we suggest you walk to the next healthcare attorney as they are many of them available who will provide you with an estimate of the fees you will likely be paying.

Back to the Case

Phillipe contacted his employer and his attorney discussed the situation with his family about his desire to leave the practice. Phillipe made a point to his employer that he was generally happy with the physicians and employees in the practice and wished to leave on good terms, but that he had to think about the happiness of his family first. Phillipe sought the counsel of a respected healthcare attorney in his community, who helped him to write a letter to all of his patients several months before his date of departure, and then made certain that he had tail coverage in the event of any lawsuit filed after he left the practice. As a result, Phillipe had a reasonably amicable separation from the practice, moved to a large community where his wife was able to obtain full time employment and they lived happily ever after!

Notice of Leaving Practice to Send to Colleagues, Professional Associations, Payors)

Dear (name of individual or agency):

It is with mixed emotion that I am [announcing my retirement from active practice; relocating my practice; etc.] as of [date]. This decision has not been made lightly, as I have enjoyed working at _____.

As of [date], Dr. _____ will be taking over my practice, as well as the bulk of my medical records. [Describe the new physician's background in 1-2 lines]. Dr. _____ can be contacted at the address below:

[Name of Physician and/or Clinic] [Address]
[Telephone number]
[E-mail]

[Use this paragraph to indicate any committees, appointments, and other positions from which you will be stepping down that could be relevant to this individual or organization, or any other message you wish to convey to referring physicians, etc.].

If you need to contact me for any reason, please don't hesitate to give me a call or send me an email and I will respond quickly.

[Your Name and/or Clinic]

[Address]
[Telephone number]
[E-mail

It has been my great pleasure to have worked with you in providing quality health care in Saskatchewan. I am grateful to have had the opportunity to meet and work alongside some wonderful and remarkable people throughout my years in practice.

Sincerely,

Dr. _____ [title]

Fig. 24.2 Notice of leaving practice to send to colleagues, professional associations, Payors).

Bottom Line

Most young physicians do not have the knowledge or the skills required for departing from a practice. It is for that reason that we suggest contacting a healthcare attorney who has experience with medical contracts before deciding to leave a practice. Leaving a practice can be a stressful time in any physician's career. A clean departure will save you headaches and possibly dollars in the immediate future and in the long run. Your careful attention to these details will ensure a smooth transition to a new practice.

References

1. Wall JD. A must-do list for the departing physician. Fam Pract Manag. 2005;12(9):54–6; James Wall is the founder and president of Wall Law Firm, P.C., based in Winston-Salem, N.C.

Resources

1. Physician Employment Contract Guide by American College of Physicians, 2017 ; https://www.acponline.org/system/files/documents/running_practice/prac-

tice_management/human_resources/employment_contracts.pdf.

2. Little KS. The exit: terminating physician employment agreements. Healthcare Law Blog; 2017; https://www.healthcarelaw-blog.com/exit-terminating-physician-employment-agreements/.

3. Leaving practice-A guide for physicians and surgeons. 2017. http://www.cps.sk.ca/iMIS/Documents/Brochures/Leaving_Practice-guide.pdf

Balancing Your Personal and Professional Lives

Ivan is an orthopedist who has been in practice for 5 years. He has a very productive and growing practice; yet he feels guilty for not spending more time with his young family. His wife has informed him that his adolescent son is having behavior problems at school. Ivan is faced with the double conundrum of feeling guilty about not spending time with his family when he is at work and feels remorse when he is with his family and not at the office or taking care of patients.

Doctors are highly motivated to be effective in their professional life but maintaining a balance with their personal lives is a challenge for all of us. How you maintain this balance will ultimately determine not only your success as a physician but also your happiness. It is common to occasionally feel discouraged about various aspects of your practice, such as the vast amount of paperwork that must be completed to care for your patients or the continued decrease in reimbursements impacting nearly every practice. Most of our colleagues are experiencing the same feelings about their practices. It is easy to become discouraged after talking to physicians who complain about their practices and complain that their family suffers because the practice consumes so much of their time. Let's remember that medicine is a noble profession that provides great satisfaction and gratification and that all that doctors need to do to be happy is to find techniques for putting balance into their careers. This chapter will discuss 10+ suggestions that may help balance the scale between your personal and professional life. Physicians who read this chapter will gain new insight into achieving balance in their practices and balance in their personal lives.

1. Always be a student. Medicine is a lifelong commitment to learning. No doctor can be on top of their game if they only use the knowledge and skills they received when they completed their education or training. Balance is achieved if you continue to follow a lifelong pursuit of knowledge. Maintenance of Certification programs for specialty boards helps to ensure that keeping current is a physician's responsibility. A medical career is a journey and not a destination. You should always make time to be a student for your entire career. Sir William Osler, honorary professor of medicine at Johns Hopkins University, recommended to physicians and students at the end of the nineteenth Century, "In order to receive the education of not a scholar, at least of a gentleman, you should read for a half hour before you go to sleep, and in the morning have a book open on your dressing table. You will be surprised how

© The Author(s), under exclusive license to Springer Nature Switzerland AG 2023
N. Baum et al., *The Business of Building and Managing a Healthcare Practice*,
https://doi.org/10.1007/978-3-031-37623-8_25

much can be accomplished in the course of a year" [1]. After all, learning new things is fun.

Options for continued learning include the regular reading of journals, attendance, and participation at specialty society meetings, or teaching the next generation of physicians. Remember, you need to be a medical student, but remember to learn about things outside of medicine through participation in book clubs, community college classes, or joining interest groups in astronomy, cooking, rock collecting, and the like. The secret of a good life is the eternal quest for knowledge. (Several learning opportunities are available at the end of this chapter.)

2. Be ethical. A recent report in a pediatric journal states "that 44.7% rated their ethics education during residency as fair or poor." The facts are that most physicians have received very little training in medical ethics. All physicians will have or will be faced with ethical decisions that we will have to make for or on behalf of our patients. Examples include end-of-life care, AIDS care, care for under-aged patients (children), the release of sensitive information, or termination of the physician/patient relationship. Balance in our lives includes making the right ethical decisions at the right times on behalf of our patients. The best advice we can offer when confronted with an ethical issue is to do what is in the patient's best interest, and you will probably make the right decision. Most state licensing boards now require that continuing medical education includes regular courses in ethics. Doctors should regard this as an opportunity to look at your patients and profession through a different and balanced lens.

3. Take active control of your finances.

Most young doctors today enter practice with nearly $250,000 of debt, which will take years to pay off. However, balance comes from having the expectation of financial security at the end of your career when you can practice because you genuinely enjoy the practice of medicine, not because you must work to earn an income. We recommend starting the saving process early to have that security and balance. Even in the face of daunting debt, you need to create a savings plan for your children's education and for your retirement long before they will need those funds for their tuition. (See Chap. 3 on Basic Personal Finance and Investing.)

4. Learn to say "no." There is no faster road to imbalance than taking on too many projects and accepting too many responsibilities. The next time you are called to join a hospital committee, become a member of a community board, or accept an invitation for an evening dinner, ask yourself these questions: Will the obligation enhance my career? Will the commitment take away from my time with my family and friends?

Will this obligation lead to balance or imbalance in my life? If the answer is that you aren't enhancing your career and if it distracts from your family time, then you should turn down these requests. Remember, it is not a sin to say no. Sometimes it is advantageous to have a mentor to rely on to help you make the decision to say no.

5. Set your priorities. Most physicians who have balance in their lives place their religion, their family, and their practice as the order of importance in their lives. Rabbi Harold Kushner, the author of "When Bad Things Happen to Good People," pointed out that "He never met a man on his death bed who said he wished he spent one more day at the office," "or saw one more patient" (italics is our addition). This is good advice, and it is never too late to spend one more day with your significant other, your children, and your grandchildren. Another saying that emphasizes this concept is, "when you climb the ladder of success, make sure your ladder is facing the right wall."

Many doctors have worked diligently and provided outstanding care for their families but have yet to remember the concept of balance. As a result, when they climbed that ladder and were medically successful, they were saddened by an unhappy marriage or children who did not turn out quite as they had hoped.

6. Find a niche. Ross Perot, entrepreneur and candidate for the President of the United States in 1992, described success as finding an unmet need, becoming an expert, and filling that unmet need. The philosopher Hegel wrote, "every occupation has reference to some want." If you can identify an unmet need and fill that need, others will be knocking on your door to be your patients or to do business with you. It is amazing how successful you can be if you focus on a single area of interest or expertise. Finding a nice applies to all areas of medicine. A primary care doctor can focus on nutrition and weight loss, an orthopedist can direct his attention to sports medicine, or a radiologist can narrow his practice to patients with head injury or back pain.

All of us have some areas that we enjoy and have expertise. It is possible to seek out those special areas and use marketing and practice promotion skills to attract those patients to our practices. When you become an expert in a narrow area, you become more efficient and productive, and focus will ultimately provide more balance.

7. Hang out with people one generation older or younger than yourself. If you are a young physician, meet older, more seasoned doctors who can mentor you, share their valuable experiences, and give you wise counsel when needed. Every young doctor needs to learn to avoid potholes when they move from training to the real world of medicine.

Find a mentor with an experienced physician who works with you to help you to develop professional goals and plans to support your growth and development.

The traditional mentor is a physician with whom you have created a formal or informal relationship to help a younger doctor become acclimated to the medical community. To have a successful mentoring relationship, meet regularly for sage advice to discuss topics of concern. Use your mentor as a sounding board to answer questions and receive feedback.

There are two ways to structure mentor relationships.

First is the formal or structured relationship. In this relationship, you arrange specific times to meet with or speak with your mentor each week or month. You can report on your progress and specific challenges in these meetings and even develop an action plan. The second type is the more common or informal relationship with the mentor.

The mentor or young doctor may check in periodically to discuss current challenges and report accomplishments without a schedule or predetermined connecting frequency.

The structured approach is better, but because physicians are busy, we recognize that sometimes a less formal structure is necessary.

In finding a mentor, select someone you admire and respect because of their age, stature, or position within the community. You want to choose a mentor with considerable expertise in your specialty or a leader in the field. The mentor should have a reputation as being a good communicator.

Look for an individual who has a caring attitude and is known for compassion and empathy with patients. You also want a positive person who is enthusiastic about their profession. Finally, look for a physician who has the time to dedicate a few minutes each month with you so that you will not feel like you are imposing on their time.

Entering private practice can be a daunting experience.

One way of softening the shock is to find a mentor who will help you learn the ropes and avoid the potholes that are sure to confront every doctor who moves from training into the real world of medicine.

Just as a mentoring relationship with an older physician benefits a younger physician, the opposite is true. The advice is to balance your friendships which will bring balance to your life. If you are a more senior physician, hang out with the Gen Xers. Contact with younger people can keep you current, energized, and on top of your game.

8. Exceed patients' expectations. To truly enjoy your medical practice, it is important to not just meet the patient's expectations but to go beyond what is expected and exceed those expectations. We suggest that you adhere to "the extra mile philosophy." This philosophy requires you to go the extra distance for your patients, exceed their expectations, and provide a little more than other doctors. Your patients will remember you for it. Many businesses, from office product suppliers to upscale department stores, have found that providing deluxe services ensures that those customers will return. Medical practice is no different from other businesses in this respect.

It is challenging to compete on price in today's healthcare market. What you can do is make sure your appointment book is full. This can be accomplished by asking and then answering two questions: (1) What do patients want? Then give them more of it, and (2) What do patients not want? Then make every effort to avoid it. It is just that simple.

9. Be a disciplined doer and a decider, not a procrastinator. Nothing adds more anxiety to our lives than deadlines and commitments we have trouble meeting. If you have several projects looming in the future, break them down into smaller projects and make a calendar marking off the completion of these little projects.

That way, you will only be left with a small project with days to complete. Discipline can bring balance to the busy professional:

(a) Clean out your inbox.
(b) Fill up your outbox.
(c) Complete your medical records before the delinquency notice arrives.
(d) Look for an endpoint to your day.

There will be a new set of mail, results, and problems tomorrow; a clean slate creates a balanced perspective. Confront those challenging decisions: a professional who can decide in a few minutes to recommend radical extirpative cancer operation to a relative stranger ought to be able to determine the new 3-year lease with a few days' reflections.

10. Have fun. The best advice to achieve balance is to take your profession seriously, not yourself. Find ways to inject a little humor into your daily activities. Start your day by listening to a humorous CD of Jeff Foxworthy, George Carlin, or an old Abbott and Costello routine. Smiling releases endorphins, and there's no better way to trigger a positive feeling in the body and reduce stress than to smile.

A smile is contagious, and you want to ensure that yours is worth catching!

Remember that medicine is the most enjoyable profession and can be the most fun and rewarding, especially if we add a dose of humor.

10+. Consider having an unplugged day.

Physicians spend excessive time on computers and watching screens on EMRs, iPads, and cell phones. It is common for a physician to start daily looking at emails and checking their computer inbox when they arrive in the office. Most physicians are tethered to the Internet and cell phone 24/7, including days when a physician is on vacation. As a result, most of us have become addicted to social media, email, texting, and apps.

There is a solution to this enslavement: it is called getting unplugged and having an electronic sabbatical.

This electronic sabbatical occurs when you are totally unplugged from the Internet, mobile phone, computer, iPad, and other electronic devices for just 1 day a week.

To prepare for your unplugged day, you can begin by thinking of a solution to move Internet or computer tasks or projects to a different day. Then answer your most important emails before the unplugged day starts. Finally, set up an automatic email responder that you will be answering emails on Monday if your unplugged day is Saturday or Sunday.

If you have a blog, post on Thursdays or Fridays to connect with your readers.

Only respond on your unplugged day if you have a Facebook account. Not be surprised if your friends still like you on Monday! Do not post on Instagram or Snapchat. Your photo can wait to go viral for 1 day!

There are other benefits of becoming unplugged. After an unplugged day when you are free from the shackles of the digital world, you will notice dramatic changes within yourself. You will think differently, act differently, and see things from a new or different perspective.

You will notice that time will slow down. You will pay more attention to the priorities of your life, and you will be more receptive to new ideas, concepts, and even new friends coming your way. Becoming unplugged will make you feel like time is in abundance.

You'll create room for ideas and insights by being unplugged for just 1 day. You'll gain real inspiration from life and circumstances that is different from the usual online inspiration. This is the best time to stimulate your creative juices.

You will soon appreciate that the positive effects of being unplugged for a day are felt long after the unplugged day is over.

As Thomas Friedman said in his book, Thanks for Being Late, the world is always in a state of acceleration. Mr. Friedman advocated taking a regular scheduled pause and reflection instead of being in a constant state of acceleration. As a result of slowing down and unplugging, you will increase the odds that you will better understand and engage the world around you and, yes, even become a better and balanced doctor.

Remember what the good book says, "Thou shalt work hard 6 days a week and rest on the seventh day." In 2018 and beyond, that means getting unplugged for just 1 day a week!

Back to Ivan

Ivan recognized that he was becoming a successful doctor but was missing balance in his life. As a result, he started scheduling time for his family just as he had a schedule for his practice. Ivan and his wife set a date night each week and even arranged an in-town vacation for just one night at a local hotel. Ivan volunteered to be an assistant coach on his son's soccer team. He decided to attend every game with the only exception of his absence as if he was in surgery. As a result, Ivan's son's behavior problems improved due to being able to spend time with his mother and father. He and his wife were back on track as a team and able to enjoy their lifestyle.

Bottom Line

No one ever said medicine was easy or fun. But it can be both and even more if you emphasize balance in your professional and personal lives. It can be done; follow these 10+ suggestions. The best ending for this chapter comes from Rabbi Harold Kushner, author of *When Bad Things Happen to Good People,* who said, He never met a man or woman on their deathbed who said, "I wish I would have spent one more day at the office." Instead, they said, "I wish I would have spent one more day with family and friends."

References

1. Kesselheim J, Johnson J, Joffe S. Pediatricians report on their education in ethics. Arch Pediatr Adolesc Med. 2008;162(4):368–73.

Further Readings

Cousins N. The anatomy of an illness as perceived by the patient. W.W. Norton; 1979.

Kushner H. When bad things happen to good people. Random House; 1981.

Friedman T. Thanks for being late. Farrar, Straus, and Giroux; 2017.

The Time for Telemedicine Has Arrived

Case Roberto

Roberto is certified public accountant (CPA) with a history of erectile dysfunction and low testosterone levels. Taking time from his busy accounting practice has been difficult. He has friends who communicate with their physicians through telemedicine. Roberto is interested in this concept and does not know how to find a doctor willing to provide virtual care.

Most doctors have practiced a simple form of telemedicine when they take phone calls from patients seeking medication refills. In these cases, physicians can either call the pharmacy to refill the medication or suggest patients make an office appointment to receive a new prescription. Physicians are not compensated for accommodating patient refills, yet the physicians are legally responsible for their actions and advice. This situation does not make for good medicine.

This is where telemedicine can enhance the communication and needs of patients who want to receive care through the technology of telemedicine. Telemedicine saves patients the time and the effort of coming to the office. A telemedi-cine visit provides a record of the interaction, making for better medicine. Many patients do not require an in-person visit to receive medical care. There is even the potential to safely provide post-operative care via telemedicine. This chapter discusses integrating telemedicine into practice with minimal time, energy, and expense.

Practices typically use telemedicine platforms to manage one or both of the following types of encounters: (1) walk-in visits through the practice's website. Patients accessing a practice through the website tend not to care which physicians they see. Their priority is usually the first available provider; and (2) appointment-based consultations, where patients schedule video chats in advance of an in-office visit, or for a quick follow-up, usually with a specific provider.

Although incorporating telemedicine into practice may seem overwhelming, it requires minimal additional equipment, interfaces easily with a practice's website and electronic medical record (EMR) system, increases productivity, and improves workflow. And patients generally appreciate the option of not having to travel to the office for an appointment.

Most patients and physicians are already comfortable with mobile phones, tablets, social media, and wearable technology, such as Fitbits. Telemedicine is a logical next step.

N. Baum et al., *The Business of Building and Managing a Healthcare Practice*,
https://doi.org/10.1007/978-3-031-37623-8_26

Getting Started

Physicians and their colleagues and staff need to become comfortable with telemedicine technology. Physicians can begin by using video communication for other purposes, such as conducting staff meetings. They should practice starting and ending calls and adjusting audio volume and video quality to ensure good reception for both the doctor and the patient.

Selecting a Video Platform

Table 26.1 provides a list of the most popular video providers and their advantages and disadvantages, and Table 26.2 shows a list of free video chat apps. Apps are available that can:

- Share lab tests, images, and other medical documents.
- Securely send documents over a Health Insurance Portability and Accountability Act (HIPAA)-compliant video.
- Stream digital device images live while still viewing the patient's face.

Physicians should ensure their implementation team has the necessary equipment, including webcams, microphones, and speakers. They should take the time to research and test out a few programs before selecting one for their practice. Consider appointing a telemedicine point person who is knowledgeable about the technology and who can patiently explain it to others. And keep in mind that video chatting depends upon a fast, robust Internet connection with sufficient bandwidth to transport a large amount of data. If your practice has connectivity problems, consider consulting with an information technology (IT) expert.

Table 26.2 Telemedicine apps

Amwell
Babylon (translation software)
Dialogue
Doctor on demand
First opinion
HealthTap
Lemonaid
MDLive
Pager
PlushCare

Table 26.1 Telemedicine video conferencing products

Products	Pros	Cons
Google + Hangout	Free	No screen sharing
Secure/Video	HIPAA compliant	
Skype	Leader voice and video	No screen sharing Requires ample bandwidth Not HIPAA compliant
Tango	Both Android and iPhone	No screen sharing
WebEx	Excellent for presentation And webinars	Decreased video performance
Zoom	Both Android, iPhone Free for <40 minutes	Minimal fee >40 minutes
CiscoJabber	**Supported on all mobile devices**	**Complicated serve requirements**

Testing It Out and Obtaining Feedback

Once a practice is comfortable using video, it is time to test it out with a few patients and perhaps a few payers. Most patients are eager to start using video for their medical encounters. Even senior patients are often willing to try consults via video. According to a recent survey, 64% of patients want to see a physician over video [1].

And among those who were comfortable accepting an invitation to participate in a video encounter, increasing age was associated with a higher likelihood to accept an invite.

Physician colleagues, medical assistants, and nurse practitioners will need some basic telemedicine skills, and physicians and staff should be prepared to make video connections seamless for patients. Usually, patients need some guidance and encouragement, such as checking their spam folder for their invites if the invites fail to arrive in their email inbox, adjusting audio settings, or setting up a webcam. Fortunately, most computers have built-in video cameras that greatly facilitate the utilization of a virtual appointment. In the beginning, physicians should make sure they build in plenty of buffer time for the unexpected, as there will undoubtedly be some "bugs" that need to be worked out.

Physicians should encourage and collect patient feedback to such questions as:

- What kinds of devices (laptop, mobile) do your patients prefer using?
- What kind of networks are they using (5G, corporate, home)?
- What features do they like? What features do they have a hard time finding?
- What do they like or not like about the video experience?
- Keep track of the types of questions patients ask and be patient as patients become acclimated to the video consultation experience.

Streaming Online Workflow

After receiving feedback from your patients, it is time to streamline the online workflow. Most physicians want to manage video visits similarly to how they manage face-to-face visits with patients. This may mean experimenting with a virtual waiting room. A virtual waiting room is a simple web page or link that can be sent to patients. Patients sign in with minimal demographic information on that page and select one of the time slots when the physician is available. Typically, these programs are designed to alert the physicians and staff when patients enter the virtual waiting room. Patients have access to the online patient queue and can start a chat or video call when both parties are ready. Such a waiting room model serves as a stepping-stone for new practices to familiarize themselves with video conferencing. This approach is also perfect for practices with a practice management system that just want to add a video component.

Influences on Practice Workflow

With good time management, telemedicine can improve the efficiency and productivity of your practice. Your daily schedule and management of patients will need some minor changes, but significant alterations to your existing schedule and workflow are generally unnecessary. One of the advantages of telemedicine is the convenience of prompt care, and the easy access patients have to your practice. This decreases visits to the emergency department and to urgent care centers. This not only decreases the cost of care but can also benefit any value-based contracts that the practice may have.

One piece of advice: consider scheduling telemedicine appointments at the end of the day when your staff has left the office, as no staff members are required for a telemedicine visit. Ideally, you should offer a set time to communicate with patients, as this avoids making multiple calls to reach a patient.

Another advantage of telemedicine is that you can provide care in the evenings and on weekends. Whereas before, you might have been fielding calls from patients during these times and not being compensated, with telemedicine, you can conduct a virtual visit from any location and any computer or mobile phone and can receive remuneration for your care.

Telemedicine and the Coronavirus

The COVID-19 healthcare crisis made implementing telemedicine essential. Patients who believed they might have COVID-19 or those who had been diagnosed needed to be quarantined. Such patients could be helped safely in the comfort of their own homes without endangering others. In fact, whether infected with COVID-19 or any other virus, patients who are febrile or have respiratory symptoms can continue to avail themselves of virtual visits. Similarly, doctors worried about infecting others with COVID-19, common colds or other minor illnesses, can safely see patients in a telemedicine network.

There are several misconceptions with telemedicine. Physicians often assume that patients prefer face-to-face visits when, in fact, many may prefer the convenience of virtual visits. More than 50% of surveyed patients about their experience with telemedicine say that online tools have helped improve their relationship with their providers [2].

Telemedicine has grown exponentially during the COVID-19 pandemic to the point where many patients now *expect* their healthcare providers to be able to conduct virtual visits. Practices that do not offer telemedicine may find their patients seeking services elsewhere. COVID-19 has motivated the increased use of telemedicine to enhance communication with patients, making it possible for patients to have improved access to healthcare during the pandemic while minimizing infectious transmission of COVID-19 to physicians and their staff [3]. Additionally, the COVID-19 pandemic motivated third-party payors such as Medicare and Medicaid to provide reimbursement for virtual visits.

Admittedly, telemedicine is not appropriate for all patients. In general, situations that do not lend themselves to telemedicine are those for which an in-person visit is required to evaluate the patient, situations where a physical examination is necessary, or those where an office procedure is needed. Additional patients for whom telemedicine may be inappropriate include those with cognitive disorders, language barriers, or for those emergency situations that warrant an office visit or a visit to the emergency department. Of course, telemedicine is always limited by the technology that the patient has at home.

Cost and Complexity

The process of implementing electronic health records (EHRs) has left a bitter taste in the mouths of many healthcare professionals because EHRs are complicated and expensive. Implementation of an EHR often results in lost productivity. Because the learning curve is so steep, many physicians have to decrease the number of patients they see before becoming comfortable with the conversion from paper charts to an EHR.

Telemedicine implementation is much less demanding and less expensive. Telemedicine is available as a cloud-based platform, which requires less information technology (IT) support and less hardware and software. The technology required for patients to participate in telemedicine is nearly ubiquitous. According to the Pew Research Center, 96% of Americans own a cell phone (81% have a smartphone), and more than half (52%) own a tablet, so the basic equipment to connect patients to providers is already in place [4].

On the provider side, the essential equipment required for a telemedicine program is a computer with video and audio capabilities and a broadband connection that is fast enough to show video in real-time and to provide high-quality viewing of any images to be reviewed. However, traditionally, most telemedicine programs required the purchase and setup of new technology and equipment and the training of staff—some of which may be outside the budgets of healthcare providers in smaller independent practices. Many physicians have technology budgets that are already stretched thin. And for patients who do not have access to a smartphone or computer with Internet access, telemedicine may not be possible.

But with new guidelines put forth by the Centers for Medicare and Medicaid Services (CMS) in March 2020, connectivity can take place inexpensively using free platforms such as Google Hangouts, Skype, Facetime, and Facebook Messenger. If a non-HIPAA-compliant platform is used initially, conversion to a HIPAA-compliant platform is recommended [5].

These platforms do not require purchasing or subscription to any expensive hardware or software. The disadvantages of these programs are the lack of documentation, the failure to be Health Insurance Portability and Accountability Act (HIPAA)-compliant, and the lack of encryption. The new CMS guidelines require the telemedicine program to be interoperable with the EHR and the billing program. Otherwise, double- and triple entry will erase the efficiency of conducting a virtual visit. Depending on the magnitude of the program, IT assistance may be needed to get started.

Licensing

Another concern or barrier is a license to participate in telemedicine. The March 15, 2020, approval of telemedicine provided that licensed physicians in the state where the patient is located did not require any additional license or permission to conduct virtual visits [6].

For questions regarding licensure, contact your State Board of Medicine or Department of Health for information on requirements for licenses across state lines (see "Resources").

Informed Consent

Like with any other aspect of providing care for patients, obtaining informed consent is important. Obtaining informed patient consent is not only a recommended practice of the American Telemedicine Association (ATA), but it is also a legal requirement in many states. It may also be a condition of payment, depending on the payer. To check the requirements regarding patient consent in your state, look at The National Telehealth Policy Resource Center's state map (see "Resources").

Some states do not have any requirements regarding consent for a virtual visit. Others require verbal consent. Even if it is not a legal requirement in your state, consider making it a part of your practice's policy to obtain written or verbal consent and document in the patient's record that permission was obtained before the virtual visit so that you are protected when using this new technology.

Because telemedicine is a new way of receiving care for many patients. It is essential to let them know how it works, including how patient confidentiality and privacy are handled, what technical equipment is required, and what they should expect in scheduling cancellations and billing policies. A sample consent form for telemedicine use is shown in Fig. 26.1.

Consent for Telemedicine Visit

I hereby consent and authorize Dr. Neil Baum and his partners, colleagues, and agents and their employed or

contracted physicians, physician assistants, nurse practitioners or other licensed health care professionals in its care

network to utilize telemedicine through its vendor systems, methods, and protocols to access, diagnose, consult, treat

and educate me and those I am authorized to represent.

I acknowledge and consent to a physician, Dr. Neil Baum, via telemedicine. I understand my eligibility to receive a

visit via telemedicine is based on the doctor's medical judgement that it is appropriate, and that the quality of care

will not be diminished using telemedicine. I understand that a telemedicine visit is distinct from an in-person visit

because I will not be in the same room as the healthcare provider, and instead, I will communicate with the doctor

through advanced communication technology using live video and audio feed.

I acknowledge that to protect my privacy, I need to choose a private location to place my telemedicine call.

<Signed>

<Patient>

<Date>

References

Fig. 26.1 Consent for telemedicine visit

Liability Insurance

Another hurdle that must be considered is liability insurance for conducting virtual visits with patients. Physicians who will offer telemedicine care to patients should request proof that their liability insurance policy covers telemedicine malpractice and that the coverage extends to other states should the patient be in another form from the state in which the physician holds a license. Additionally, physicians who provide telemedicine care should check with liability insurers regarding any requirements or limitations to conducting a virtual visit with their patients and should document them. For example, the policy may require that the physician keep a written or recorded record of the visit in the EHR. If that is the case, using Skype, Facebook, or Google for the virtual visit, which does not include documentation, would be less desirable.

Privacy

Certainly, there is concern about privacy, and HIPAA compliance is critical to telemedicine success. Because of the COVID-19 emergency, on March 1, 2020, physicians became able to communicate with patients and provide telehealth services through remote communications without penalties [7].

With these changes in the HIPAA requirements, physicians could use applications that allow for video chats, including Apple FaceTime, Face- book Messenger video chat, Google Hangouts video, and Skype, to provide telehealth without the risk that the Office for Civil Rights would impose a penalty for non-compliance with HIPAA rules. When using these platforms, the consent for patients should mention that these "public" applications potentially introduce privacy risks. This motivates physicians to consider programs that promise encryption, privacy, and HIPAA compliance, such as Updox, Doxy.me, and Amazon Chime. It is also important to recognize that a virtual visit could result in colleagues (if the patient is in an office setting) or family members (if the patient is in the home environment) over-hearing conversations between the healthcare professional and the patient. Therefore, we suggest that patients conduct virtual visits in locations where they feel assured of privacy.

Compensation for Telemedicine

The most significant barrier to virtual health adoption has been compensation for telemedicine visits. Both commercial payers and CMS have been slow to enact formal policies for telemedicine reimbursement. Common misconceptions that providers cannot be reimbursed for telemedicine appointments or that compensation occurs at a reduced rate have persisted, thus making telemedicine economically unappealing. The good news is that this is changing. Legislation in most states is quickly embracing virtual health visits because of the COVID-19 pandemic [8]. In fact, as of January 1, 2020, telemedicine services are no longer considered "optional" coverage in Medicare Advantage plans [9].

Additionally, patients can utilize telemedicine without additional insurance cost. CMS now allows telemedicine as a standard, covered benefit in all plans, enabling beneficiaries to seek care from their homes rather than requiring them to go to a healthcare facility [10].

In the past, telemedicine was restricted for use in rural areas or when patients resided a great distance from their healthcare providers. Starting March 6, 2020, and throughout the COVID-19 public health emergency, Medicare allowed payments for professional services furnished to beneficiaries in all areas of the country in all settings regardless of location or distance between the patient and the healthcare provider [11].

In addition, since March 15, 2020, CMS expanded access to telemedicine services for all Medicare beneficiaries—not just those who have been diagnosed with COVID-19 [12].

The expanded access also applies to pre-COVID-19 coverage from physician offices, skilled nursing facilities, and hospitals. This means that Medicare will now make payments to physicians for telemedicine services provided in any healthcare facility or in a patient's home. Patients do not always need to go to the physician's office.

The facts are that there are now parity laws stating that commercial payers and CMS are required by state law to reimburse for telemedicine—often at the same rate as that for a comparable in-person visit. On the commercial side, there has been an increase in commercial parity legislation that requires health plans to cover virtual visits in the same way they cover face-to-face services. (To stay abreast of state-by-state changes in virtual health reimbursement, the Center for Connected Health Policy and the Advisory Board Primer are valuable resources. See "Resources,") Suppose the provider performs and documents the elements of history and decision-making, including the time spent counseling, and records the visit as if a face-to-face visit occurred. In that case, clinicians have a billable evaluation and management (E&M) visit.

Virtual Services for Medicare Patients

There are three types of virtual services you can provide to Medicare patients: (1) Medicare telehealth visits, (2) virtual check-ins, and (3) e-visits.

Medicare Telehealth Visits

Largely because of the COVID-19 pandemic, Medicare patients may now use telecommunication technology for services that previously occurred with in-person communication. The physician must use an interactive audio and video telecommunications system that permits real-time communication between the physician and the patient. The patient should have a prior established relationship with the physician with whom the telemedicine visit occurs [13].

The Current Procedural Terminology (CPT) codes for virtual visits using synchronous audio/visual communication are:

- 99,201–99,295, *Office visit for a new patient*
- 99,211–99,215, *Office visit for an established patient.*

Important modifiers for telemedicine visits include:

- Modifier 02 for POS (place of service) for telehealth Medicare,
- Modifier 95 for commercial payers.

(A list of all available CPT codes for telehealth services from CMS can be found in "Resources,")

Virtual Check-Ins

CMS allows established Medicare patients to have a brief communication with physicians the traditional way using a telephone or live video. These short virtual visits, usually 5–10 minutes in duration, are initiated by the patient. The virtual check-in aims to determine if an office visit, a test, or a procedure is indicated. Medicare pays for these "virtual check-ins" (or short communication technology-based services) for patients to communicate with their physicians and avoid unnecessary trips to the office. These brief virtual check-ins are only for established patients. If an existing patient contacts the physician's office to ask a question or determine if an office visit is necessary, the physician may bill for this brief visit using code G2012.

E-visits. Established Medicare patients may have non-face-to-face patient-initiated communications with their physicians without going to the physician's office. These services can be billed only when the physician has an established relationship with the patient. The services may be billed using CPT codes 99,421 to 99,423. Coding for these visits is determined by the length of time the physician spends online with the patient:

- 99,421: *Online digital evaluation and management service, for an established patient,* 5–10 minutes spent on the virtual visit
- 99,422: 11–20 minutes
- 99,423: ≥ 21 minutes

Since March 15, 2020, relaxation of the HIPAA restrictions for telemedicine, it is now possible to have a virtual visit with a patient using one of the free, non-HIPAA-compliant connections. This type of visit is no different than a telephone call but with an added video component. Many physicians who want to start the telemedicine process with their patients will avail themselves of the free video communication offered by Google Hangouts, Skype, Facetime, and Facebook Messenger. Using these free technologies, a physician can have an asynchronous visit with a patient (the store and forward method of sending information or medical images). The service takes place in one direction with no opportunity for interaction with the patient. Asynchronous visits are akin to video text messages left for the patient. By contrast, a synchronous or real-time video visit with a patient is a two-way communication that provides medical care without examining the patient.

Using Triangulation

There are some downsides to telemedicine visits. First, virtual visits on Skype, FaceTime, and other non-HIPAA-compliant methods are not conducted on an encrypted website. Second, no documentation is created for the doctor-patient encounter. Finally, unless the physician records these virtual visits and submits the interactions to the practice coders, there will be no billing and thus no reimbursement for the visits. In this scenario, physicians are still legally responsible for their decision-making, prescription writing, and medical advice but do not receive compensation for their time and medical advice.

This can be remedied by using "triangulation," which involves: 1. the physician, 2. the patient, and 3. a scribe or medical assistant who will record the visit. Before initiating the virtual visit using triangulation, it is imperative to ask the patient for permission if your medical assistant (or any other person in the office who functions as a scribe) will be listening to the conversation. It is important to explain that the person is there to take accurate notes and enter the notes into the EHR. Also, the scribe or assistant will record the time, date, and duration of the visit, which is a requirement for billing purposes. The scribe may also ascertain that the visit is appropriately coded and entered into the practice management system and that a bill is submitted to the insurance company. By using triangulation, you have documentation that consent was obtained, that the visit took place, that notes were taken, and that the patient's insurance company will be billed for

the visit (see Fig. 26.2 for a sample documentation form).

Which CPT Codes Should I Use?

The answer depends on several factors, but a good rule of thumb is to use the same codes that you would use for an in-person appointment (CPT codes 99,211–99,215 for an established patient visit and 99,201–99,205 for a new patient visit). These are the most common CPT codes for outpatient office visits, whether face-to-face or synchronous virtual visits (via a real-time interactive audio and video telecommunications system).

For example, the reimbursement for code 99213 ranges from $73 to $100. You may wonder how to achieve the complexity requirements for a level-3 office visit without a physical examination. Whether as a face-to-face or virtual visit, documentation for these encounters requires 2 of 3 of the following components:

- Expanded problem-focused history,
- Expanded problem-focused exam (not accomplished with telemedicine),
- Low-complexity medical decision-making,
- At least 15 min spent face to face with the patient if coding is based on time.

If a physician reviews the results of a recent lab test for a patient and adjusts the dosage of prescribed medication, writes a prescription, and spends 15 minutes communicating with the patient, they have met the complexity requirements for a code 99213. Because Level 3 and 4 visits (99,214 and 99,215) require a comprehensive physical examination, it is necessary to document the time spent with the patient (code 99214 requires 25–39 minutes of consultation, and code 99215 requires ≥40 min).

Virtual Visit Documentation Form

Date: ____/____/____ Time Start ____A.M./PM

Total Time of Visit ___min

Patient Information

First Name_____   Last Name _____

DOB ____/____/____Phone _____

Email_____

Mode of Communication

  Telephone__   Text__   Video Chat__ Instant Messenger__   Other__

Diagnosis _____

Etiology_____

Symptoms

Clinical Findings

Prescriptions Provided

Treating physician_____

Signature_____

CPT Code_____

Date entered in EMR_____

  Additional notes_____

Fig. 26.2 Sample documentation form

Some Final Billing and Coding Advice

Always confirm telemedicine billing guidelines *before* conducting telemedicine visits. Consider starting a phone call to a payer armed with the fact that the payer is required to offer parity between telemedicine and face-to-face visits. Then ask which specific billing codes should be used.

Before providing telemedicine services, it is necessary to make the patient aware of the cost, if any, of the virtual visit. Payment arrangement should be completed *before* the delivery of the service.

Until you become comfortable with the coding and billing process for telemedicine, consider using a telemedicine platform with a built-in rules engine that offers recommendations for each telemedicine visit based on past claims data. These systems help physicians determine which CPT code to use and which modifiers are appropriate for the various insurance companies. The rules engine enables you to submit a clean claim that is less likely to be denied and more likely to be paid. Some vendors are so confident that their rules engine will match the service with the proper CPT code and modifier that they guarantee full private payer reimbursement for telemedicine visits, or the vendor will reimburse the claim.

An Example

A visit with an existing patient using telemedicine using CPT codes: 99211–99,215. These are the most common CPT codes for outpatient physician offices, either face-to-face or remote telemedicine visits. The reimbursement for 99,213 has a national average of $73. But how can you achieve the complexity requirements for a level 3 office visit without a physical exam? The documentation for these encounters requires *two of three* of the following components:

1. Expanded Problem Focused History.
2. Expanded Problem Focused Exam (of course, that cannot be accomplished by using a telemedicine visit).

3. Low Complexity Medical Decision Making.
   or
4. 15-min spent face to face with the patient if coding based on time.

For example, if a physician reviews the results of a recent lab test for a diabetic patient and adjusts the diabetic medication, this visit meets the complexity requirements for a 99,213.

Using the GT Modifier

The GT modifier indicates a service was rendered via synchronous (a live communication between doctor and patient) telecommunication. The rules engine provides modifier recommendations for each appointment based on past claims data to help providers determine which modifier is most appropriate.

Modifier 95

Modifier 95 is a modifier to be used when billing private payers to indicate services were rendered via synchronous telecommunication. The rules engine provided by your vendor is a good resource for selecting the appropriate modifier for your claim.

The good news is that in most states, Medicaid covers telemedicine services. Like billing E&M codes for telemedicine, Medicare requires billing the standard CPT code and adding the GT modifier.

Take-home message on reimbursement for telemedicine:

Whatever telemedicine service you use, always confirm the payer's billing guidelines before engaging patients with telemedicine visits. Perhaps you can start the call to the payer armed with a copy of this chapter that reminds the payer that the payer is required to offer parity between telemedicine visits and face-to-face visits. Then ask which specific billing codes you should use and whether they recognize the GT modifier.

Back to the Case

Roberto surveyed his patients, and several were eager to participate in virtual visits. He subscribed to an encrypted, HIPAA-compliant video-conferencing program. Roberto started regularly conducting telemedicine visits at the end of his workday. He soon discovered that telemedicine was efficient and productive. The feedback from his patients was favorable, and now, he holds three to five virtual visits a day.

Bottom Line

Patient-driven care is the future, and telemedicine is part of that. Patients want to have ready access to their healthcare providers without having to devote hours to a medical encounter that could be completed in minutes via telemedicine. It is not a matter of "if" but rather "when" to incorporate telemedicine as a communication and practice tool. The sooner, the better.

References

1. Gardner MR, Jenkins SM, O'Neil DA, et al. Perceptions of video-based appointments from the patient's home: a patient survey. Telemed J E Health. 2015;21:281–5.
2. Eddy N. Patients increasingly trusting of remote care technology. Healthcare IT News. 2019;22; https://www.healthcareitnews.com/news/patients-increasingly-trusting-remote-care-technology-says-new-report.
3. Hollander J, Carr BG. Virtually perfect? Telemedicine for COVID-19. N Engl J Med. 2020;382:1679–81.
4. Pew Research Center. Internet and Technology. Mobile Fact Sheet. 12 Jun 2019. https://www.pewresearch.org/internet/fact-sheet/mobile/.
5. American Medical Association. AMA quick guide to telemedicine in practice. *AMA*. https://www.ama-assn.org/practice-management/digital/ama-quick-guide-telemedicine-practice.
6. Center for Connected Health Policy. Federal and state regulation updates. https://www.cchpca.org.
7. https://www.whitehouse.gov/presidential-actions/proclamation-declaring-national-emergency-concerning-novel-coronavirus-disease-covid-19-outbreak/.
8. Center for Connected Health Policy. Quick glance state telehealth actions in response to COVID-19. https://www.cchpca.org/sites/default/files/2020-05/state%20telehealth%20actions%20in%20response%20to%20covid%20overview%205.5.2020_0.pdf.
9. Medicare.gov. https://www.medicare.gov/sign-up-change-plans/types-of-medicare-health-plans/medicare-advantage-plans/how-do-medicare-advantage-plans-work.
10. Centers for Medicare and Medicaid Services. CMS finalizes policies to bring innovative telehealth benefits to Medicare Advantage. 2019. https://www.cms.gov/newsroom/press-releases/cms-finalizes-policies-bring-innovative-telehealth-benefit-medicare-advantage.
11. Centers for Medicare & Medicaid Services. Medicare telemedicine health care provider fact sheet. https://www.cms.gov/newsroom/fact-sheets/medicare-telemedicine-health-care-provider-fact-sheet.
12. Centers for Medicare & Medicaid Services. Medicare telehealth frequently asked questions. https://www.cms.gov/files/document/medicare-telehealth-frequently-asked-questions-faqs-31720.pdf.
13. American Hospital Association. Coronavirus update: CMS broadens access to telehealth during Covid-19 public health emergency. *AHA*. https://www.aha.org/advisory/2020-03-17-coronavirus-update-cms-broadens-access-telehealth-during-covid-19-public-health.

Resources

1. COVID-19 and Telehealth Coding Options as of March 20, 2020. https://www.ismanet.org/pdf/COVID-19andTelehealthcodes3-20-2020Updates.pdf.
2. Federation of State Medical Boards. US States and Territories Modifying Licensure Requirements for Physicians in Response to COVID-19. 2020. https://www.fsmb.org/siteassets/advocacy/pdf/state-emergency-declarations-licensures-requirementscovid-19.pdf.
3. Center for Connected Health Policy. Current State Laws and Reimbursement Policies.
4. https://www.cchpca.org/telehealth-policy/current-state-laws-and-reimbursement-policies/.
5. Centers for Medicare and Medicaid Services. List of Telehealth Services. Updated April 30, 2020. https://www.cms.gov/Medicare/Medicare-General-Information/Telehealth/Telehealth-Codes.
6. American Medical Association. AMA quick guide to telemedicine in practice. Updated May 22, 2020. https://www.ama-assn.org/practice-management/digital/ama-quick-guide-telemedicine-practice.

Case Abner

Abner, a neurologist, was consulted to see one of his patients in the ICU. The patient had a recurrent deep venous thrombosis despite rivaroxaban therapy. The patient had recently been placed on phenytoin for complex seizures. Abner was not aware of the connection between the antiepileptic drug and the anticoagulant. Phenytoin and rivaroxaban are metabolized similarly and phenytoin can induce the enzyme that metabolizes rivaroxaban leading to lower levels of the medication. What can Abner do to prevent that kind of drug-drug interaction?

Now more than ever, physicians will need to be more efficient to remain more productive. A few years ago, physicians saw low volumes of patients and were able to spend time educating patients about their medical condition and helping them understand the importance of being compliant. Now doctors need to see larger volumes of patients and will be spending less time with each patient and will not have the luxury of lengthy explanations about their health and providing them with one-to-one educational discussions. Nowadays, patients rely on the Internet and other sources, such as social media, to obtain medical information. As a result, patients are often less compliant regarding their medications. When compliance has been decreased, the outcomes are often less desirable. In the recent past, the formula for practice productivity was low patient volumes, substantial reimbursements in a fee-for-service arrangement, and good doctor-patient relationships. Today the situation is reversed: large patient volumes, decreased reimbursements for the same services performed a few years ago, and less time spent with each patient. Physicians are now forced to see more patients compared to a few years ago. As a result of spending less time with patients, there is less opportunity to educate patients about the importance of compliance, the adverse drug events associated with medication, and instructions on dosing. Patients may be less compliant because they have less information about their medical condition, and this may portend a deterioration in patient outcomes.

Adherence to therapies is a primary determinant of treatment success. Medication nonadherence in patients leads to substantial worsening of disease, death, and increased healthcare costs.

Several factors are likely to impact adherence.

Medication adherence is defined by the World Health Organization as "the degree to which the person's behavior corresponds with the agreed recommendations from a health care provider" [1]. Though adherence and compliance are synonymous, adherence differs from compliance. Compliance is the extent to which a patient's behavior matches the prescriber's advice [2]. Compliance implies patient obedience to the physician's recommendations. However, adherence signifies that the patient and physician collaborate to improve the patient's health by integrating the physician's medical opinion and the patient's lifestyle, values, and preferences for care [3].

There are several types of nonadherence. The first is primary nonadherence, in which providers write prescriptions but the medication is never filled or initiated. This type is commonly called non-fulfillment adherence [4].

The second type of nonadherence is called non-persistence when patients decide to stop taking a medication after starting it without being advised by a health professional. Non-persistence is rarely intentional and happens when patients and providers fail to communicate about therapeutic plans.

Unintentional nonadherence arises from capacity and resource limitations that prevent patients from implementing their decisions to follow treatment recommendations (e.g., problems accessing prescriptions, cost, and competing demands) and sometimes involves individual constraints (e.g., poor inhaler technique, problems remembering doses). Intentional nonadherence arises from the beliefs, attitudes, and expectations influencing patients' motivation to begin and persist with the treatment regimen [5].

The third type of nonadherence is known as non-conforming; this type includes a variety of ways in which medications are not taken as prescribed; this behavior can range from skipping doses to taking medications at incorrect times or at incorrect doses.

An extensive review of the literature reveals that in developed countries, adherence to therapies averages 50% [6]. Approximately half of this nonadherence is intentional, while the remainder occurs because patients are either unaware that they are not taking medications as prescribed, or the regimen is too demanding. Adherence rates are typically higher among patients with acute conditions than those with chronic conditions.

Studies reveal that patients with chronic illnesses take only ~50% of medications prescribed for those conditions [7].

The consequences of nonadherence are a waste of medication, disease progression, reduced functional abilities, lower quality of life, increased use of medical resources such as nursing homes, hospital visits, poor outcomes, and hospital admissions [8]. Economic studies reveal that poor adherence to prescribed regimens can result in serious health consequences, supported by various studies. For instance, in a study by Anon, it was shown that the risk of hospital readmission was more than double in patients with diabetes mellitus, hypercholesterolemia, hypertension, or congestive heart failure who were nonadherent to prescribed therapies compared with a general population. Studies conducted among Chronic Obstructive Pulmonary Disease patients have shown that poor adherence to drug therapy and disease management leads to emergency hospitalization [9].

Medication nonadherence can have negative consequences not only for the patient but also for the provider. The potential burden of medication nonadherence outcomes on healthcare delivery makes it an important public health concern. Additionally, with value-based contracts, nonadherence can lead to reimbursement penalties [10]. Hence, helping patients take their medicine appropriately avoids the higher risk of severe relapses, antibiotic resistance, and preventable hospitalizations.

Influencers of medication adherence.

Barriers to the effective use of medicines specifically include poor provider-patient communication, inadequate knowledge about a drug and its use, not being convinced of the need for treatment, fear of adverse effects of the drug, necessity for long-term drug regimens, complex regimens that require numerous medications with varying dosing schedules, cost, and access barriers [11].

Adherence to drug therapy varies with the patient age group also. In children, adherence to drug therapy is affected due to their dependence on an adult caregiver. The literature concerning adherence reports in elderly patients reports that compliance rates range roughly from 38 to 57% with an average rate of less than 45% [12].

A significant reason for nonadherence is the failure of the physician to communicate the proper use of the medication and the patient's inability to remember the physician's advice. Studies report that 40-60% of patients needed help to correctly report what their physicians expected of them 10–80 minutes after receiving the information. Yet another study said that over 60% of patients interviewed immediately after visiting their doctors misunderstood the directions regarding prescribed medications [13].

Nonadherence can also occur when the medication regimen is complex, which could include improper timing of drug administration or administration of numerous medications at frequent or unusual times during the day. Most deviations in taking medication occur because of the omission of doses (rather than additions) or delays in the timing of doses [14].

Patients often become non-compliant with chronic diseases like hypertension or elevated cholesterol levels. These two conditions are often unpleasant, even without strict compliance with the medication regimen. Estimates of medication nonadherence illustrate that the nonadherence percentage is most significant when the patients are symptom-free. However, when medication was to be taken over a long period, compliance rates dropped dramatically to around 50% for either prevention or cure [15, 16].

One major factor influencing adherence is the patient's ability to read and understand medication instructions. Patients with low literacy may have difficulty understanding instructions, resulting in decreased adherence and poor medication management [17]. Gender may influence adherence-compliance rates. For instance, women may be better at adhering to their medication regimens than men. This may be particularly so for drugs that treat behavioral health conditions, such as antidepressant medications [18].

Improving medication adherence.

Unfortunately, patients do not volunteer that they are non-compliant with their medications. The simplest way of measuring adherence is from the patient's self-report [19].

1. Medication costs.

The cost of drugs can often be solved by contacting pharmaceutical companies for medications at a reduced or no cost to the patient. We suggest asking the patient about their compliance with the medication. Ask patients if cost is an issue or if the instructions need to be clarified.

A systematic approach that could be instituted in improving medication adherence is as follows:

Whenever possible, involve patients in decision-making regarding their medications, so they have a sense of ownership and are partners in the treatment plan. Whenever possible, use a simple regimen based on patient characteristics

2. Communicating with the patient:

Explain key information when prescribing/dispensing a medicine.

Address the key information about the drugs (what, why, when, how, and how long).

Explain the common side effects and those that patients should know. Patients become more worried, leading to nonadherence due to side effects not being discussed in advance.

Provide medication calendars or schedules that specify the time to take medications, drug cards, medication charts, medicine-related information sheets, or specific packaging such as pill boxes, blister packaging, and special containers indicating the dose time.

3. At follow-ups:

Monitoring medication adherence should occur with subsequent follow-up. This is an opportunity for healthcare providers to identify the underlying causes of patient nonadherence. With this information, an appropriate interventional strategy can be instituted.

One of the major reasons that patients become nonadherent is forgetting to take their medications. Results of a study conducted showed that 49.6% of patients mentioned forgetfulness as one of the major non-intentional reasons for nonadherence [20]. Forgetfulness can be resolved by recommending reminders, i.e., telephone, e-mails, text messages to cellular phones, and alarms. Involving the patient's caregivers would be another way of combating nonadherence due to forgetfulness.

Medication nonadherence may also occur because patients perceive it to be unnecessary or because of their fears and beliefs related to the adverse effects of drugs. Hence, providing clear medication-related information to patients is essential to improve adherence, including addressing the key information of what, why, when, how, and how long. Patient medication counseling can be supplemented by providing detailed written information about medications. Succinctly written instructions, including drug cards, medication charts, or any written material in a plastic sheet or laminated sheet, also help improve adherence, especially for elderly patients who find it difficult to comprehend much of the information provided during medication counseling.

Patients' fears and concerns about adverse drug reactions can be alleviated by educating patients regarding common side effects of the drugs they are taking, how to prevent an adverse drug reaction, if possible, and convincing the patient of the need for treatment. The complexity of the drug regimen is found to negatively affect medication adherence. When possible, reduce the frequency of administration and/or the number of different medications. If applicable, replace them with combination products. An example is treating men with benign prostate gland enlargement (BPH) by combing an alpha-blocker and a 5-alpha-reductase inhibitor in one tablet or capsule.

4. An underutilized resource for enhancing medication compliance is the involvement of pharmacists in conducting an annual medication audit. There are two options: targeted interventions consisting of a 5-15′ in-person or telephone conversation with patients. This brief visit allows pharmacists to explain adverse drug events to patients. The other option is annual medication reviews consisting of a 45-minute in-person audit of the patient's clinical information and a review of all of the patient's medications, including over-the-counter medications. The patient-pharmacist communication is central to optimizing patient adherence [21]. Comprehensive medication management is a patient-centered approach to optimizing medication use and improving patient health outcomes delivered by a clinical pharmacist working in collaboration with the patient and their healthcare providers [22]. This is a win-win-win situation that benefits patients, doctors, and pharmacists. Now the doctor can offload an annual drug review to the pharmacists, who can spend more time with the patient and help motivate compliance.

Assessing children's adherence can be done by asking for the help of a caregiver (school nurse or teacher). Among the various methods of questioning the patient, patient diaries and assessment of clinical response are all relatively easy to use but asking the patient can be susceptible to misrepresentation and tends to result in the healthcare provider overestimating the patient's adherence.

Electronic monitors capable of recording and stamping the time of opening bottles, dispensing drops (eye drops), or activating a metered dose inhaler for asthma can also measure adherence. The disadvantage of this method is that the measure of adherence is not accurate as the patients may open the container and not take the medication, take the wrong amount of medication or take multiple doses out of the container at the same time [16].

Back to the Case

Abner recognized that drug-drug interactions were possible with the existing prescribing methods used in practice. Abner used Hippocrates.com to check on the possibility of drug-drug interactions. Abner also created FAQs to give to each patient receiving a prescription on the most prescribed drugs, identifying possible drug-drug interactions. As a result, patients were informed and received valuable information on their medications and the possible interactions with their existing medications, and the adverse drug events for those medications.

Bottom Line

A treatment's effectiveness depends on the medication's efficacy and the patient's adherence to the therapeutic regimen. Patients, physicians, and healthcare systems all have a role in improving medication adherence. A single method cannot improve medication adherence. Instead, a combination of various adherence techniques should be implemented to improve patients' adherence to their prescribed treatment.

Patient medication nonadherence is a major medical problem. There are many interrelated reasons for non-compliance. Though patient education is the key to improving compliance, compliance aids, proper motivation, and support are also shown to increase medication adherence. Healthcare professionals should identify strategies to improve medication adherence within the limits of their practice, eventually enhancing therapeutic outcomes. It should be a multidisciplinary approach that needs to be carried out with the support of all involved in medication use.

References

1. Dobbels F, Van Damme-Lombaert R, Vanhaecke J, De Geest S. Growing pains: nonadherence with the immunosuppressive regimen in adolescent transplant recipients. Pediatr Transplant. 2005;9(3):381–90.
2. Horne R. Compliance, adherence, and concordance: implications for asthma treatment. Chest. 2006;130(1):65S–72S.
3. Spiro H. Compliance, adherence, and hope. J Clin Gastroenterol. 2001;32(1):5.
4. Gellad WF, Grenard J, McGlynn EA. A review of barriers to medication adherence: A frame work for driving policy options; http://www.rand.org/pubs/technical_reports/2009/RAND_TR765.pdf.
5. Horne R, Weinman J, Barber N, Elliott RA, Morgan M. Concordance, adherence and compliance in medicine taking: a conceptual map and research priorities. London: National Co-ordinating Centre for NHS Service Delivery and Organisation NCCSDO; 2005.
6. Carter S, Taylor D, Levenson R. A question of choice- compliance in medicine taking. From compliance to concordance. 3rd ed. London: Medicines Partnership; 2005; www.medicines-partnership.org/research-evidence/major-reviews/a-question-of-choice.
7. Haynes RB, McDonald HP, Garg AX. Helping patients follow prescribed treatment: clinical applications. JAMA. 2002;288(22):2880–3.
8. Sullivan S, Kreling D, Hazlet T. Noncompliance with medication regimens and subsequent hospitalizations: a literature analysis and cost of hospitalization estimate. J Res Pharm Econ. 1990;2:19–33.
9. Garcia-Aymerich J, Barreiro E, Farrero E, Marrades RM, Morera J, Antó JM. Patients hospitalized for COPD have a high prevalence of modifiable risk factors for exacerbation (EFRAM study). Eur Respir J. 2000;16(6):1037–42.
10. National Council on Patient Information and Education. Enhancing prescription medicine adherence: a national action plan. 2007. http://www.talkaboutrx.org/documents/enhancing_prescription_medicine_adherence.pdf.
11. Tarn DM, Heritage J, Paterniti DA, Hays RD, Kravitz RL, Wenger NS. Physician communication when prescribing new medications. Arch Intern Med. 2006;166(17):1855–62.
12. Sackett DL, Snow JC. The magnitude of compliance and non-compliance. In: NRB H, Taylor DW, Sackett DL, editors. Compliance in health care. Baltimore: John Hopkins University Press; 1979. p. 11–22.
13. Meichenbaum D, Turk DC. Facilitating treatment adherence: a practitioner's guidebook. New York: Plenum Publishing Corp; 1987.
14. Burnier M. Long-term compliance with antihypertensive therapy: another facet of chronotherapeutics in hypertension. Blood Press Monit. 2000;5(Suppl 1):S31–4.
15. Jimmy B, Jose J. Patient medication adherence: measures in daily practice. Oman Med J. 2011;26(3):155.
16. Praska JL, Kripalani S, Seright AL, Jacobson TA. Identifying and assisting low-literacy patients with medication use: a survey of community pharmacies. Ann Pharmacother. 2005;39(9):1441–5.
17. Ward A, Morgan W. Adherence patterns of health in men and women enrolled in an adult exercise program. J Cardiac Rehabil. 1984;4:143–52.
18. Walsh JC, Mandalia S, Gazzard BG. Responses to a 1-month self-report on adherence to antiretroviral therapy are consistent with electronic data and virological treatment outcome. AIDS. 2002;16(2):269–77.
19. Adisa R, Alutundu MB, Fakeye TO. Factors contributing to nonadherence to oral hypoglycemic medications among ambulatory type 2 diabetes patients. Pharm Pract. 2009;7:163–9.
20. Golin CE, MR DM, Gelberg L. The role of patient participation in the doctor visit. Implications for adherence to diabetes care. Diabetes Care. 1996;19(10):1153–64.

21. American College of Clinical Pharmacy, McBane SE, Dopp AL, Abe A, Benavides S, Chester EA, Walker S, et al. Collaborative drug therapy management and comprehensive medication management—2015. Pharmacotherapy. 2015;35(4):e39–50.

22. Gellad WF, Grenard J, McGlynn EA. A review of barriers to medication adherence: A framework for driving policy options. http://www.rand.org/pubs/technical_reports/2009/RAND_TR765.pdfmultiple-doses in another container.

Case Bernice

Bernice joined a large group practice after completing a residency in family medicine. She was seeing 15–20 patients each day. She was overwhelmed by adult patients, parents of her pediatric patients, paperwork, and her interaction with the office manager. She noted that she was experiencing insomnia, gaining weight, and periods of tachycardia. Her partner complained that she was bringing her work home and was not fully present at the dinner table, in the evenings, and on weekends. She didn't know what to do or whom she should turn to for help.

This chapter will discuss how mindfulness works and suggestions for learning how to use mindfulness\meditation to help conquer anxiety.

What Is Mindfulness?

Mindfulness meditation is the practice of purposely focusing your attention on the present moment—and accepting it without judgment [1]. Mindfulness is focusing your attention on experiencing the present without judgment from the past or worries about the future. Mindfulness is now being examined scientifically and is a key element in stress reduction, overall happiness, and a non-medical approach to anxiety.

Historically, mindfulness has roots in Buddhism and has been used for millennia to help control anxiety and depression. Most religions include some type of meditation techniques that help shift a devotee's thoughts away from their work or source of anxiety and move toward an appreciation of the moment and consideration of life's bigger picture.

Dr. Jon Kabat-Zinn, Ph.D., founder and former director of the Stress Reduction Clinic at the University of Massachusetts Medical Center, helped to bring the practice of mindfulness meditation into mainstream medicine and demonstrated that practicing mindfulness can bring improvements in both physical and emotional issues as well as positive changes in health, attitudes, and behaviors [2].

Mindfulness can enhance a person's well-being by increasing their capacity for a positive work experience and a satisfying life. Being mindful makes it easier to savor the pleasures in life, helping you become fully engaged in all of life's activities, and creating a greater capacity to deal with adverse events. Doctors who practice mindfulness find they are less likely to get caught up in worries about the future or regrets over the past. These doctors are less preoccupied with concerns about success and self-esteem. They can better form deep connections with others, including their patients, coworkers, family, and friends.

Mindfulness techniques have been demonstrated to improve physical health [3]. In addition to reducing anxiety, mindfulness can help relieve stress, lower blood pressure, improve sleep, and even lower blood pressure. Mindfulness is helpful for physicians and is beneficial for our patients who experience anxiety and symptoms caused by stress and anxiety.

In recent years, mental health experts have recognized that mindfulness is an important element in treating several mental health problems, including depression, substance abuse, post-traumatic stress disorders, eating disorders, couples' conflicts, anxiety disorders, and obsessive-compulsive disorders. These are many of the same issues and problems affecting doctors experiencing these mental health issues [4].

How Does Mindfulness Work?

Some experts believe that mindfulness works by helping people to accept their experiences rather than negate those feelings. Negative feelings can cause emotional havoc on a doctor and impact their relationships with their patients.

There is good evidence that mindfulness results in changes in the brain and decreases the body's production of hormones such as cortisol, which can suppress the immune system when increased.

Research suggests that mindfulness leads to non-judgmental and acceptance of any negative experience, which is associated with positive psychological and improved physical outcomes [5].

There is now a significant body of research documenting changes in the brain associated with mindfulness practice. A 2014 review of brain imaging studies found eight brain regions consistently altered in those who regularly meditate, [6]. including areas important for:

- Self-awareness of thoughts and emotions (frontopolar cortex/BA 10).
- Body awareness (sensory cortices and insula).
- Memory (hippocampus).
- Self and emotion regulation (anterior and midcingulate; orbitofrontal cortex).

- Communication between parts of the brain (superior longitudinal fasciculus; corpus callosum).

The brain imaging studies are consistent with research that tracks the participants' changing perceptions and looks at their behaviors or physiological measures, such as brain wave activity or stress hormones such as cortisol and epinephrine. This suggests that mindfulness can positively affect our thoughts and feelings, including reducing fear and anxiety.

In addition, mindfulness is associated with changes in connections between regions in the brain. Specifically, the connections weaken between the fear-responsive amygdala and the rest of the brain. With meditation and mindfulness training, those connections between the emotionally-regulating prefrontal cortex and the rest of the brain are strengthened. These changes suggest that mindfulness lessens reactive and fearful responses, which are part and parcel of the causes of anxiety.

It is common for doctors to feel pressure and to always portray a positive attitude. Having a positive attitude as a solution to stress, anxiety, depression, and panic attacks is unrealistic. The practice of medicine is often associated with sadness, depression, guilt, fear, and anxiety. These are normal attitudes and experiences that we all face as physicians. Trying to ignore these feelings or not talking about these feelings and thoughts with others can make us feel isolated and even ineffective as a physician. Some physicians may feel guilty or blame themselves when they can't stay positive, adding to their heavy emotional burden.

Getting Started with Mindfulness

There is more than one way to practice mindfulness. Still, the goal of any mindfulness technique is to achieve a state of alert, focused relaxation by deliberately paying attention to your thoughts and sensations without judgment. This allows the mind to focus on the present moment.

For most beginners who are learning mindfulness, you will often begin by focusing on your breath. There are multiple techniques of breathing, and we recommend either having an instructor\guide or having one of the many CDs that provide directions for concentrating on your breath. You will also find the book *Breath* by James Nestor [7] as an excellent resource for learning a breathing method. (There are suggestions for mindfulness CDs at the end of this chapter).

For the most part, mindfulness breathing should take air in through the nostrils and exhale through the nostrils or the mouth. Inhaling through the nose is important because the nose filters the air, heating it, and moistens the air for easier absorption. One of the easiest methods for beginners is to alternate nostril breathing. This is accomplished by placing your thumb over one nostril, inhaling through one nostril, pausing briefly, then placing the index finger on the opposite nostril, exhaling, and then repeating these five to ten times.

When you breathe deeply, the air coming in through your nose fills your lungs, and you will notice that your chest expands, and your abdomen rises. There is good scientific reason for taking a full breath and expanding the chest *and* the abdomen. Both lungs hold about 3000 mL of air. When resting or doing sedentary activities, we inhale and exhale only 500 mL of air. As a result, most of our lung capacity isn't used, and stale air containing card dioxide accumulates in the lungs. By taking a deep breath and exhaling as much air as possible, we remove the carbon dioxide and increase the oxygen delivered to the bloodstream.

Another technique used by the Navy SEALs is called "box breathing." This is accomplished by inhaling to a count of four, hold your breath for a count of four, exhale for a count of four, and hold for a count of four and then repeat. By repeating the box breathing for five or six rounds will lead to relaxation and is especially effective before sleeping.

Regardless of the mindfulness technique you select, you will usually find that your attention begins to wander after a few seconds. Mind wandering happens to nearly every mindfulness beginner. It is challenging to stay focused, and our minds are easily distracted. When you find your mind wandering and not focused on breathing, slowly bring your attention back to your breath. This refocusing on your breath is a process that can be learned. It is almost like exercise and strength training. You can't expect to work out once and have a muscular body or a six-pack. To increase your muscular strength, you must continue the exercise even when distracted. After repetition and focusing on the exercises, muscular strength will occur. The same repetition and refocusing apply to mindfulness breathing. You can become proficient at breathing exercises with repetition and bringing the mind back to your breath.

Another method of staying focused is using a word, phrase, or mantra. Some mindfulness beginners find it easier to maintain attention by slowly repeating a meaningful word, phrase, or mantra. A mantra is a single word or phrase that helps the mind from wandering. Repeating your word or mantra out loud can help take your wandering thoughts back to your breathing exercise. Any word or phrase can be used that is meaningful to you. Examples of a mantra are the Hindu\ Budhist ohmmmmmmm, a Judeo-Christen ahhhhmen, the Arabic saaalaam, or the Hebrew word sha'mmmmmma.

Take three and call anyone in the morning!

You can achieve relaxation at any time of day using petal breathing. This is accomplished by sitting, standing, or even laying down.

Close your eyes and place your thumb on your four fingers like a closed flower. Take a deep breath, inhale through your nose, and open your hand as if the petals of the flowers are opening to the sun (Fig. 28.1). Then exhale and allow the thumb to return to the tips of the fingers as if the flower's petals are collapsing and coming together. Repeat this three times, and you will often find you can achieve relaxation and remove the stressful situation you are experiencing. Petal breathing is effective when you recognize you are becoming anxious and your stress level increases. Merely taking 10–12 s to do a few petal breaths is all that is necessary to dissipate the tension.

Finally, total body relaxation using the body scan.

This is a technique that incorporates focusing on breathing and visualization. This technique

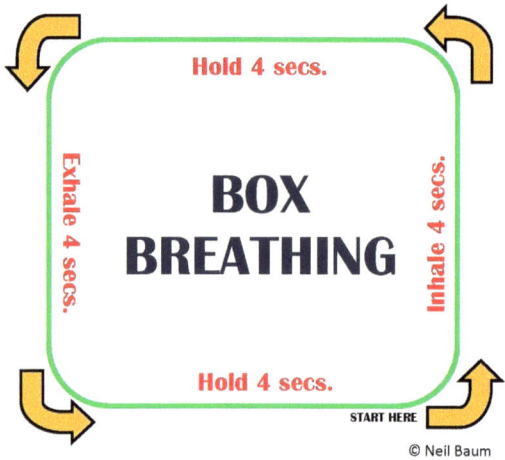

Fig. 28.1 Box breathing used by the Navy Seals to stay calm and focused

helps you become attuned to your body and aware of the connection between your mind and body.

Performing a body scan is quite simple. Start by concentrating on one part of your body at a time. Then focus on that muscle or boy party. Imagine those muscles as being warm and relaxed. You should feel any tension melt away.

As a guide, follow these steps, which are adapted from Dr. Herbert Benson and Aggie Casey's book *Mind Your Heart* [8].

- Sit or lie down. Breathe deeply, allowing your abdomen to rise and fall as you exhale. Breathe this way for 2 min before you start.
- Concentrate on your right big toe. Imagine the atoms in your toe and focus on the space between each atom. Imagine your toe feeling open, warm, and relaxed.
- Now shift your focus to each of the other toes on your right foot, visualizing them one by one. Again, notice the sensations of your toes and envision them as open, warm, and relaxed.
- Slowly shift your focus to your foot, moving mentally from the ball of your foot to the arch, then the top of the foot.
- Now work your way up your leg, turning your attention to your ankle, calf, knee, thigh, and

hip. Take your time, slowly working through each area. For each body part, envision the atoms and the space between those atoms. Picture each muscle feeling open, warm, and relaxed.

- Allow your right leg to relax, sinking into the support of the floor.
- Now repeat these steps, focusing on your left foot and leg.
- Next, become aware of your back. Does it feel tight or tense? Pay attention to each vertebra and the space that surrounds it. Let each vertebra feel light and spacious. Slowly work your way up your back, relaxing each muscle there.
- Gradually, move on to your abdomen and chest. Picture your organs and the space between them. Allow your belly to feel light and open.
- Become aware of your right thumb and then your remaining fingers. Envision each finger one by one, then slowly work your way through your hand and arm: relax your palm, wrist, forearm, elbow, upper arm, and shoulder.
- Feel your right arm relax and warm, spacious, and light.
- Do the same thing with your left hand and arm.
- Think about your neck and jaw. Yawn. Allow each part of your face to relax, working through your jaw, eyes, and forehead. Shift your attention to the top and back of your head.
- Let your whole-body sink into your chair or bed. Does it feel light and relaxed? Focus on your breath. Imagine yourself breathing in calm and peace. As you breathe, imagine any remaining tension being expelled from your body.
- If any part of your body is still tense, focus your breathing in that area, releasing tension from that spot as you exhale.
- Sit or lie quietly for a few minutes, noting how light and spacious your body feels. Then open your eyes slowly. Take a moment to stretch at the end of the body scan.

Getting Started on Your Own

Bernice, described at the beginning of this chapter, is typical of the experience of many physicians who become quickly overwhelmed with the practice of medicine. Doctors often state that they can't easily concentrate on their breath or relaxation techniques when other thoughts cloud the effort to be mindful. That is normal, and all that is required is to slowly drift back to concentrating on your breath, body, or word\mantra. Some types of meditation primarily involve concentration—repeating a phrase or focusing on the sensation of breathing, allowing the multiple thoughts that inevitably arise to come and go. Meditation techniques and other activities such as tai chi or yoga can induce the well-known relaxation response, which is very valuable in reducing the body's response to stress.

We might also add that mindfulness is therapeutic for our patients with various emotional and physical complaints. Mindfulness may lessen the emotional experience of pain. Patients with chronic pain who engaged in meditation reported the unpleasantness of pain is less connected than normal to the prefrontal cortex (where emotions are processed). This suggests that mindfulness may lessen the emotional experience of pain.

Using brain imaging tools, such as fMRI, scientists have shown that the threat response, which begins in a region of the brain known as the amygdala, is calmed in meditators. Researchers at Stanford and Harvard have found that meditation reduces the density of neurons, hence the activity in the amygdala, and increases neuron density in the prefrontal cortex, which is an important area for regulating emotions. In essence, the reactive fear center of the brain shrinks, and the more thoughtful response center of the brain grows [9].

Back to the Case

Bernice shared her situation with one of her senior partners. Her senior associate understood the situation and recommended a mental health expert, who had a reputation for helping physicians conquer anxiety. Bernice had weekly visits with the therapist. The psychiatrist prescribed XXXX, plus XXXX, to help with the acute situation. The therapist also recommended that Bernice participate in a mindfulness program. Bernice was provided with CDs and an app for working on her breathing and meditation exercises. Bernice learned that she could use petal breathing when she was becoming anxious about certain events in the practice that precipitated feelings of anxiety and was able to abort these panic attacks. Bernice also shared that her insomnia also improved.

Bottom Line

Modern medical practice can affect you both physically and emotionally. We recommend you consider engaging in mindfulness and meditation if you are experiencing these symptoms. Certainly, there is a role for mindfulness and meditation for doctors experiencing anxiety, an excess of negative thinking, or even depression. This is an option that is not expensive, has no side effects, and has a history of being helpful.

Questions to ask your partner's doctors

1. Are you familiar with mindfulness and meditation?
2. Do you think it will work in my situation?
3. What kind of a doctor, counselor, or therapist do I need to see?
4. Does insurance cover mindfulness treatments?
5. Do you have any idea how successful meditation or mindfulness is?

References

1. Horne Ludwig S, Kabat-Zinn J. Mindfulness in medicine. JAMA. 2008;300(11):1350–2. https://doi.org/10.1001/jama.300.11.1350.
2. Kabat-Zinn J. A study in happiness—meditation, the brain, and the immune system. Mindfulness. 2018;9(5):1664–7. https://doi.org/10.1007/s12671-018-0991-3.
3. Creswell JD, Lindsay EK, Villalba DK, Chin B. Mindfulness training and physical health: mechanisms and outcomes. Psychosom Med. 2019;81(3):224. https://doi.org/10.1097/PSY.0000000000000675; PMID: 30806634; PMCID: PMC6613793.
4. Fendel JC, Bürkle JJ, Göritz AS. Mindfulness-based interventions to reduce burnout and stress in physicians: a systematic review and meta-analysis. Acad Med. 2020;96(5):751–64. https://doi.org/10.1097/ACM.0000000000003936.
5. Wenzel M, Rowland Z, Kubiak T. How mindfulness shapes the situational use of emotion regulation strategies in daily life. Cogn Emot. 2020;34(7):1408–22. https://doi.org/10.1080/02699931.2020.1758632. Epub 2020 May 6
6. Falcone G, Jerram M. Brain activity in mindfulness depends on experience: a meta-analysis of fMRI studies. Mindfulness. 2018;9(5):1319–29. https://doi.org/10.1007/s12671-018-0884-5.
7. Nestor J. Breath: The new science of a lost art. Penguin; 2020.
8. Benson H, Casey A. Mind your heart: A mind/body approach to stress management, exercise, and nutrition for heart health. Simon and Shuster; 2004.
9. Pittman CM, Karle EM. Rewire your anxious brain: How to use the neuroscience of fear to end anxiety, panic, and worry. New Harbinger Publications; 2015.

Case Than

Than has spent the past 5 years working in a concierge internal medicine practice in a large Pacific Northwestern city. Although she finds her work rewarding, she is frustrated with the complex and disjointed systems of care available in her community. Specifically, she is discouraged with the lack of preventive services available to her patients. She knows that patients are coming into her practice with advanced diseases that could have been more efficiently managed had they presented earlier. She is also concerned about patients in her community who cannot afford the level of care that she is able to provide. Than is thinking of changing careers to work for a large commercial not-for-profit insurer in her community. She has a minimal understanding for providing care for a population of patients, rather than focusing on individual patients, but needs to learn more about this concept of medical care.

Population health refers to the concept of providing care for an entire population of patients, either through a public health entity, a practice, an insurance plan, or a health plan. Examples of global population health programs include efforts to increase screening and vaccination for COVID-19, efforts to reduce air pollution, and efforts to reduce cardiovascular risk factor such as smoking cessation, weight loss, or choosing healthy foods for a community. Incumbent upon successful population health programs is coordination between healthcare practitioners, the community, and payors.

David Nash described four pillars of population health: chronic care management, quality and safety, public health, and health policy. Chronic care management is critical to the appropriate use of health resources. Approximately 90% of US healthcare expenditures are for the management of chronic conditions and nearly 50% of the population is affected by a chronic disease [1]. Chronic care management is best facilitated by a team of people dedicated to modifying behaviors, educating patients, and facilitating access to healthcare providers in a given community. Part of chronic care management is assuring that patients are receiving care in the most appropriate setting. One of the most expensive places to receive medical care is the emergency room. Unnecessary emergency room visits in the United States are estimated to cost over $47 billion per year [1]. Obviously, a major facet of population health is not only reducing emergency room visits but also assuring access to lower cost facilities such as doctor's offices and urgent care centers which leads to decreased cost and increased efficiency of care delivery.

Medical errors are unfortunately common in the United States and contribute not only to death and disability but also contribute to increased medical costs. Improving healthcare quality and safety, like chronic care management, requires a team of individuals who work to improve systems of care to minimize errors. Quality and safety teams typically use protocols and workflows to standardize processes to minimize the potential for error. They also have systems to investigate medical errors and near misses. By analyzing and collecting data, quality and safety teams are able to develop systems to reduce the likelihood of a repeat adverse event.

Public health by its very nature addresses the health of populations. The response to the COVID-19 pandemic exemplified the disconnect between public health and clinical medicine found in the United States and also uncovered the problems that occur with improper funding of public health. Delays in diagnostic testing, disruptions in the supply chain for personal protective equipment, and lack of preparedness for mitigating viral spread such as social distancing are all examples of the disconnect. To best care for populations, environmental health experts, epidemiologists, and health administrators need to be involved and work alongside clinicians. Public health teaches us the importance of prevention and can help identity problems with access and quality of healthcare. Population health is best accomplished at the intersection of clinical medicine and public health.

Providing adequate care for populations involves not only public health but also involves establishing health policies that directly affect the care of the community. Laws affording care to marginalized populations, laws enforcing public health measures, and policies dictating care paradigms can help to provide care for a population. Although physicians are not typically involved in public policy, this is an area that has the greatest impact on population health. Moving forward, it is beneficial to establish pipelines so that physicians can be involved as policy makers. The Centers for Medicare and Medicaid Innovation established the Initiative to Support Promising Research (INSPIRE) as a means for academic and community physicians to contribute their knowledge and expertise towards public policy surrounding Medicare. Additionally, many medical societies now offer experiential training in dealing with government and policy making.

So how does this affect a healthcare practice? Pay-for-performance (P4P) is an alternative to reimbursement for healthcare services that are based on volume (numbers of office visits, tests ordered, procedures performed, etc.). In a P4P, healthcare providers are reimbursed for behaviors that positively affect the health of their patients. This includes providing preventive health services such as vaccinations in children or keeping blood pressures or blood sugars in a certain range. P4P systems are designed to improve the care of populations. In spite of early enthusiasm, the evidence that P4P improves healthcare outcomes has been unfortunately modest. A growing trend in healthcare reimbursement is an extension of P4P termed "value-based care." In a value-based system, like traditional P4P, reimbursement is dependent on health outcomes rather than the volume of services provided. Reimbursement is also dependent on the proper utilization of tests and procedures to control cost. Using the equation that Value = Quality divided by cost, value is best when quality is high and cost is low. In a value-based contract, physicians are typically granted a bonus for providing quality care in a cost-efficient manner and are typically penalized for care falling below a given threshold. To be most effective, value-based care requires a team to gather and record patient outcome data and an electronic system to record data. In a value-based payment system, the accurate attribution of patient and physician is a critical first step to ensure that providers are being rewarded and de-incentivized appropriately. It is important to ensure the proper collection and recording of interventions and outcomes. It is estimated that within several years, value-based care will be the dominant reimbursement system in the United States. To best manage patients under a value-based system, social and economic conditions found in the population such as water quality, education, and access to care must be considered. Access to healthy foods and access to public transportation to get to physician appointments are critical predictors of favorable health outcomes. Additionally, in any population, preventive services such as vaccination and screening are important to minimize serious late-term complications of chronic illnesses and providing these services must be incentivized.

In the practice of population health and value-based care, information systems are necessary. These systems need to be interoperable such that data acquired on one platform can ideally be inputted (or transferred) into another platform. The data collected must include important social determinants of health to allow for analyzing and improving care for complex patients with chronic diseases. In addition to data collection, data analytics are useful in predicting healthcare utilization and in predicting risks to health so that preventive measures can be undertaken in a timely fashion. Finally, an information system can be used to "gamify" healthcare to reward positive behaviors and to provide electronic encouragement for positive outcomes such as weight loss or medication compliance.

In the past decade, the Centers for Medicare and Medicaid Services (CMS) established value-based programs in order to better care for individuals and populations and at a lower cost. The five original programs included an end-stage renal disease program, a hospital-based purchasing program, a physician value modifier program, (Marc, what is a value modifier program? Does it require more description?) a hospital readmission reduction program, and a hospital acquired condition reduction program. CMS expects that all traditional Medicare beneficiaries will be in a value-based care model by 2030. Unfortunately, it is still too early to tell if value-based programs are effective in improving patient outcomes at a lower cost.

Back to the Case

Than decided to take a position with the insurance company. She decided that caring for a population of patients rather than caring for individual patients was more satisfying. She felt that participation in population health could make a bigger difference in health outcomes and would provide her with more satisfaction.

Bottom Line

Value-based care is the next logical extension in reducing healthcare costs. Providing incentives for patients and physicians for medical compliance and favorable outcomes and having the systems to collect and analyze data are critical for a value-based system to work. Additionally, value-based care and the accompanying reimbursement systems should result in better care for populations of patients.

Reference

1. Nash DB. The population health mandate. A broader approach to care delivery: Boardroom Press; 2012; http://populationhealthcolloquium.com/readings/Pop_Health_Mandate_NASH_2012.pdf.

Case Sebastian

Sebastian is an internist with more than 2000 active patients. He noted that he spends less time with each patient and more time entering data into his electronic medical record. Sebastian has noted that he works more than 60 h a week, takes work home, and spends less time with his family. He does not have time for exercise and has gained twenty pounds in the last 2 years. He feels that he is on a trajectory to burnout. What might he do? One popular option has been the consideration of concierge medicine.

What Is Concierge Medicine?

Concierge medicine is also known as *retainer medicine*, is a private relationship between a patient, and usually a primary care physician in which the patient pays an annual fee or retainer. This may or may not be in addition to other charges beyond basic medical exams. In exchange for the pre-paid retainer, doctors agree to provide highly personalized care and on demand access. In some cases, the physician will even come to your home or place of business.

Concierge primary care is defined by the American College of Physicians as "any practice that directly contracts with patients to pay out-of-pocket for some or all of the services provided by the practice, in lieu of or in addition to traditional insurance arrangements, and/or charges an administrative fee to patients, sometimes called a retainer or concierge fee, often in return for a promise for more personalized and accessible care[1]."

This model of medicine has been referred to as retainer medicine, membership medicine, cash-only practice, and direct to consumer care. While all very similar in concept, they can vary widely in their structure, payment requirements, and form of operation. It is estimated that fewer than 800 US providers practice concierge medicine, but numbers are growing each year mostly due to high deductibles and co-insurance and access to high quality care. We also have what many have described as a perfect storm setting us up for a massive shortage of high-quality caregivers which will no doubt accelerate the movement to concierge medicine.

So, what is this perfect storm? It is a simple math problem, but one that will have major consequences if we don't come up with solutions. The number of elderly people per 100 working age people will nearly triple from 20 to 100 in

---

[1] Doherty R. Assessing the Patient Care Implications of "Concierge" and Other Direct Patient Contracting Practices: A Policy Position Paper From the American College of Physicians. Ann Intern Med. 2015;163(12):949-952. doi:10.7326/M15-0366

1980 to 58 in 100 in 2060. In short, our health-care demands are outpacing our workforce supply at a time when the United States is expected to see a massive decline in primary and specialty care providers. Some estimates show we could see a decline in excess of 100,000 physicians by the year 2032. Our population is also living much longer, resulting in even more demand on our caregivers. As a result of this demand, it will likely set up an opportunity for those who can afford it to buy their way to preferred access. This would be akin to purchasing a first-class ticket or membership to a country club to avoid the wait times for tee off for a round of golf. That said, the idea of supply and demand is one of the very basics of economics and what drives market demand. Supply is created by the sellers, while buyers generate demand. Anytime you have a market where the demand is high, and the supply is low, you can expect innovation and opportunity seekers to fill in the gaps as a response to the demand.

Even consumers who have employer provided healthcare coverage may find concierge medicine appealing. Today, many consumers have deductibles as high as $5000 to $10,000 per year. So, unless they end up needing major medical services, they are basically a cash paying patient. Patients who are younger with less health issues may find this approach less expenses even if they continue purchasing healthcare coverage from their employers. And not surprisingly, doctors who go into concierge medicine will generally be extremely selective as to who they will accept as members. Logically speaking, a younger, healthier membership generally translates to less consumption of the provider's time and efforts.

It should also come as no surprise that concierge medicine can also be controversial. Some view this as a system for the wealthy and privilege. Some even speculate this will only make our access problem to providers more expensive because these models are generally designed to reduce the patient load for a provider. However, one could argue this is a convenient way for providers to reduce their administrative burdens to free up more time for patient care. Recent studies have found that often times providers are spend-ing a mind-bogging 10 h per week in administrative tasks and many end up taking work home with them that goes unaccounted for. We have also recently introduced EHRs that allow for direct electronic patient engagement without any compensation for the provider's time to respond to these messages.

When you examine the economics, it appears to be win/win for the consumers and the providers. The typical employed primary care provider can expect to earn a salary between $125,000 and $150,000. They will generally be expected to work 4–5 days a week and will see between 20 and 30 patients per day and will usually have several hours of charting and documenting at the end of the 8-h day. The typical panel size is an average of 2300 patients. While this is not an unreasonable salary, it can be very misleading when you factor in the number of hours and the high cost of medical school. In 2016, Dr. Neil Baum famously wrote a blog[2] comparing a doctor's salary to that of a UPS driver. Surprisingly, the incomes were almost identical once you reconciled for working hours, medical school debt, malpractice, continued education, compliance, and the risk and liabilities associated with the delivery of care. And this was not intended to draw sympathy for physicians. Money is not the only driving force to become a provider, but it does illustrate how and why a provider might feel undervalued and would look for other alternatives to earn a living. For example, under the concierge model, the same provider can manage just 100 healthy families for an annual fee of $5000 per family and make $500,000 and do far less work. They could do this without any billing staff or expensive EHR systems and could even to it almost 100% virtually or by making house calls.

Ironically, the basic concept and premise of concierge medicine are rooted in the original house call. In the early years of medicine, we had community doctors, black bag in hand, and traveling to a patient's home to provide medical care was very common up to the mid-twentieth century. In fact, Fig. 30.1 depicts one of the most

---

[2] If doctors wanted to be wealthy, they would have become UPS truck drivers (kevinmd.com)

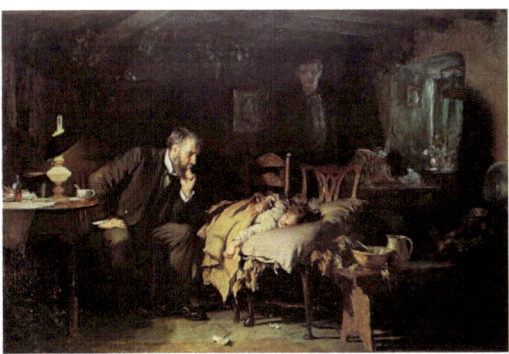

Fig. 30.1 The Doctor - by Luke Fildes, 1891

famous paintings in the world by Luke Fildes depicting a Victorian doctor observing the critical stage in a child's illness while the parents gaze on helplessly from the periphery. The scene for the painting is the home of the helpless child. The painting depicts the concentrated focus of the doctor on the child and shows the patient as a person and individual and the doctor as a compassionate caregiver with empathy for the patient's suffering. Less notice is how the parents, especially the father, have relinquished all their trust and confidence in the doctor to save their child. This is a very powerful image, and it portrays the special bond between patients and providers. This paining is frequently used as an illustration in medical journals and at medical conferences to portray the values of the ideal physician and the inadequacies of the medical profession. One

famous quote about the painting comes from a surgeon, Dr. Mitchell Banks: "What do we not owe to Mr. Fildes for showing to the world the typical doctor as we would all like him to be shown—an honest man and a gentleman, doing his best to relieve suffering?" He continued: "A library of books written in your honor would not do what this picture has done and will do for the medical profession in making the hearts of our fellow men warm to us with confidence and affection".

Back to the Case

Sebastian was approached by a national concierge medicine company. The company arranged a focus group with twenty-five of his existing patients. The survey from the focus group indicated that his existing patients wanted more of his time and more access to care. He signed up with a national company. The company suggested that he reduce his patient volume to 500 patients. This allowed him to spend more time with his patients, provided them with greater access to care, reduced the stress of practice, lost twenty pounds, and found that he was home for dinner.

Bottom Line

History has a way of repeating itself. Although some direct-to-consumer care may exist, the demand for concierge medicine is likely to increase. The limits are the amount of money consumers are able and willing to pay.

Case Hassan

Hassan was a member of a large multi-specialty group practice and occasionally had the office manager check his online reviews. The office manager only periodically checked the doctors' online reviews. Hassan had only five reviews, to his surprise, and two of the reviews consisted of negative experiences the patients had with his office. Hassan wanted to improve his online reputation but didn't know what to do.

"It takes 20 years to build a reputation; it can be ruined in just five minutes." Warren Buffet.

A physician can have their reputation tarnished by just one patient who has had a negative experience with the practice. The Internet has replaced the Yellow Pages for patients to obtain information about individual practices and the services they offer. Research has emphasized that 61% of American adults look online for health information [1]. Every physician must eventually deal with a disgruntled patient, and some unhappy patients may choose to share their displeasure through an online review. This chapter will define online reputation management and provide you with techniques and steps to easily manage and control your online ratings. You don't want to take your reputation for granted, and you want to be proactive in protecting your most valued asset, your reputation.

In today's Internet-savvy world, paying attention to how your patients can affect your online reputation is necessary. Online reputation management, or ORM, is the art of making your name and your practice look their best on the Internet. The Journal of the American Medical Association reported that 25% of US adults consulted online physician rating sites, and more than 33% of online viewers went to a physician or avoided one based on the ratings [2].

Consumers are now using online dating sites to evaluate physicians. A 2008 Wall Street Journal Harris Interactive poll found that 91% of those surveyed would prefer online information about doctors provided by their health plan(s), and 87% expressed interest in providing feedback to health plan sites for physician rating [3].

One of the most common urologic conditions reviewed on the Internet is the treatment of prostate cancer. A significant number of patients, especially those men younger than 65 years with prostate cancer, access the Internet to obtain cancer information. The authors suggested that urologists and radiation oncologists should be familiar with this important resource to help patients access appropriate material [4].

Risks of Ignoring Your Online Reputation

What appears on the Internet remains on the Internet forever. In this Internet era, your exposure is much greater, and negative comments can go viral and may be seen by thousands of potential patients. The reality is that just a few negative reviews can ruin your reputation, which has taken years to build.

If someone has had a negative experience or is unhappy with their treatment, they may find multiple online review sites and tell the Internet world about their negative experience. Unfortunately, patients pleased with their experience rarely bother to place a positive review. Malicious comments are often anonymous, or the writer may use a false name, thus making it impossible for the physician to attempt to reach out in a personal and conciliatory manner. Additionally, in such cases, there is often no way to verify if the review originates from an actual patient or is the handiwork of a competing physician or angry employee [5].

A survey of 500 physicians pointed out how precarious and fragile are our online reputations. The study concluded that most physicians are rated on at least one physician review website. While most physician ratings and reviews are favorable, composite scores are typically based on a few reviews and, therefore, can be volatile [6].

Of course, online reviews can be helpful to practice, which is always trying to improve and provide a better quality of care to the patients. For example, online reviews critical of office personnel and procedures can be helpful if they spur a physician to pay more attention to office performance, thus producing happier patients who will write more positive reviews in the future.

Another report from a German study emphasized that patients may be making decisions to select a physician based on their positive reviews. Their study showed that 65% of patients surveyed had chosen a particular physician based on positive ratings. The authors concluded that "neither health policymakers nor physicians should underestimate the influence of physician-rating websites"[7].

In today's Internet-savvy world, you must recognize that your patients can easily affect your ORM. There are many review websites where your patients can express their experience with you and your practice. These include www. RateMDs.com; www.vitals.com; www.ZocDoc. com; www.HealthGrades.com; www.ucompare-health.com, CitySearch.com, and Google Plus and www.Yelp.com.

These review sites allow patients to rate a physician on:

- How your staff has treated a patient,
- Patient wait time,
- The doctor's diagnosis,
- The doctor's attitude,
- The level of trust in the doctor's decisions,
- The patient's treatment and their results.

Some unscrupulous doctors may post negative comments about their fellow doctors to put their competition in an unfavorable light. Fortunately, this doesn't happen very often.

How Can You Control Your Online Reputation?

First, it is incumbent on you to monitor your online reputation. If someone has posted a negative review, respond to those comments directly on the review site. This response to negative reviews does not violate privacy laws if you do not mention the patient's name or details that identify the patient. You can explain aspects of your practice without confirming or denying that the dissatisfied reviewer was or is a patient. We suggest that you don't mention anything specific regarding a patient's condition.

If you feel the online review is unjustified, you can dispute it with the review site.

Review sites may consider that a patient is ranting and will remove the negative comment.

Next, you can set up alerts such as Google Alerts (www.Google.com/alerts), and we suggest that you or someone on your staff Google your name or the name of your practice at least once a month to check the review sites and read all of the comments, both positive and negative. However, this is a reactive solution, and we suggest that you consider a proactive approach.

Don't wait for a bad review to show up before starting to solicit positive reviews.

Dr. Robert Wachter, Chairman of the Department of Medicine at the University of California, San Francisco, said, "Whether we like it or not, our online reputation is becoming the main prism through which we will be known—to colleagues, to friends, to patients, to prospective employers…. With this realization comes the recognition that we can no longer afford to be passive observers of our online persona" [8].

As large and unwieldy as the Internet is, you have a lot of control for monitoring and controlling feedback from your patients and what you can do with the feedback you receive. This proactive approach does require you or your staff to set up a system to continually request feedback/testimonials from your patients [9, 10]. This is where most medical practices fail. There is no system in place to solicit positive reviews. It can be as simple as having a quick meeting with the doctor and staff, mentioning that the practice will now request patient testimonials. There are two places you want to have patient reviews posted. The first is on your website, and the second is on the review sites.

Patient Testimonials on Your Website

The best time to obtain a patient's feedback is when the patient offers a compliment about the physician or the staff. Everything is still fresh in their mind; they are probably happy with the outcome and more receptive to providing a testimonial. This proactive approach is a system to follow when placing testimonials on your website:

1. Testimonials should be on the front page of your website and every subsequent page. They should be visible to the website visitor when they first view the page without scrolling down the page to find them. Your testimonial is worthless if the website visitor doesn't see it or doesn't take the time to find it.

2. Testimonials should be in italics using quotation marks.

   Doing this makes it look like someone posted a comment rather than having it look like just another part of your website page.

3. Your testimonial should have a headline in bold and italics. The headline should be the testimonials' keywords that resonate with the reader. For example, if, within the body of the testimonial, the patient says, "I can now function in a normal manner," or "I had been to several doctors, but you were the only one that cured me,"; these become the headlines introducing your testimonials.

   Here's an example:

   "You Turned My Life Around"
   "I had a surgical procedure, and it was a game-changer. You turned my life around, Dr. Baum! Thank you!"

4. Have the main testimonials page on your website and pick out different headlines from each testimonial so it would appeal to a diversity of prospective patients. We suggest having a button directing the viewer to the testimonial page or placing the button on the left side of the home page. The website visitor may not read the entire testimonial, but they will at least read and scroll through the headlines.

5. Testimonials are far more believable and credible if the patient signs them. An anonymous testimonial or a testimonial merely signed "J.D." doesn't carry credibility unless the patient's full name is included.

Put Patient Feedback Surveys on Your Website.

Another way to encourage your patients to give you their feedback or testimonial is to have a "patient feedback survey" on your website. The doctor or the staff asks the patient if they would go to your website and complete the survey. Many patients will agree to this suggestion, but very few will leave the office and follow up and complete the survey. A far more effective way is to request that they complete the survey while still in your office. Have your receptionist hand the patient an iPad after their appointment and ask them if they would take a couple of minutes to complete your feedback form on your website.

Ask Patients to Post Their Testimonials on Review Websites.

Asking patients to post on review sites is less effective, as most patients will not take the time or effort to follow through. So, you must make it as easy and as fast as possible.

You can accomplish this by providing your patient with instructions on what to do and how to do it.

The first step is to provide your patient with a feedback form that has four or five questions that they answer. (A sample form is in Fig. 31.1) Giving your patients the questions will elicit an emotional response that helps the patient describe their experience with you and your practice.

If you let the patient create a testimonial on their own without specific questions to answer, you merely receive a bland or neutral comment such as: "I'm happy with my results" or "She is a nice doctor."

Next, provide your patient with a step-by-step process, direct them to rating websites, and provide instructions to navigate the website to enter their feedback. Providing a review is often a daunting task for your patient, so your instructions should be clear and straightforward.

Thank you for helping us to serve you better

Was it easy for you to obtain an appointment in this office?
_____Yes   _____No

Is your general impression of this office favorable?
_____Yes   _____No

Was the office staff friendly and concerned?
_____Yes   _____No

Did the doctor adequately answer your questions?
_____Yes   _____No

Would you recommend this office to someone else?
_____Yes   _____No

Do you have any additional comments?

Fig. 31.1 Card given to patients to rate their experience with the practice

Back to the Case

Hassan was, a well-respected physician, one of the best in his field, noticed that the number of new patients had decreased drastically, and he didn't know why. Upon examining his online reputation with the review sites, he found that his reputation had plummeted because there were four negative reviews and no positive reviews. We suggested that he begin soliciting positive reviews from his patients, which he and his staff were able to accomplish easily in just a few weeks. Upon further examination of his online reviews, there was a significant increase from two to more than four stars.

Bottom Line

The good news is that a damaged reputation can be repaired. Don't get caught with one or two unhappy patients ruining your well-deserved reputation. We highly recommend that you not wait for a negative review to appear on the review sites. You start collecting positive reviews so that any negative reviews can be diluted by the many positive reviews you so rightfully deserve.

The most precious asset a doctor has is their reputation. We spend our entire medical lives protecting that asset. A patient using the Internet and their First Amendment right to free speech can ruin our reputation with a click of the mouse. We can protect our reputation by practicing good medicine and taking good care of our patients. We can protect our online reputation by using the techniques described in this chapter.

References

1. Fox S, Jones S. The social life of health information. Pew Internet & American Life Project, 2011. http://www.pewinternet.org/2009/06/11/the-social-life-of-health-information/.
2. Kuehn BM. More than one-third of U.S. individuals use the internet to self-diagnose. JAMA. 2013;309(8):756–7. https://doi.org/10.1001/jama.2013.629.

3. Harris Interactive. Are there fair and reliable ways to assess healthcare quality? 2008. http://www.harrisinteractive.com/NewsRoom/PressReleases/tabid/446/ctl/ReadCustom%20Default/mid/1506/ArticleId/351/Default.aspx.

4. Smith RP, Devine P, Jones H, DeNittis A, Whittington R, Metz JM. Internet use by patients with prostate cancer undergoing radiotherapy. Urology. 2003;62(2):273–7.

5. Escoffery RM, Bauer JG. Manage your online reputation—or someone else will. Aesthet Surg J. 2012;32(5):649–52.

6. Ellimoottil C, Hart A, Greco K, Quek ML, Farooq A. Online reviews of 500 urologists. J Urol. 2013;189(6):2269–73. https://doi.org/10.1016/j.juro.2012.12.013; Epub 7 Dec 2012.

7. Emmert M, Meier F, Pisch F, Sander U. Physician choice-making and characteristics associated with using physician-rating websites: a cross-sectional study. J Med Internet Res. 2013;15(8):e187; CrossRefMedlineOrder article via InfotrieveGoogle Scholar.

8. Pho K, Gay S. Establishing, managing, and protecting your online reputation: a social media guide for physicians and medical practices. Phoenix, AZ: Greenbranch Publishing; 2013.

9. Conner C. Protecting your online reputation: 3 key tasks your business must complete in 2014. Forbes; 2013; http://www.forbes.com/sites/cherylsnappconner/2013/12/09/protecting-your-online-reputation-3-key-tasks-your-business-must-complete-in-2014/.

10. Dolan PL. 5 ways to manage your online reputation. American Medical News, 2011. http://www.amednews.com/article/20110912/business/309129966/4/

Case Dr. Mendoza

Doctor Mendoza is the managing partner of multispecialty group practice. The practice has a website that was cobbled together from the practices tri-color, threefold brochure that was created years ago. Doctor Mendoza recognizes the importunate of medical marketing and is not sure how to proceed. He received several marketing proposals from marketing firms but remains confused on how to proceed. This chapter will describe a one-page marketing plan that will serve as a marketing roadmap for the practice.

Marketing can be a complex and confusing endeavor. Most physicians and practices have little or no experience or training in marketing and practice promotion. The process is simplified by creating a one-page marketing plan. This plan is easy to create, easily modified, and will almost certainly produce results. This chapter will provide you with the nine components of a one-page marketing plan that will be easy to create and implement into nearly every medical practice.

Today, marketing in medical practices is ubiquitous. Who would've ever thought that great medical establishments such as Mayo Clinic, Cleveland Clinic, and Kaiser Permanente embark on a marketing strategy for their institutions? Marketing consists of attracting new patients to the practice and then providing them with a stellar patient experience followed by a system to keep the patient within the practice and make them into raving fans. This can be accomplished with a one-page marketing plan.

Every profession, including healthcare, has a well-thought-out plan that is created, distributed to the staff, and followed meticulously. This is true in the airline industry where pilots follow a flight plan as well as in the military when soldiers follow an operation plan. Marketing is not a subject that is taught in medical school and most physicians and office managers are clueless when it comes to marketing and practice promotions. We have seen many practices that hire a marketing consultant who provides an assessment of the practice in a slick business plan which identifies the needs and wants for marketing the practice. This very expensive, multipage plan is put on a shelf and never looked at again and, more importantly, never implemented. The result is a waste of precious marketing dollars that doesn't work for the practice.

We are suggesting that you consider creating a one-page marketing plan that results in taking action and you are likely to see more patients enter the practice as a result of this approach to medical marketing.

© The Author(s), under exclusive license to Springer Nature Switzerland AG 2023
N. Baum et al., *The Business of Building and Managing a Healthcare Practice*,
https://doi.org/10.1007/978-3-031-37623-8_32

The Circus and Marketing

Historically, physicians think that marketing is merely advertising and requires an outlay of lots of money. Let's look at marketing as thinking about the circus coming to town. If the circus is coming to town and there is a sign saying, "Circus Coming to the Showground on Saturday," that is advertising. If the sign is on the back of an elephant that strolls into town, that's promotion. If the elephant walks through the town's flower bed in front of city hall and the newspaper writes a story about the debacle, that's publicity. However, if the mayor offers his observation of the elephant and laughs about the elephant, that's public relations. Now if the town's citizens show up at the circus and buy a ticket to see the show, that's sales!

The one-page marketing plan consists of nine elements which are divided into three phases. (Fig. 32.1) There are three phases of every marketing plan: (1) identifying a target market and follow-up on any potential patients needing the services of the practice, (2) providing the patient with educational materials before they enter the practice and the patient is given an outstanding experience, (3) after the patient leaves the practice they continue to return regularly, and, more importantly, become raving fans who tell others about the wonderful experience they had with the doctors and the practice.

Phase Number 1: Before the Patient Enters the Service Cycle.

It is at this stage that the future patient doesn't know anything about you or your practice. If you can create an awareness of your practice, you have accomplished the first and very important part of the patient cycle. This phase is a magnet or the hook that entices the patient to provide information about him\herself and that the patient will avail themselves of phase two or when they become part of your practice.

Phase Number 2: During this phase, the patient becomes a patient and has an experience with the practice. If that experience is positive, the patient is likely to remain in the practice and will segue to phase 3.

Phase Number 3: After you and your practice have participated in the care of the patient and

that the patient had a positive experience, you will want them to tell others about that positive experience. The patient has interacted with your staff from the time they made the phone call to the practice, until the moment that you have ended the doctor-patient relationship, they pay their bill, leave with educational material, and all of their questions have been answered. Your marketing has made promises of providing access to the practice, that timely follow-up was achieved, and all of the patient's questions were answered at the time of the visit. Now the patient has a favorable relationship with the doctor and the staff and is very likely to refer others to the practice.

You will notice in Fig. 32.1 that each phase of the one-page marketing plan consists of three components. Let's look at the three components of the first phase with practical examples of each component that will hopefully lead not only to adding more patients to your practice but will also maintain the loyalty of those patients who are already in your practice.

First Component of the Before Phase of the One-Page Marketing Plan

The goal of this component is to make it possible for your patients to know you and your practice. When you create a message to prospective patients and have demonstrated even a modicum of interest, you have to continue to connect with the prospective patient to motivate him\her to enter the practice.

This usually begins by identifying your target market. Let's be very honest, it is nearly impossible or unreasonable to target everyone with what you do and how you do it so that everyone enters your practice. Phase one also means avoiding a mass marketing plan such as TV, radio, or newspaper with bland comments about your outstanding services, or first in the area to offer such a service or treatment.

The "PVP" approach is used to identify your ideal patient. This consists of "personal" enjoyment, "value" to the marketplace, and "profitability."

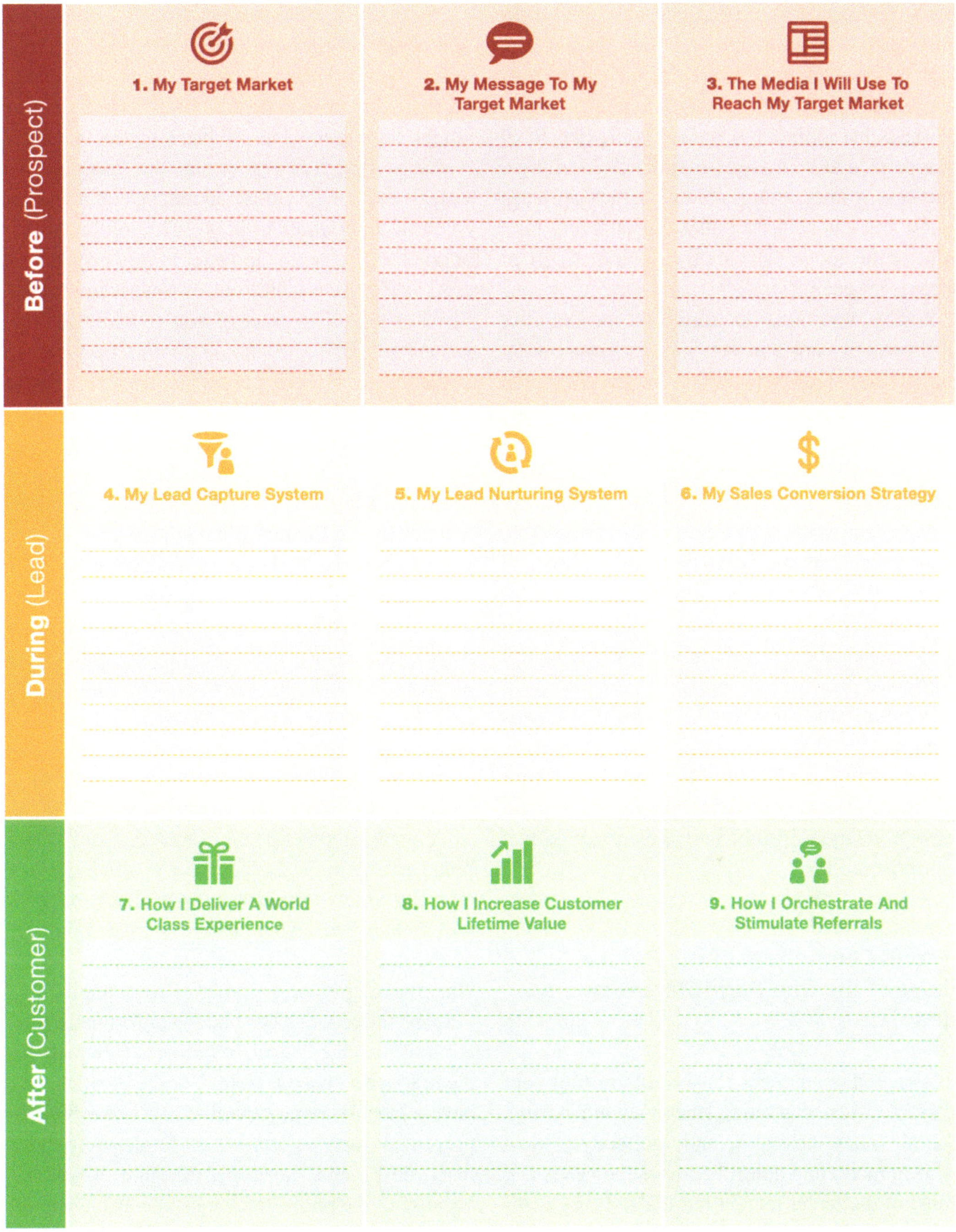

Fig. 32.1 One-page marketing plan. (Source: Used with permission from Success Wise and available at 1pmp.com)

Personal enjoyment is the enjoyment you have providing care for a certain type of patient. For example, if you are a primary care doctor, do you enjoy helping patients achieve their ideal weight and help them with their diet, nutrition, and the use of supplements. If you are an orthopedic surgeon, you may have an interest in sports medicine and helping weekend worriers overcome injuries of the middle age and seniors who engage in sports. Another example is the urologist who offers treatment for middle-aged men with difficulty with urination and erectile dysfunction. Each practice can find an area or niche that they enjoy, and this identifies a target market.

The value to the marketplace is the benefit of your service to your target market. If your target market is women with problems achieving pregnancy, you can be certain that this is a very high value to the couple who are trying desperately to become pregnant.

Finally, you must determine the profitability of providing care and services for your target market. You want to avoid any target where the fees you charge are not worth the effort or the expense of your marketing programs. You want to avoid at all costs having a target market that is not profitable.

Next, you want to learn as much as possible about your target market. If you have a medical practice that is dependent upon referrals from other physicians, then you want to know as much as possible about your target marketing of physicians.

A simple worksheet for the purpose of identifying the hot buttons of referring physicians is shown in Fig. 32.2. This brief survey of your existing and potential referring physicians can provide valuable insight into their practice and their private life.

Second Component of the Before Phase of the One-Page Marketing Plan

This second component consists of crafting your message. Most marketing messages are boring, like all other messages, and ineffective. Most medical marketing doesn't address the needs and wants of the target market but instead lists platitudes that don't work to attract patients. The practice logo and a laundry list of the diseases and conditions that are treated and the procedures that are performed are ineffective. We call this "me too" marketing that is likely the same as all the other practices in the community. So why are you wasting your precious time and dollars?

We'd like to recommend that you develop a unique service proposition or USP. What is it that makes you different and special and that distinguishes you from others who are also trying to attract the same kind of patients that you are reaching for? Let's look at the example of water—one of the most abundant commodities on earth. In contrast to many areas of the world, in our country, most tap water is free and safe to drink, yet there are millions of Americans paying $1.69 or more for a liter of bottled water such as Evian®, Fiji,® or Smart Water®. The price of bottled water is 20% more than the same volume of Budweiser beer, 40% more than the same volume of milk, and three times the cost of gasoline! Now that's the power of your USP: motivating people to pay more for water than what is available for free at the tap. What is your USP so that you can become the Evian of healthcare?

Most of the choices we make—from the coffee shop we frequent for our jolt of java to the company that provides the medical supplies for our medical office—are based on having a USP. Doctors may not even be aware of it, because subliminal suggestions, social media, and word-of-mouth marketing can be as contagious as a multi-million-dollar advertising campaign.

A medical practice is a business and needs brand recognition. In fact, if a practice doesn't take the time to build a unique brand, patients will seek care elsewhere and may create opinions of the doctors and the practice that may not be what the doctors or the practice were hoping for. Perhaps the practice has had the unfortunate situation of just one "negative online review" giving the practice a one-star rating" or the practice may have a label or reputation that can't be erased or prevented such as long wait times, unfriendly front desk, and can't get through by phone because of the phone tree, are some examples. As in other businesses, the most successful hospitals and practices usually have a strong USP that clearly differentiates them from all others that provide similar services.

We recommend that you identify your USP and craft your message to your target market emphasizing what makes your practice special

Fig. 32.2 Identifying hot buttons for referring physicians

1. NAME_____ D.O.B._____

2. TELEPHONE NUMBER(W)_____ (H)_____

   FAX NUMBER:_____ E-MAIL:_____

3. ADDRESS (W)_____

   (H)_____

4. EDUCATION:_____

5. SPECIAL AREAS OF INTEREST:_____

   _____

6. HOBBIES AND RECREATIONAL ACTIVITIES:_____

   _____

7. MARITAL STATUS:_____ PARTNER:_____

8. CHILDREN:_____

   _____

9. CONVERSATIONAL INTERESTS:_____

   _____

10. DINING PREFERENCES:_____

ADDITIONAL NOTES:_____

and different. The goal of your USP is to answer the question, "Why would a potential patient prefer to become a patient in your practice than a similar practice in the area?" It is a fact that most patients find out about your USP after they have become part of your practice. What we want to emphasize is that your USP is to be used to attract patients before they have entered your practice.

Third Component of Phase One or Reaching Potential Patients Using Social Media

John Wanamaker, a media mogul, once said, "Half the money I spend on advertising (practice promotion) is wasted; the trouble is I don't know which half." That comment was made over 50 years ago when tracking of marketing efforts was in its infancy. Today, technology is readily available to track our marketing effectiveness quickly, inexpensively, and easily.

For the most part, this cannot be accomplished in-house especially in small- to medium-sized practices that don't have a marketing expert on board. To determine the success of your marketing using the website and social media analytics, you will probably need to hire an expert who specializes in medical marketing and is familiar with your target market and the media that you use to reach that market whether it is print advertising, direct mail, Internet, or social media. If you are going to be successful in marketing and promoting your practice, you will want to have a return on your marketing expenditures.

An example of measuring the return on your marketing investment assume you use a direct mail campaign and send out 100 letters. The cost of printing and mailing your 100 letters to potential patients is $300. Your response to those 100 letters was ten potential patients or a 10% response rate. From the ten who responded, only two called for an appointment or a 20% closure rate. Carrying out the calculation a little further, you acquired two new patients at a cost of $300 or $150 for each new patient from the marketing effort. If each new patient had medical services of $200, you made 50 dollars for each new patient. If you are in primary care and the patient stays with you for ten or more years, the return on your investment is going to be huge, especially if the patient has a good experience and tells others about you and your practice.

The take-home message is just getting your name out there or word of mouth promotion, you'll do much better by concentrating on getting the name of potential patients in here or in your practice.

The second phase of the one-page marketing plan is to understand what happens when you receive leads from your marketing efforts. You will need to develop a system of follow-up and how to keep in touch with potential new patients.

In prehistoric times (probably the Paleolithic age), the man (most likely a male member of the clan\tribe) woke up every morning and collected his primitive weapons and headed out to hunt for food for his clan or family. On a successful day, he would come back with a deer or antelope and the family was able to eat. However, I am sure there were days when he returned empty-handed, and the family might go hungry. There was pressure every single day to hunt successfully as the life of the clan depended on it.

Contrast the daily hunter with the farmer or when the hunter-gathers became involved in agriculture. The farmer planted seeds, and the clan would wait weeks or months later for the wheat, barley, or corn to become ready for harvesting. From planting to harvesting, the plot of land

needed to be watered, weeds removed, and the crops tended to on a regular basis.

What does the hunter-farmer story, which is perhaps the most significant single development in human history, have to do with one-page medical marketing? Our observation when it comes to practice marketing, most physicians behave more like hunters rather than farmers. They take their threefold brochure and electronically convert the content and then hire a high school student to paste it into a website template and declare, "Our practice has a website." Another example is the practice hires a marketing firm that has little or no experience in medical marketing to create a logo and write a newsletter and add some meaningless slogan like "state of the art technology" and then claiming to be a leader or expert in the area and send it out for a few months but without any follow-up to any potential patients who contact the practice for more information and are disappointed and state, "Marketing doesn't work." Merely "getting the word out" or "getting the practice name out there" is going to be futile and a waste of time and money.

Most medical practices are clueless about the purpose behind practice promotion and effective marketing. These practices and doctors believe that marketing consists of primarily of getting the word out, getting recognized, or creating a buzz about the doctors or the practice. If you ask doctors the goal of their marketing, they will state they are interested in more patients and\or more procedures. This hunting approach is akin to flushing water down the toilet. Successful medical practices that truly understand practice promotion describe marketing as keeping existing patients and attracting new patients who are interested in your area of interest or expertise. This kind of marketing is the long haul or farming approach versus the instant one or the hunting approach to practice promotion.

The successful practice identifies potential patients and enters them into a database and then follows up with additional educational material on a regular basis or provides useful products that are a constant reminder of the practice so that when "the time is right" and the patient needs to avail themselves of your services, your practice will be remembered, and they will call for an appointment and become members of your practice. Now your practice is building value that will serve as a magnet to attract new patients to your practice and will also keep your existing patients within your practice.

Mankind made progress by moving from hunter-gathers to farmers. However, farming did require regular care and attention to the crops. The same applies to your practice promotion and marketing efforts. You can't create just one newsletter, one blog, or one social media submission and have the phone ring off the hook. It requires constant and frequent offerings so that when the time comes for the potential patient to need your services, your practice and your name will be easily recalled, and you will have captured a new patient from your marketing efforts.

The next step in your one-page marketing plan is to create a database system for organized follow-up to any potential patients. For example, if you make a presentation to a lay audience and you collect the names, address, and email addresses, then you must have a process for connecting with all of those people who were in your audience. The likelihood of giving a single talk to a church group or a service club will result in a significant number of those in the audience will become patients.

Let's apply some numbers to having a database system. For example, you have a monthly support group for a medical condition that is in your repertoire or in your strike-zone of medical care. At any given time or on average 3% of those attending, the program might be highly motivated and ready to call for an appointment. There is an additional 7% who are very amenable to becoming a patient and then there may be another 30% who are interested in your services but not now. Then there's 30% who are not interested at all and finally, the reality is that there is 30% who just come to the meeting for the coffee and the cookies and aren't ever being interested in becoming patients even if you wouldn't charge them. If you measure your marketing by new patients that contact your practice right after the program, the 3%, you are missing out on the other 97%. You must be a farmer and continue to take care of your field, or those who may eventually need your services at a future date. You need a system to continue to reach out to those who you can possibly identify as potential patients. Now, by going from the 3% who are immediately interested to nearly 40%, you are multiplying the effectiveness of conducting a support group by 1233%. Now that's what we call a real return on your investment (ROI).

Therefore, it is imperative to keep track of your potential patients with a customer relationship management (CRM) system. You will want all of your leads of potential patients to be entered into your CRM.

(Fig. 32.3 is a list of software programs for healthcare practices that offer CRM)

Next, comes nurturing your leads.

Most medical practices have an attitude of "one and done." They write a blog, add an article to their website, or send out a newsletter. Nothing happens after one or two attempts and the statistics on the success of nurturing your leads in all areas of marketing and practice promotion is that 50% of practices will give up after one contact with a potential patient; 65% give up after two, and 80% give up after three attempts [1].

With each interaction with the patient, you have an opportunity to create a negative impression, a neutral impression, or a knock their socks off mind-blowing impression. Most practices accept the negative or neutral impression. The really successful practices create a shock and awe approach so that whenever the patient needs the services the practices offer, they will be quickly remembered and they will make that call to become patients in the practice.

A shock and awe approach is best when a physical package is mailed to the potential

Zendesk (Zendesk.com)
Salesforce (Salesforce.com
Monday.com (Monday.com)
Scoro (Scoro.com)
Hubspot (Hubspot.com)
NetSuite (NetSuite.com)
Nutshell (Nutshell.com)
Qucikbase (Quickbase)
Freshworks (Freshworks)

Fig. 32.3 Healthcare CRM programs

patient. This provides information or surprises that are so unique that the recipient cannot forget where it came from and who was the sender.

Examples of a shock and awe package might include a book on a medical topic. This is even more meaningful if you have written the book. For example, if I give a program on impotence\erectile dysfunction, I send them a copy of a book I wrote on the topic.

Of course, I could save on postage if I gave out copies to those in the audience right after an evening program on the topic. It is far better to send a copy of the book a few days later. I usually will distribute a sign-in sheet and tell the audience that if they sign the sheet with their name, home address, and email address, I will send them a copy of the book. I almost every member of the audience provides this information to receive a copy of the book.

Another "present" in the shock and awe package is a DVD or CD that introduces the doctors in the practice, a tour of the office, and testimonials from a few patients.

If you have articles that appeared in the local or national media, send copies to the patients as this enhances your credibility.

It's also effective to send papers or articles that you have written which appeared in professional journals which add to your expertise.

The least effective are scratch pads, pens, magnetic refrigerator calendars, or mousepads with the name of the practice, contact information and logo. These are given out by other practices usually at the point of service and your trinkets will not stand out amongst the "tschokas" from other practices.

I think the best shock and awe packages contain a handwritten note from the doctor expressing interest in the potential patient and offering to be available and to answer any questions.

In summary, a shock and awe package should (1) give potential patients an amazing and unexpected surprise that is valued by the recipient, (2) demonstrate your expertise in a particular medical area and that you are a trusted authority in your field, and (3) move the potential patient closer to picking up the phone and making a call to your office if they are in need of your services.

Our message is that a shock and awe package provide you with a huge competitive advantage. It's ethical, it's easy, and it's effective.

It is common for those not skilled at marketing to put their toe in the water before becoming fully immersed in the river. They will often send out one or two newsletters from the practice and fail to receive new patients from their efforts and then cease all marketing endeavors. Our take-home message is that an attitude of "if you build it, they will come" may apply to baseball fields but not to marketing and practice promotion. A newsletter like all others is screaming "me too," and you may be left with competing on price which is a losing marketing plan.

A true story about a virtuoso violinist, Joshua Bell, emphasizes the importance of context. Joshua Bell is one of the best concert violin players in the world. As an experiment sponsored by the Washington Post, Mr. Bell wore a baseball cap and sunglasses, played for 45 min, on a 300-year-old Stradivarius violin worth $3.5 million at a Washington DC subway station during rush hour on January 12, 2007. Over a thousand people passed by Bell; however, only seven people stopped to listen to him play, and only one person recognized him.[1] Just a few nights before his performance in the subway station, he played at the Kennedy Center and the cost of each ticket was $100. He had a hat placed conspicuously to collect tips and received a grand total of $32. Here was a virtuoso who would receive $1000 per minute to play in front of a sold-out audience.

This is no surprise; the social context in which a behavior occurs affects how it is interpreted. The very same talented musician, playing the exact same music on the same violin, in one instance he earns $32 an hour, and in another context, he earns $60,000 per hour. What made the dramatic difference? I believe it was positioning.

If you are a professional musician and think of yourself as a subway performer, your audience\

---

[1] You can watch this amazing story of Joshua Bell in the Washington DC subway station on YouTube: https://www.youtube.com/watch?v=LZeSZFYCNRw

patients will pay you accordingly. On the other hand, if you position yourself as a professional concert performer, you attract a totally different customer\client\patient and get paid accordingly. Our take-home message is that the public will accept you at your own appraisal of yourself.

If you believe you provide superior service, you have the possibility of positioning yourself at a much higher level. You can offer your service at a much higher price and attract a higher quality of patient. Don't try to compete on price because there will always be someone who will charge less than you do and then you reduce your price even more and ultimately the quality of your service will deteriorate.

We want you to think in terms of providing value to your patients. We would like you to think in terms of providing useful material that educates potential patients and enhances the trust that potential patients will have with you and your practice. It is necessary to think of the pain points patients are experiencing and how you can provide a solution to that problem. If you are a primary care physician who is focused on being an obesity expert and you can help patients lose weight, and more importantly, help them keep the weight off, then offer that information on a regular basis to potential patients. If you are an orthopedic surgeon, specializing in sports medicine, provide information on injuries incurred by weekend warriors and focus on prevention of soft tissue injuries. If you are a urologist and your area of interest and expertise is erectile dysfunction, speak to your patients about non-medical, non-surgical solutions to this common problem impacting millions of middle-aged men.

We believe the road to conversion is paved with expertise and education. You must see yourself as virtuoso violin player playing on one of the world's finest violins and in this context, you are a creator of great value, a resource of good health that will positively change the lives of patients who become part of your practice.

The third phase of the one-page marketing plan is creating raving fans who will promote your practice to others. If you define tribe, you will find that it is a group of people connected to one another by a leader who serves as the connec-

tor. Outstanding practices lead tribes of raving fans. If your practice has raving fans, you have special patients who are promoters and cheerleaders for your practice. Your raving fans will enhance your marketing message and escalate your reputation beyond what you might be able to do alone.

To create these raving fans, it is necessary to continually impressing your patients about your stellar services. Practices with raving fans will try to foster a lifetime relationship with their patients. These practices that attract raving fans will make it slam dunk easy for them to interact with the doctors and the practice. These practices have a system in place that allows them to frequently and consistently create a stellar experience. It is necessary to have a strategy for building a following of raving fans and make every effort to take very good care of them. You must consider that each raving fan creates exponential results because each patient doesn't add revenue on their first visit, but it's repeated revenue as this patient serves as magnifier for creating new business for your practice.

Delivering a World-Class Patient Experience

There's an advantage of being small, flexible, and having the ability to make decisions quickly. Large practices and large groups are stymied by their bloated bureaucracy, which have layers and a hierarchy of people that need to sign off on any decision that needs to be made. Smaller practices have the advantage of being agile and can respond to patients' needs and make decisions quickly and much faster than large organizations. More importantly, small practices can micromanage the doctor-patient relationship. As a result, the patient doesn't find themselves adrift in a sea of other patients and the practice has an opportunity to offer a personal and customized interaction that is conducive to creating a raving fan.

The first step in creating a raving fan is to find out what your patient wants. It is imperative to think about not only what the patient wants but what the patient needs. For example, in an IVF practice, the woman wants to become pregnant and have a baby. Every woman who enters the practice wants that result. Now how can you give her hopefully what she wants but, if not, what she needs? It is necessary to understand both needs and wants. The needs and wants may be overlapping but often they are completely separate. Our challenge is to motivate patients to do what they need to do to achieve the results they want and need. This is the topic compliance which is often difficult to achieve. The take-home message is that we want our patients to achieve the results both the doctors and the patients want. The benefit of reaching this goal is that the patients who achieve their goals will spread accolades to others who are likely to become patients in your practice. We've found the best way to encourage compliance is to divide the process into bite-sized morsels so that the whole process doesn't seem so daunting.

In this age of technology, you have an opportunity to make healthcare frictionless. For example, make it easy for patients to make an online appointment. This is particularly important and attractive to millennials. Another friction point is for making payments to the practice. When this can be made easy and quick, your practice will be attractive to patients. Another method of reducing friction regarding payment is to provide prices of your services. There should be no secret about the cost of visits and procedures that you offer and should be readily available to patients. Receptionists should be able to quickly quote the cost of each service the patient is likely to encounter. These prices should also be posted on the website. It is of interest that in 2021 the government will require hospitals to disclose their prices that they have negotiated with insurers [2]. The purpose of any new technology that is implemented into your practice should serve the purpose to eliminate friction.

Increasing Patient Lifetime Value

First, it is important to understand the lifetime value of patient to your practice. The calculation for LTV is the average value of an appointment multiplied by the average appointments per year multiplied by the average number of years a patient is likely to remain in your practice.

The calculation of the lifetime value = $V \times N \times Y$ where,

V = Average Value of Appointment

N = Average Number of Appointments Each Year

Y = Average Number of Years They Visit Your Practice

For example: if you are an middle-aged otolaryngologist and your average patient is seen three times a year and each visit is worth approximately \$150, and stays within your practice for 6 years, then the average lifetime value of your patients would be $3 \times \$150 \times 6$ or \$2700.

A classic story is Russell Conwell's Acres of Diamonds. (available online at https://www.google.com/books/edition/Acres_of_Diamonds/O44DAAAAYAAJ?hl=en&gbpv=1&printsec=frontcover) The story is about farmer living between the Tigris and Euphrates rivers who wanted to find diamonds so badly that he sold his farm, left his family, and went off on a search that took him all over the world to search for diamonds. His search was futile and ultimately led to extreme poverty including the loss of his family. The new owner of his farm discovered a mother lode of diamonds on the farm that he had purchased from original owner. The moral of this story is to dig first on your own property when seeking a treasure or more succinctly look first at what you already have. If you apply that to your marketing efforts look at your existing patients and see that they have a stellar experience before reaching out for new patients. Numerous studies have shown that it is far easier to satisfy an existing patient than the time, money, and energy required to attract new ones. Those studies indicate that a person is 21 times more likely to buy from a business\practice they've already used compared to one they have never visited [3]. There can be plenty of productivity from your existing or past patients and there are diamonds right in your own practice.

Nearly every practice has dozens and perhaps hundreds of patients who have fallen through the cracks and have missed appointments for follow-up examinations. In this pandemic era, there are large numbers of patients who have been fearful of coming to the doctor and have skipped follow-up appointments.

More than a third of adults report they've delayed or forgone healthcare either due to fear of COVID-19 infection or their physician offering limited services during the pandemic [4].

An even larger portion (40.7%) of respondents with one or more chronic conditions reported they've delayed or forgone care, while 56.3% of respondents with both a physical and a mental health condition have failed to follow-up with their doctor [5].

Black adults were more likely (39.7%) to report forgoing or delaying care than Hispanic (35.5%) or White (34.3%) adults and more likely to report forgoing or delaying multiple types of care with 28.5% compared to 22.3% and 21.1% respectively. (Ibid).

The most common type of medical care delayed or forgone was visiting their primary care physician or specialist with 20.6% and receiving preventive health screenings or medical tests with 15.5% [6].

Respondents with one or more chronic health conditions like hypertension, diabetes, respiratory illness, heart disease, cancer, kidney disease, and mental health disorders made up the vast majority (76%) of those who have delayed or forgone healthcare [6].

Delaying and forgoing care isn't without its dangers as 32.6% of respondents say that doing so has worsened one or more of their health conditions or limited their ability to work or do other daily activities, according to the report. (Ibid).

This would be a perfect time to institute telemedicine for those patients who have missed appointments. A primary care doctor probably has numerous patients who need follow-up cholesterol testing and blood pressure monitoring. A urologist certainly has patients with low-grade bladder cancer who need follow-up office cystoscopies. Men who are using testosterone for hypoandrogenism require monitoring of the hemoglobin\hematocrit and PSA levels.

How to keep these existing patients in the loop or within the practice? We suggest sending the patients reminders by email, SMS, or even snail mail. It is possible with modern technology to send reminders automatically to patients who are likely to need follow-up appointments.

You can make your practice user-friendly by making your practice accessible. Tell existing patients that they can have same day or next day appointments. Another convenience is to offer early morning, late afternoon, evening, or weekend appointments. If you are delivering extra value that your competitors do not provide, your existing patients will continue to remain loyal members of your practice.

We suggest developing a reactivation campaign. This consists of going through your patient database and identifying patients who need to return to the practice. You need to give them a strong reason to return to the practice. An example would be type 2 diabetic patients who are using finger sticks multiple times a day and you can offer them one of the small wearable devices that transmits glucose readings to their mobile phones.

When the electronic contact method fails, then consider calling the patients and ask them why they haven't returned. Let the patient know you care about them and their health. Tell them you want them to return to the practice and make it convenient for them to re-enter the practice. Ideally a reactivation should not be necessary. But there are going to be situations such as the pandemic, hurricanes, floods, and other natural disasters making it difficult for patients to return to the practice. However, a reactivation campaign can be your acres of diamonds and significantly increase the lifetime value from your existing patients.

The basics of conducting a reactivation campaign begin with looking at your patient database and retrieving names of patients who haven't returned for follow-up. Next create a strong offer to entice them to come back. In most healthcare practices, returning is beneficial to their health and failure to come back may cause deterioration in their health and well-being. Finally, if they do call for a follow-up appointment, send them a thank you note indicating that you are looking forward to seeing them.

It is important to stay connected with your patients who haven't followed up. Let them know that you are concerned about them, that you're available, and you will find that they will handsomely reward you by reactivation into the practice. On the other hand, if you don't reach out to them, then they will forget you and their health may deteriorate.

Repetition will lead to repeat visits and loyalty from patients. One contact is not likely to keep your name and the name of your practice for recall when patients may need your services. By sending patients regular reminders, newsletters, and emails, you become a familiar name and more likely they will be calling for an appointment when they need your services. Reaching out to patients in your data base can be easily automated with current technology to do the heavy lifting. This technology allows you to easily keep in touch and continue to develop and maintain a relationship through your customer relationship management (CRM) system. Maintaining that connection can be as simple as a monthly postcard or text message.

Orchestrating and Stimulating Referrals

Several decades ago, the concept of marketing and spreading the word was relegated to "word of mouth" or what we call "hopeium" where the doctor and the practices "hope" that patients who have had a favorable experience will walk out of the practice and tell others about that positive experience. That's a "sit and wait' approach to building and maintaining a practice. That approach may have worked a few decades ago but that's a passive approach and you may wait a very long time for it to work, while others are taking a more active approach and creating raving fans who do the marketing and practice promotion on your behalf.

The attitude of asking for referrals is often considered beneath us and akin to begging for business. It is possible to initiate the process by simply asking patients whom you have delivered

an outstanding care and have had a favorable result to share that experience with others including their primary care doctor. However, you need to give them the ammunition necessary to be your publicist.

For example, a patient returns for a follow-up semen analysis after a vasectomy, and he is sterile with the outcome he and his partner desired. A follow-up with a letter mentioning that you would appreciate if they would share their experience with other men who need the procedure. You might include several packets that provide education material on vasectomy and offer their friends a free consultation if they would consider having the male sterilization procedure. These satisfied patients will know others in a similar situation and in need of family planning and will very likely share their vasectomy experience.

Remember, it is human nature to be attracted to people with the same likes, interests, and situations as themselves. Also, no man is looking to have a vasectomy. However, he is looking for a solution for a specific problem, i.e., no more children. The effective approach is to identify the problem and offer a solution that will solve that problem.

This process acknowledges them and appeals to their ego as nearly everyone likes being acknowledged. Rather than appear to be asking for a favor, you might consider offering something of value that they can share with their family and friends. This process is far more effective taking an extra dose of "hopeium"!

Back to the Case

Dr. Mendoza developed a comprehensive marketing plan for his practice and enjoyed the benefits.

Bottom Line

The one-page marketing plan is not a sprint but a marathon. Outcomes and gratification are deferred but it all begins with a plan of action. The one-page marketing plan is an effective approach to medical marketing that is well within the reach of every medical practice regardless of size, location, and current level of marketing and practice promotion.

There's a popular Chinese proverb that says: "The best time to plant a tree was 20 years ago. The second-best time is now." Basically, this means that if you want success and growth tomorrow, the best time to act is now. So, consider start planting your one-page marketing page today!

References

1. Moncrief WC. Are sales as we know it dying… or merely transforming? J Pers Sell Sales Manag. 2017;37(4):271–9.
2. Wheeler C, Taylor R. New year, new CMS price transparency rule for hospitals. Health Aff. 2021; https://www.healthaffairs.org/do/10.1377/forefront.20210112.545531/.
3. Gallo A. The value of keeping the right customers. Harv Bus Rev. 2014; https://hbr.org/2014/10/the-value-of-keeping-the-right-customers.
4. Czeisler MÉ, Marynak K, Clarke KE, et al. Delay or avoidance of medical care because of COVID-19–related concerns — United States, June 2020. MMWR Morb Mortal Wkly Rep. 2020;69:1250–7. https://doi.org/10.15585/mmwr.mm6936a4.
5. Claxton G, Damico A, Rae M, Young G, McDermott D, Whitmore H. Health benefits in 2020: premiums n employer-sponsored plans grow 4 percent; employers consider responses to pandemic: the annual Kaiser Family Foundation employer health benefits survey of the cost and coverage of US employer-sponsored health benefits. Health Aff. 2020;39(11):2018–28.
6. Gonzalez D, Zuckerman S, Kenney GM, Karpman M. Almost half of adults in families losing work during the pandemic avoided health care because of costs or COVID-19 concerns. Urban Institute; 2020; https://www.urban.org/research/publication/almost-half-adults-families-losing-work-during-pandemic-avoided-health-care-because-costs-or-covid-19-concerns#:~:text=Almost%20half%20(45.5%20percent)%20of,about%20exposure%20to%20the%20coronavirus.

33

Surveying Your Practice: Cost-Effective Methods of Identifying the Needs and Wants of Your Patients

Case Reginald

Reginald noticed that his staff reported that patients complained about the long wait times to obtain an appointment. Patients also complained of waiting in the reception area and the exam room for the doctor or medical assistant. Patients complained that phones were not answered quickly and that the calls were often answered rudely. Reginald also noted that his online reviews were often scathing and were nothing he was proud of. Reginald was at a loss for what he should do.

Start by listening to your patients' impressions of your practice. When you listen, you will learn what patients want and give them more of what they want, and you will know what they don't like and make every effort to avoid what turns them off. As a result, you will improve your patients' quality of care. Look at your practice through the lens of your patients. An even better method is to ask your patients what they think. In this chapter, we introduce techniques to look at your practice from the point of view of your patients. These will help you assess your current standing with your existing patients and referring physicians. A healthy practice always needs to attract new patients. However, you also must keep the patients you already have. Even full or closed practices should evaluate their services periodically and listen to their patients. Changes always occur, and the cup may not "runneth over" forever. Besides, if your patients and staff are satisfied, your work will be more enjoyable, and you will be home for dinner!

Today, knowing the needs and expectations of your patients and referring physicians is critical. This information is available by surveying your practice. A survey will also provide an update on your practice's strengths and weaknesses. This information is readily available to your patients. Patients are a valuable source of information and can help you improve the quality of care you provide. What better place to begin evaluating your practice than to ask what your patients think of you and the service you provide?

Five effective techniques for determining how patients perceive your practice and for evaluating your performance and reputation:

1. Conduct personal interviews
2. Conduct patient surveys
3. Create a focus group
4. Use a suggestion box
5. Survey your peers

"Those who enter to buy, support me. Those who come to flatter, please me. Those who complain, teach me how I may please others so that more will come. Those only hurt me who are displeased but do not complain. They refuse me permission to correct my errors and thus improve my service." Retailing Pioneer Marshall Field

© The Author(s), under exclusive license to Springer Nature Switzerland AG 2023
N. Baum et al., *The Business of Building and Managing a Healthcare Practice*,
https://doi.org/10.1007/978-3-031-37623-8_33

Personal Interviews

Ask your patients about their experiences with you and your office staff. This method is the least popular for acquiring information because patients often feel "put on the spot" and will not reveal true feelings during a face-to-face inquiry.

However, informal conversations with your patients can reveal information about your practice. Patients are more likely to respond honestly to specific rather than general questions. You might ask a patient:

- Do you think the time you spent in the reception area (not the "waiting room") was excessive?
- Would you like us to call or fax your prescription to the pharmacy so it will be ready for you when you arrive to pick it up?
- Are you likely to use our website to schedule your appointments with our office and receive reports and lab results without coming in or calling us?
- Would you be interested in having the ability to email questions or concerns to the nurse or the doctor?
- Would you like an electronic copy of your medical record?
- If we had a nutritionist available, would you use their services?
- Would you like us to contact you by phone, text messaging, or email?
- Would you like to pay your bill online or at the time of service?

When you ask questions such as these, you show concern for your patients' time and pocketbooks, and the answers will probably be helpful. You could also conduct a survey focusing on how promptly you see patients and how long they wait in the reception area or exam room before seeing a physician.

Patient Surveys

Written patient surveys are the most popular method for obtaining patient feedback. You can give written surveys to patients during their office visits or send the survey to their email. The advantages of sending the survey via email are that the patients can remain anonymous and complete the survey at their leisure. The disadvantages are that once patients leave the office setting, they are not likely to return them.

What to Ask

The survey should be short and require no more than 3–5 min to complete. The survey should be limited to both sides of a single 8 1/2 × 11-inch piece of paper or just one or two screens if they complete the survey online. Begin with an opening paragraph that outlines the purpose of the survey (i.e., to evaluate your practice's strengths and weaknesses and ultimately provide better healthcare for your patients) (See Figs. 33.1 and 33.2). Yes/no or multiple-choice questions are the easiest to quantify.

Suggested questions include:

- Do I see you on time for your appointments?
- Is my office staff friendly and courteous?
- Are my office hours convenient?
- Is it easy to make an appointment?
- Do my staff and I return phone calls in a timely fashion?
- Would you like me to provide you with the opportunity to purchase your medications in the office if the prices were competitive with local pharmacies?

We do not suggest you ask any questions regarding your fees because most patients consider medical fees too high. Finally, you can conclude with an open-ended question: What can I do to make your experience with my office more pleasant?

Whom to Include

Choose a cross-section of patients if you choose to email your survey. Include some active and inactive patients and patients who have left your practice. Also, consider various age groups, from millennials to older, retired patients.

Dear Patient:

My staff and I want to provide you and your family with the highest quality healthcare possible. To help us evaluate our effectiveness, we would like your opinions of my practice.

Your answers and suggestions on the following questionnaire will help us continue to improve the healthcare we provide you. Please take a few minutes to give us this important information and return it to us in the enclosed stamped, self-addressed envelope.

Thank you,

Dr. Neil H. Baum and staff

Fig. 33.1 Sample Cover Letter to Accompany Patient Survey

Suggested questions include:

• Do I see you on time for your appointments?

• Is my office staff friendly and courteous?

• Are my office hours convenient?

• Is it easy to make an appointment?

• Do my staff and I return phone calls in a timely fashion?

• Would you like me to provide you with the opportunity to purchase your medications in the office if the prices were competitive with local pharmacies?

Fig. 33.2 Suggested questions to use in a brief survey

Customizing the Survey

Instruct patients to return the survey to your p email address. If the survey returns to your office and contains critical or negative comments regarding your office personnel, the survey may not reach your attention. If patients experience problems with your staff, you want to be made aware of those issues. Another option is to use an electronic survey with SurveyMonkey.com.

Implementing the Survey

We recommend that you survey your patients at least once every 2 years. According to the American Medical Association, one good rule of thumb is to study at least 20% of your existing patients (Bujang MA. A Step-by-Step Process on Sample Size Determination for Medical Research. Malays J Med Sci. 2021 Apr;28(2):15–

27.) or a minimum of 200, whichever is greater. It is also good to survey inactive patients because you will often obtain important information about your practice. You may learn why they are no longer patients or don't return for follow-up care. The physician should personally review all the surveys. Keep an open mind as you do this, remembering that the purpose is to improve your practice. Even though you may get criticisms, most comments will probably be positive. But it's the criticisms that will help make improvements to your practice. (Find quote from Chicago Department store president).

Tabulating the Results

We recommend that you keep your surveys simple. Most of them have yes or no answers. Easy-to-complete surveys make tabulating the results easy and less time-consuming. Tabulation counts the number of responses received and the number of yes or no answers for each question.

Using the Results

You have worked hard to devise a concise patient survey. Several patients have emailed them to you. Do not relegate these valuable letters to your email's "black hole." Those survey comments and answers are a gold mine. Now, you must address the concerns. Your practice will stand out not only with those who took the time to answer the survey but also with the rest of the patients already in your practice.

It is also essential to prioritize the comments received from the survey. If your survey shows that an overwhelming percentage of patients feel they were waiting for long periods, then that problem must be addressed first. On the other hand, if only one or two people claim your office hours are inconvenient, that issue can be lower on the list. A staff meeting is the best time and place to address the survey results. For instance, a survey revealed complaints about delays in the office. This is an opportunity to brainstorm possible solutions. A solution might consider inviting a local dentist with a reputation for being on time with their patients to a "lunch-and-learn" program. The dentist may provide suggestions for improving time management in your office. You are likely to find ideas from that meeting regarding the scheduling of patients and how to manage urgencies and emergencies.

One response from a survey was that a patient had a late afternoon appointment on several occasions and found that the patient's restroom was untidy. The office manager looked at this for a few days and discovered that the wastepaper baskets were overflowing with paper towels and that a urine specimen cup had spilled and was not cleaned up. Now, the staff checks the restroom right after lunch and again in the middle of the afternoon. The goal was to ensure that the patient who had the last day's appointment encountered the same clean restroom as the first patient in the morning. Without a survey, this problem might have gone unnoticed.

Focus Groups

With a focus group, the most important step is the selection of participants. An effective focus group consists of a cross-section of diverse, opinionated, and vocal individuals who are willing to honestly assess your practice. When selecting participants for a focus group, choose patients who are keen observers and patients who are also complainers. Avoid "yes" men and women. The purpose of the focus group is not to hear how wonderful you are. It is really to troubleshoot your practice, which is why you want vocal, articulate complainers as your participants.

Invitations and Reminders

Once participants for the focus group are selected, the best results will occur if the doctor or office manager calls each patient and personally invite them to assist in evaluating your practice. Then send an email note that includes the purpose of the focus group and an agenda that you would like the participants to think about before the meeting (see the sample email invitation in Fig. 20.1). The day before the focus group, have your office staff call and remind the participants of the meeting.

Fig. 20.1 Mailing list

It is convenient to hold the meeting in your reception room. We suggest limiting the discussion to 90 min. Provide coffee, soft drinks, and dessert. Pay the parking fees or in the case of participants who prefer not to drive at night, taxi fare to and from the meeting. Ask permission to tape-record the meeting, so you are not distracted by having to take notes.

Running the Meeting

After introductions, briefly reiterate your reasons for inviting participants to your office. Solicit examples from them of excellent customer service. Request ideas for improvement based on their experiences at other medical offices and businesses. Ask open-ended questions, not questions that are merely answered by yes and no.

Weekend office hours may not be practical for some physicians. For example, one focus group revealed that several patients were interested in evening and weekend office hours. One solution was to have Saturday morning hours when one of the doctors was on call. The other doctors in the practice agreed with this idea. Now, weekends are covered, and one doctor can see patients in their office.

We also learned that patients preferred to avoid paying to park under our building. Another finding from one of the participants claimed that most other hospitals and doctor's offices did not charge for parking services. This problem was solved by validating parking for office appointments.

Another focus group finding was that patients needed help knowing where to go to pay their bills and schedule their subsequent appointments. This feedback demonstrated the need for better signage. The solution to the signage problem was to provide signs at the business office and wherever the exit signs appeared in the office.

Follow-Up

After conducting a focus group, consider sending or emailing each participant a thank-you note. It is essential to let each person know you appreciate their time and their opinions. Whenever the focus group generates a change, acknowledge that their suggestions were implemented.

Suggestion Box

The suggestion box is a time-honored and inexpensive method of obtaining valuable feedback about patients' experiences in the office. Consider placing a suggestion box in the reception area. Place a sign on the suggestion box stating, "Please let us know what we can do to improve our service to you." Include pencils and 3 x 5 index cards. The patients have the option of signing their names or remaining anonymous. The

essential responsibility is to check the suggestion box *daily*. Do not treat the suggestion box as fluff or window dressing. Take it seriously and make it a functional part of your ongoing practice survey techniques.

If patients sign their names, call them, thank them for their suggestions, and respond to them within a day or two of their office visits. Let them know the follow-up on their suggestions, especially if you implement one of their ideas.

Survey Your Peers

Finally, you want to evaluate or survey your referring physicians. A written or verbal survey can determine your colleagues' experiences and opinions. Holding an informal meeting is the easiest and most comfortable method. For this method to succeed, the feedback must go both ways. In addition to soliciting critiques of your practice, you should provide your colleagues with constructive comments regarding their practices. Most physicians will be pleasantly surprised by how valuable this type of candid conversation with peers can be.

For example, while field testing a computerized referral letter with colleagues, the response was unanimous approval of the concept. Subsequently, a few colleagues adopted the idea of the computerized letter for their practices.

A survey of colleagues does not have to be as formalized as a written patient survey. You can select physicians with whom you feel comfortable. Ask them to meet you for lunch or for coffee.

You want to know if the reports are arriving in a timely fashion. We suggest approaching a cross-section of colleagues: some older physicians, some contemporaries, and a few younger physicians. You want to ask whether they received feedback from the patients they sent to you and your practice. Ask if you can do anything to make your practice more user-friendly.

For example, a physician related that one of his pet peeves was that the office would call him to discuss a patient, and the doctor was on hold for 15–30 s before the staff placed the doctor on the line. "Look," he said, "this is just one of my quirks. I can't explain it, I know it isn't necessarily right, but it galls me. Know that that's one of my quirks. Please respect it and be on the phone when your office calls me." That way, whoever places the call to this doctor must be sure that the caller is immediately available to take the call. We also record this information on each physician's WIN sheet (WIN is short for 'What's Important Now', which I adapted from Harvey Mackay's 66-question customer profile) (See Fig. 33.3)

These discussions with your peers can be informal. Explain to your colleagues, "Look, we send patients back and forth. I want to get better, and I can only do that if you give me feedback on how I'm doing. If there's anything I can do to improve the practice and give you better service, please let me know?"

Fig. 33.3 The WIN Sheet or What's Important Now

The WIN Sheet

1. NAME_____   D.O.B._____

2. TELEPHONE NUMBER(W)_____ (H)_____

   FAX NUMBER:_____ E-MAIL:_____

3. ADDRESS (W)_____

   (H)_____

4. EDUCATION:_____

5. SPECIAL AREAS OF INTEREST:_____

   _____

6. HOBBIES AND RECREATIONAL ACTIVITIES:_____

   _____

7. MARITAL STATUS:_____ PARTNER:_____

8. CHILDREN:_____

   _____

9. CONVERSATIONAL INTERESTS:_____

   _____

10. DINING PREFERENCES:_____

ADDITIONAL NOTES:_____

Consider using this list of questions:

- If you need a consult immediately, is your patient seen on time?
- Is my office-friendly to your patients?
- Do I get my referral notes back to you on time?
- Do you feel that my office is user-friendly?
- Are there any problems you are having that I need to know about?

The take-home message is letting colleagues know you are serious about enhancing your service to their patients. Send a follow-up thank-you note to those physicians who agree to provide feedback.

We suggest repeating this process every 6–12 months to keep up with what referring physicians think about your practice. At a minimum, survey the physicians who refer the most patients to your practice. In primary care, consider surveying the specialists you refer to frequently. We suggest you track your best referral sources if you are a specialist. Suppose you notice a good referral source who previously sent three to five patients a month has not sent you a patient in a few months. Set up a meeting with that doctor or office to see if there is a problem and what you can do to remedy it. For example, if a referring physician had not sent any patients for several months, contact that physician and ask if there was a problem. You might discover that the referring physician's office staff had difficulty arranging appointments at your office for their patients. Suppose the physician commented that their patients were very busy and couldn't take time off for medical appointments. Perhaps you can provide their office with your back-office telephone line, which is a direct line to the scheduler, and offer their patients same-day appointments. You might inform the referring physician that you now provide telemedicine appointments when it is unnecessary to examine the patient (see Chap. 26 on telemedicine) You probably cannot offer that service for all referring doctors, but you may make an exception for a good referral source.

Asking the Platinum Question

Whether one of your patients or your colleagues, you need to ask what Ed Koch, the previous mayor of New York City, the platinum question. The mayor would routinely walk the streets and asked New Yorkers the platinum question: "How'm I doin'?" How can I get better?" [1].

> **Back to the Case**
> *Reginald started making a survey of his patient's experience with his office. Reginald learned what his patients were experiencing when they called his office for an appointment. He hired a focus group evaluator who conducted several focus groups of his existing patients. The survey results and the feedback from the focus groups were evaluated. Reginald discovered what could be done to resolve many of the complaints and took action to correct the problems. As a result, his patients were happier, his staff less stressed, his online reviews improved, and Reginald was more content with his practice.*

Bottom Line

When you solicit honest feedback from your patients and referring physicians, you may get surprises. If you listen and learn from their responses and implement their suggestions, you will improve the quality of the care you give and the quality of your bottom line!

References

1. Remembering Ed Koch, Economist, February 2, 2013.

Cybersecurity and Ransomware-Managing Threats and Protecting Patient Data

34

Case Dr. Lavine

Dr. Lavine is enjoying his Saturday morning when he gets a call from his answering service indicating one of his patients is having a severe allergic reaction to a medication. Dr. Lavine immediately attempts to sign into his electronic medical records system so he can see a complete list of medications the patient is taken. This is where his nightmare begins. Instead of getting into his EHR, he is redirected to a CryptoLocker website demanding a ransomware payment to unlock his system. As terrifying as this sounds, Dr. Lavine knew this day would eventually come so he secured all his data in second location not connected to his network. He also had a backup stored on a removable hard drive kept in his personal safe at his home. As a result, Dr. Lavine did what any doctor would do first, he logged into his back-up server and took care of the patient, then he told the cyber criminals to go pound sand. He did not have to pay the ransomware demand because he had a secure back up of his data. He did, however, have the unfortunate duty of reporting his data breach to the Office of Civil Rights (OCR) since it affected more than 500 individual patients. He also had to notify all his patients about their data had been compromised by cyber criminals.

Abstract: Until recently, cyber threats were problems for larger organizations and issues mostly read or heard in the news. However, after years of attack, these larger organizations have spent millions fortifying their IT infrastructure, making medical practices and hospitals the new soft targets for these criminals. Cybersecurity awareness and prevention have been the IT department's worry. Now, the attacks are so debilitating that cybersecurity has become a crisis and a crisis management issue.

In addition to cybersecurity now being part of crisis management, it also has significant compliance stipulations. The Health Insurance Portability and Accountability Act (HIPAA) security rule requires that healthcare entities covered by HIPAA conduct a security risk analysis (SRA) of their organization. Non-compliance can result in harsh penalties and fines for not complying with these rules.

In the following pages, we address the problem of cybersecurity breaches, sources of threats, the Chief Information Officer's (CIO) responsibilities, working with third-party vendors, and conducting privacy and security risk analyses. The information will help your organization take proactive steps to gain ground in developing and maintaining a healthy cybersecurity posture. There is much catching up to do.

Cybersecurity Breaches on the Rise

Healthcare cybersecurity is a growing concern, as evidenced by the steady rise in hacking and IT security incidents in recent years. Many healthcare organizations have struggled to defend their network perimeter and hold cybercriminals at bay. Now, more than ever, healthcare providers must protect multiple connected medical and non-medical devices. Additionally, the number of Internet of Things (IoT) devices that are integrated into the healthcare industry has exploded. Data is the new currency, and cybercriminals will stop at nothing to gain access to this valuable commodity. These offenders are developing more sophisticated methods and techniques to attack healthcare organizations and increase their chances to cash in on this data by holding it at ransom or selling it on the black market.

The 2019 HIMSS Cybersecurity Survey [1] provides valuable insight into US healthcare organizations' information security experiences and practices undergoing hacking and compromises. In polling over 160 US-based health information security professionals, the findings reflect the following:

- A pattern of cybersecurity threats and experiences is discernable across US healthcare organizations. Significant security incidents are nearly universal in US healthcare organizations with many of the events initiated by bad actors leveraging email to compromise their target's integrity.
- Many positive advances are occurring in healthcare cybersecurity practices. Healthcare organizations appear to be allocating more of their information technology (IT) budgets to cybersecurity.

- Complacency with cybersecurity practices can put cybersecurity programs at risk. Certain responses are not necessarily bad cybersecurity practices but may be an early warning signal about potential complacency seeping into the organization's information security practices.
- Notable cybersecurity gaps exist in critical areas of the healthcare ecosystem. The lack of phishing tests in certain organizations and the pervasiveness of legacy systems raise serious concerns regarding the healthcare ecosystem's vulnerability.

External Attacks

According to the Office for Civil Rights (OCR) at the U.S. Department of Health and Human Services (DHS), approximately 15% of healthcare providers reported a data breach due to a hacking of hospital IT systems in the past 24 months (Table 34.1). The remainder of the victims were other healthcare organizations, such as physician practices, ambulatory surgical centers, mental health facilities, rehabilitation facilities, and others. Further, approximately two-thirds of non-acute and vendor organizations reported experiencing a security incident in the past 12 months.

Source: HIMSS 2019 Cybersecurity Survey [1].

Unfortunately, many healthcare organizations have been slow to respond to cybersecurity threats and generally lag other industries in prevention. Cybersecurity budgets are increasing, and healthcare entities purchase new cybersecurity technologies, yet healthcare entities still struggle to thwart attacks and keep their networks proactively secure.

Table 34.1 Recent security incidents in healthcare

Recent significant security incident	2019					2018
	Hospital (%)	Non-acute(%)	Vendor(%)	Other(%)	Total(%)	Total(%)
Yes	82	64	68	76	74	76
No	14	33	30	20	22	21
Don't Know	4	3	3	4	4	3

Insider Threats

In addition to cybersecurity attacks from external actors, healthcare organizations continue to deal with challenges inside their organizations. Securing healthcare data and managing an effective cybersecurity program can be daunting. According to a recent Verizon Data Breach Investigation Report, 58% of healthcare PHI breaches are by insiders [2]. The report states that healthcare was the only industry where internal actors are the greatest threat.

Healthcare data is primarily used internally but shared with various individuals to facilitate the coordination and delivery of care. This activity is complicated to accomplish in and of itself, and to secure the data while ensuring access to those who need it adds a layer of complexity. Even with the increased transition to electronic health record (EHR) systems, paper records are causing data security problems, according to the Verizon study. Hard copy documents were the assets most often involved in incidents entailing error. Healthcare organizations, therefore, should consider instituting an effective risk management program that invests in comprehensive data breach detection measures. This program would include table-top exercises and reviewing Internet of Things (IoT) security as just a few prevention and detection requisites. Additionally, it is mandatory for healthcare leaders to ensure that internal staff has adequate cybersecurity training and resources to ensure the appropriate precautions to protect sensitive data from compromise by internal and external bad actors.

Cybersecurity and Today's Healthcare CIO

Among other regulatory compliance requirements, cybersecurity continues to be top-of-mind for healthcare chief information officers (CIOs), chief information security officers (CISOs), executives, and boards. Healthcare entities continually face the challenge of balancing tightly secure, protected health, and financial information by providing easy authorized access within

Table 34.2 Key areas to take proactive measures

Security area	Considerations
1. Network perimeter security	• Also known as a demilitarized zone (DMZ), perimeter security addresses the boundary between the private, locally managed, and owned side of a network and the public and externally managed network such as the Internet. The DMZ is one of the highest security risks that must be assessed, tested, and addressed continually
2. EHR system security	• Passwords, audit trails, dual authentication, role-based security profiles
3. End user authentication	• We have seen a continual rise in the number of legitimate users logging on to an organization's wired or wireless network to access protected health information. This escalation increases the amount of network traffic to monitor for unauthorized access. CIOs need assurance that all log-in attempts are monitored and acted upon accordingly. Some CIOs have implemented a single-sign-on (SSO) solution to control and resolve these issues. Whatever solution the organization deploys, it must test, document, and resolve authentication issues continually
4. User identity	• More organizations are implementing a virtual desktop infrastructure (VDI) in their EHR environments. It often becomes difficult to capture and audit user identities in these environments, which further raise security risks
5. Internet-of-things ("IoT")	• We see an exponential number of items (devices) becoming computer-based and linked to the Internet. IoT apparatuses such as biomedical, security cameras, and HVAC systems must be identified, continually monitored for security risks, and managed

Source: Coker Group

and across the organization, including external entities. As CIOs seek ways to achieve this delicate balance, they are trying to move from a reactive to a proactive position in several key areas, including the following (Table 34.2):

Merely complying with privacy, security, and confidentiality regulations is no longer sufficient. Violating these regulations often results in tens or hundreds of thousands of dollars in fines, not to mention potential destruction of an organization's information assets, an adverse patient outcome, or negative publicity. CIOs must proactively secure and monitor their networks, applications systems, and data while conducting periodic security audits.

As the number and complexity of IT systems, devices, and users increase, forward-thinking CIOs welcome third-party advisors to conduct ongoing security audits, assessments, and penetration tests using human interaction with specialized automated tools to conduct and report these security activities. The existence and compliance with updated privacy and security policies are under closer scrutiny along with employee behavior and habits in complying with these policies. Additionally, updated cybercrime and security education and training must be implemented on an ongoing basis.

CIOs are expected to develop and implement a cyber defense strategy to protect their healthcare organizations and patient information. Those CIOs who openly assess their vulnerabilities, prioritize their actions, and continually monitor and manage their security risks are in the best position to help their organizations grow efficiently, effectively, and safely.

Third-Party Vendors

If dealing with your own security threats was not a substantial challenge, you must also ensure all your business associate (BA)[1] partners are compliant. Many organizations mistakenly assume a signed Business Associate Agreement (BAA)[2] is

sufficient for ensuring that third-party vendors are compliant and responsible for their breaches. While having a BAA is a critical first step, it is unsatisfactory in and of itself. There are three common misconceptions about the BAA.

1. The third-party vendor or person doing work for the hospital/practice is not storing PHI data; therefore, they are not considered a BAA. This presumption is false. If they have access to data, they qualify as a BA and must sign a BAA.
2. All third-party vendors use encryption and offer a privacy statement. Again, false. They still have access to the data, and encryption is not always a 100% safeguard.
3. The vendor has a BAA with the hospital and practice; any subcontractors or partners are under the same BAA. False. As soon as PHI is entered in the vendor's system, they are automatically deemed a business associate. Further, any subcontractors working on behalf of the vendor or the practice are also considered business associates. The latest rules state that covered entities (YOUR PRACTICE/HOSPITAL) MUST obtain satisfactory assurances from their business associates no matter how far down the chain the information flows. Everyone involved needs to be under a BAA, and it is your responsibility to make sure they are.

Many security breaches happen because primary vendors use unidentified, down-the-chain resources who are not directly contracted with the hospital/practice. In some cases, these are individuals who may come from staffing agencies and/or work as freelancers. They will usually be unaware of policies or standards. They carry no insurance and would have no means of protecting anyone if they cause a breach, so there would be little to no recourse. Further, they may not even be in the United States. Therefore, here are several tips to reduce security threats when working with third-party vendors:

---

[1]A "business associate" is a person or entity, other than a member of the workforce of a covered entity, who performs functions or activities on behalf of, or provides certain services to, a covered entity that involves access by the business associate to protected health information.

[2]Covered entities must ensure that they have a current HIPAA business associate agreement in place with each of their partners to maintain PHI security and overall

HIPAA compliance. These partnerships are known as business associate agreements (BAAs).

- All subcontractors require preapproval. Under no circumstances can any vendor use subcontractors without prior permission.
- Vendors must disclose all existing subcontractors and require each to sign the BAA provided by the hospital/practice and present proof of insurance. If covered under the primary vendor's insurance policy, require evidence.
- All vendor contracts should require provisions about cybersecurity breaches. Specifically, the vendor must be responsible for their mistakes and the cost to remediate the issue.
- The BAA should have a breach notification requirement mandating the vendor to notify of any incidents.
- There should be a data return policy and/or destruction requirement.
- System access should have a start and end date. Most systems today allow for setting an expiration date.
- Require the right to audit and inspect adherence to these policies at any time.
- Have vendors provide evidence of their security risk analysis, compliance certifications, and proof of staff privacy training.
- Revisit policies and the BAA after each major upgrade, new release, and version change as these events are when new contractors are often introduced.
- Consider adopting contract management software to help manage and track key dates and documents as these BAAs are updated annually.

Responding to a Breach/Incident

Responding to a cybersecurity breach/incident can be terrifying. These ordeals are challenging to manage because the criminal is often invisible and unstoppable once they control a network. In some cases, you do not learn about the incident for months or even years later. In other cases, it will be a brute force attack, and the criminals will disable a network or conduct a ransomware attack demanding money to return the data. In any event, here are some short- and long-term responses you will need to consider:

During an Attack

- Immediately disconnect the entire network from the Internet to block any other access and data transfers.
- Quarantine all infected devices. These will be needed for the investigation.
- Find out who has been infected or impacted. An example may be everyone who clicks on the suspicious link/email. It is critical that NO one receives punishment for making a mistake; otherwise, people may conceal their mistakes out of fear of losing their jobs. This information is crucial to properly respond, so do not make anyone feel uncomfortable about coming forward.
- Immediately loop in all vendors and IT staff so they can start their investigation.
- Bring in counsel familiar with cybersecurity regulations and incident response protocols. From this point forward, all communication must go through counsel; otherwise, you can forfeit your client/attorney privilege. Counsel will help you determine if you need to call in the authorities, notify patients, contact the media, and provide additional guidance.
- Conduct a comprehensive investigation and document everything. Start pulling together all your policies and network diagrams as the investigators will need this information.
- Contact your cybersecurity insurance, who will likely have their experts join the investigation.
- Do not assume this is a breach. In most cases, these turn out to be just an incident, not an actual breach. You will have 60 days to investigate before you are required to respond based on the findings. (If you can reasonably show there was not a breach, the incident does not require a report to the ONC.)

After the Incident

Depending on the type of breach and the circumstances, you may need to self-report. Each incident is different, so it would not be possible (or appropriate) to provide specific recommendations.

Moreover, these guidelines have changed, so we recommend following the official HHS/HIPAA official website for guidance on responding to a breach. Here is the link https://www.hhs.gov/hipaa/for-professionals/breach-notification/index.html

The Impact on Covered Entities

Organizations that maintain thorough and well-documented HIPAA compliance and risk management programs reduce their risk of financial exposure to civil monetary penalties from HHS/OCR. Preserving the appropriate privacy and security documentation necessary to satisfy compliance with key HIPAA security rules is critical. This also includes conducting a security risk analysis (SRA) to help covered entities avoid the fourth and highest-level of liability: "willful neglect--not corrected." The SRA should be performed at least annually and include assessing the covered entity's technology infrastructure and information security policies and procedures. The SRA should consist of a remediation plan to outline the actions to address any weaknesses in the organization's security program.

The use of risk analysis and risk management tools, such as the ones leveraged by Coker Group, can be a significant resource in assessing and managing any gaps identified through the SRA process. Risk analysis tools can provide a method of documenting each recognized risk event or vulnerability point in the organization, including those with business associates. They also serve as a repository of your organization's security remediation efforts and evidence in the event the covered entity is subject to an audit from the Office of Civil Rights (OCR). This detailed documentation validates that a covered entity has an effective risk management program and may help prevent the "not corrected" status associated with the $1.5 million annual limit.

Also, OCR has stated that it will be actively auditing organizations that do not report any breaches. Therefore, covered entities with the most accurate security risk analysis and comprehensive breach detection program will reduce the likelihood of the imposition of fines and penalties because of a security audit or breach.

Disaster Recovery (DR)

After the crisis the practice will start the recovery process. This is when you will likely discover any major gaps. Depending on how much you had to self-report, you may be required to go over a corporate integrity agreement with the OCR as part of your penalty. If this is the case, do not ignore this as it could make the penalty much more sever. You will need to demonstrate a good security posture going forward and open the practice up to outside inspections to verify you have taken proper measures to prevent future breaches. As you go into recovery mode, here are things to consider…

- Step One: Find out how long will it take to restore the data.
- Step Two: Once you get attacked, Criminals will almost always come knocking on the door again. Make sure the vulnerabilities exploited in the previous attack are no longer a threat
- Step Three: Identify who will need to help you recover (IT experts, legal experts, insurance agents)
- Step Four: Start pulling all your documentation together. It will be needed for the investigation and the recovery team
- Step Five: Contract all your vendors
- Step Six: Start preparing for the notifications if the breach was in excess of 500 records.
- Step Seven: Have all communicate go through your attorney so you can secure client/attorney privilege
- Step Eight: Find out if any of the equipment needs to be replaced or repaired
- Step Nine: Sweep all the firewalls and networking equipment to make sure the hackers did not leave open any back doors
- Step Ten: Quarantine all the machines and server infected until the can be fully wiped and restored

Most of this chapter covered how to respond to a cyber security crisis, so let's end with some tips on how to avoid one.

Simple Tips

- Keep your computers up-to-date with the latest antivirus software.
- When in doubt, don't click on any files or links
- Use strong passwords and change them frequently
- Limit staff to only the access they need
- Consider cloud technology so you don't have to worry about protecting servers
- Education, Education, Education. Create a culture of compliance and patient privacy.
- Stop using Gmail accounts and yahoo accounts. Use a corporate grade email such as Microsoft Exchange.

Advanced Tips

- Hire someone to hack the practice. This is called penetration testing or white hacking. The best way to know if the practice is secure is to attempt your own breach from the outside
- Launch your own Phishing attack to see if employees are properly trained to spot fake emails.
- Deploy cyber prevention tools such as insider threat monitoring and net nannies that can watch for dangerous intruders
- Deploy vulnerability scanning tools that can search the entire network for known threats
- Consider having cyber security experts like Coker complete a third-party audit
- Put encryption on all devices, including mobile devices
- Lock-down your wireless network
- Complete the SRS annually (This is required by HIPAA).

Bottom Line

The 2019 HIMSS Cybersecurity Survey findings suggest that healthcare organizations' cybersecurity initiatives are moving in the right direction with some degree of uniformity. However, we still have a long way to go in comparison to other industries. While the progress is positive, budgets allocated to cybersecurity are still inadequate to deal with all the emerging cybersecurity threats

> **Back to the Case**
>
> *As awful as this sounds, Dr. Lavine was lucky and was even complemented by the OCR for his proactive efforts to keep the cyber criminals from profiting from their attack. If more practice would take these measures, these criminals would simply go aways as this would be a waste of their time and effort. He also discovered during his investigation the breach was caused by one of his vendors and was able to hold them legally and financially accountable since he had them sign a business associate agreement (BAA), per HIPAA policy. Unfortunately, most practices think this can never happen and do not take proactive measures. Here is an example of the CryptoLocker screen that popped up when he logged into his EHR.*

that most healthcare organizations face. Moreover, the lack of knowledgeable cybersecurity personnel also continues as a detriment to progress.

Legacy systems and lack of staff awareness continue to present a problem in need of innovative approaches. Overall, healthcare organizations are moving in the right direction, but bad actors continue to stay one step ahead in the game.

Coker Group and its partners have developed a comprehensive and cost-effective approach to conducting a risk analysis that meets the nine essential elements required by The Office of Civil Rights (OCR). For additional information on Coker's comprehensive cybersecurity risk analysis, contact us at 800.345.5829 or email info@cokergroup.com.

References

1. HIMSS. 2019 HIMSS cybersecurity survey. HIMSS; 2019; https://www.himss.org/sites/hde/files/d7/u132196/2019_HIMSS_Cybersecurity_Survey_Final_Report.pdf. Accessed 30 Oct 2020.
2. Snell E. Health IT security. 58% of healthcare PHI data breaches caused by insiders. Health IT Security. 2018. https://healthitsecurity.com/news/58-of-healthcare-phi-data-breaches-caused-by-insiders.

Case Raquel

Raquel has never seen a computer gadget she could resist. She was the first to adopt electronic billing, then electronic records, then electronic patient communications. When COVID-19 hit, Raquel was taking full advantage of virtual care and created the first digital front door in his community allowing patients to get checks in without any human contract. Talk about social distancing! Artificial Intelligence (AI) has now caught the attention of Raquel and she is all too eager to jump in but has found getting started a bit perplexing. Like most trendsetters, they accept the lack of product maturity as a tradeoff for early adoption, but is AI a product? Is it a platform? Who creates and owns it? Who owns what it can learn from Raquel's input?

Present-day headlines can very quickly change the entire dynamics of a topic in an instance. In June of 2022, while writing this chapter, an AI engineer working for Google by the name of Blake Lemoine claimed that one of the company's chatbots had become "sentient" [1]. Unsurprisingly, the engineer was immediately suspended shortly after going public with these statements. The story made national headlines and has since called into question the ethics of machine learning, specifically as it relates to the ethics of using AI to emulate human behavior. If the claim holds any truth, this would be an unheard-of-achievement, one historically thought to be impossible. It would mean the technology is progressing to such an extent that it is becoming conscious or self-aware. Google denies these claims and with having suspended the engineer, further speculation of attempts to discredit and downplay the claim was raised. It should be noted that other AI experts agreed with Google that this was not possible. However, the question that then presents itself is where should the lines be drawn for AI?

There is much to unpack as one dives down the rabbit hole of ethics and boundaries. This is especially true as the role of information technology in healthcare continues to increase and becomes part of the innovative efforts to optimize patient care. This will be discussed in greater detail in this chapter.

The adoption of artificial intelligence (AI) in healthcare is on the rise and is solving a variety of problems for patients and providers. According to Forbes, there has been a 14-fold increase in AI start-ups since 2000, and investing is up sixfold, topping out at over three billion [2].

But what really is artificial intelligence? These are some of the defining characteristics as we know them today:

© The Author(s), under exclusive license to Springer Nature Switzerland AG 2023
N. Baum et al., *The Business of Building and Managing a Healthcare Practice*,
https://doi.org/10.1007/978-3-031-37623-8_35

- For there to be AI, there must first be intelligence. Intelligence is the ability to acquire and apply knowledge and skills, to interact (whether it is through means of speech. Sight, motion, manipulation) and reason, to learn and adapt, and finally to be able to think abstractly as measured by objective criteria (e.g., testing).
- The term "artificial intelligence" is an umbrella term for any machine capable of perception, logic, and learning. Today, there are two types of AI:
- Machine Learning—Employs algorithms that learn from data to make predictions or decisions, and its performance improves when exposed to more data over time. In some cases, this may be a simple "if, and, do what" programmed logic. For example, if a patient is a child, the logic/decision will flow toward outcomes applicable to children. (See Fig. 35.1 for an illustration of "if, and, do what" programming logic.)
- Deep Learning—Uses many-layered, neural networks to build algorithms that find the best way to perform a task on their own based on vast sets of data. Deep learning will typically

improve over time by adding all past outcomes to the logic for future decisions. (See Fig. 35.2 for an example of deep learning logic.)

While we do not see AI taking over all human activity, the ethics and risks of machine involvement in patient care over traditional methods have yet to catch up to the technology. Of greater concern is the overall impact AI will have on society and the inequality shift AI is expected to cause. Specifically, AI is expected to eliminate 40% of all repetitive jobs over the next 20 years. Examples include call centers, patient check-ins, registration, triage, collections, AR follow-ups, campus delivery services, and many more. In March of 2019, UPS launched a new service using drones to transport blood and other medical supplies between the various buildings at WakeMed Raleigh's medical campus in North Carolina [3]. The speed at which the drones delivered the samples was significantly faster compared to humans and this difference could truly prove to be a matter of life and death. While this was a positive use of AI, several courier jobs on campus were instantly eliminated. One could

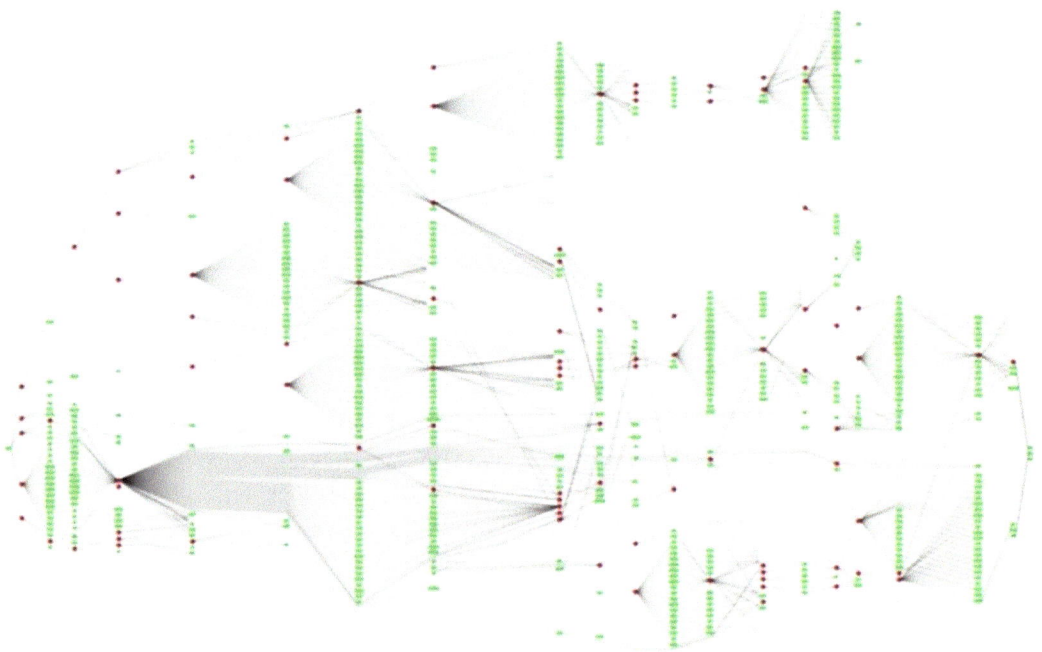

Fig. 35.1 If, and, do, what logic

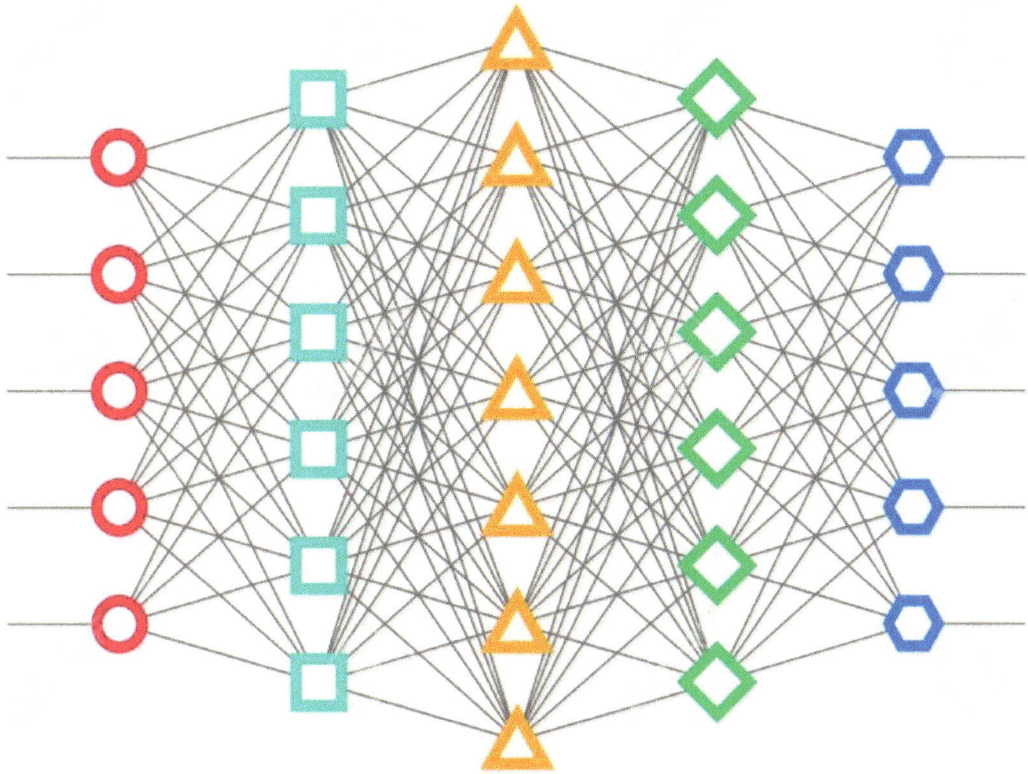

Fig. 35.2 Deep learning illustration

argue that a few drone developer jobs were added, but it is a reality that those employed in what would be considered low-skilled or lower-wage jobs were replaced by technology, and the ratio of jobs eliminated to created is far greater.

There are many examples throughout history where innovation has created winners and losers in the job market. One famous example was the massive amount of horse manure (15 kg of manure per day, to be exact) that was deposited on the streets of New York City in the late 1800s. At the height of the problem, over 170,000 horses were defecating in the city daily. In fact, the iconic elevated staircases (stoops) seen throughout New York today were born out of the efforts to keep manure from accumulating at the front door of the homes. This manure crisis created hundreds of jobs for people willing to remove excrement off the streets. Farmers from neighboring cities and states started monetizing services to haul this away and utilize this as free

fertilizer. There was an entire industry of jobs created to deal with this issue. Then, at the beginning of the twentieth century, the proliferation of automobiles replaced horses as a means of transportation, resulting in these jobs becoming eliminated.

Uber is a more modern example of how the entire taxicab industry forever changed, seemingly overnight. Netflix wiped out Blockbuster. The examples are endless and while this is not a new phenomenon, AI has the potential of eliminating millions of low-skilled jobs almost instantly. Unlike Uber and Netflix, however, it has taken more time for AI to catch up as a force of change. This in turn has given people the time to consider re-training for other job opportunities and, alternatively, to adapt to the new circumstances. For example, many taxi drivers now work for Uber and report higher incomes as independent contractors. Despite legitimate concerns, this should not deter us from exploring the benefits of

AI, especially as our society continues to change. Rather, it is necessary to become more informed on the topic in order to better understand both the benefits and risks associated with AI.

As we look into the future of AI, consider this scenario:

You are sitting in an exam room waiting to be seen by a provider. On the counter is an AI listening device, programmed to record the conversation you are about to have with your physician. This recording is being converted into metadata and will be used to make thousands of calculations and/or predictions based on the conversation it is picking up between you and the physician. After the exam, the AI device may support the physician's decision-making and/or trigger additional action items, such as ordering the test the physician discussed with you. The AI device may also warn the physician of a dangerous drug-to-drug interaction because the AI device is aware of what you have purchased over the counter. Or the data has been combined with other caregivers who are also using similar AI listening devices. Maybe you have forgotten to mention some over-the-counter supplements to your physician, but the AI device is also considering all your recent Amazon purchases and already knows you take fish oil. Fish oil can act as a blood thinner and should be discontinued before surgery. What about the information from Google? Google reports that it already has access to 70% of our credit card transactions, so it would not be unheard of for this data to be aggregated. In fact, if you spend any time on social media, you already know Big Tech has profiled and targeted you based on your spending habits. The innovators of these listening devices more often than not are created by tech companies who care more about collecting large quantities of data as their business model. Most likely, the AI listening device in the exam room will be provided by a business such as Google or Amazon, so it can be linked to the Google database of prior transactions, allowing the real-time conversation with the provider to be reconciled with other key data elements impacting your care. A case in point: Google already knows you recently booked a trip to South America, so it triggers a reminder for travel shots. The possibilities are endless.

So, does this make you feel a bit frightened, or shocked perhaps? Are you nervous about the type of information that gets picked up? Alternatively, does it make you feel more confident knowing there is a second set of ears, albeit electronic ones, helping you with decision-making? What about the matter of genetic testing? What if this data gets combined with AI software to better understand past medical history from relatives you know little about?

How does this impact providers? Are providers comfortable with their conversations being recorded by these third-party AI listening devices? Who is responsible for leaks or unintended uses of the data collected? On the positive side, could this be a great way to defend against a malpractice claim given how easy it can be for anyone to make up false claims? It would also be a great way for an elderly patient to share their visit with a caregiver who could not attend the visit in person. Again, the possibilities are endless and so are the benefits and risks.

According to an article published by Fierce Healthcare, about one in every ten patients (10%) secretly record their conversations with their providers [4].

While the above scenario may sound hypothetical and even improbable, truth be told, it is already happening.

A great majority of people have utilized GPS apps such as Google Maps or Waze. Have you ever experienced apps making real-time suggestions, such as offering new routes based on a set of circumstances like a construction or traffic jam? Have you ever understood the dynamics behind this? The answer is simple: Your phone is now a tracking device. It acts as a beacon that is communicating with other devices in the same area. Some apps even allow you to share helpful information with other drivers, such as advance warnings of police radar traps.

Have you ever noticed the way Facebook and other social media apps seem to know your hobbies, travel preferences, and even political affiliations, making recommendations based on these preferences? Have you ever seen an ad pop up in your newsfeed after visiting a new place or restaurant, even though you did not disclose your location? These are all examples of AI-based on crowd-sourcing data and/or accessing existing databases. There are also many data collection agencies that sell our data, and we often unknowingly release our data on many of the social media platforms. For example, if you check-in to nightclubs regularly, the Internet might assume you love to socialize, while others may think you have a drinking problem. All kidding aside though, we do give up a lot of personal information in exchange for these technological benefits. You might even feel that this is an invasion of privacy, but most of us unknowingly consent to give up this data when we agree to use third-party apps or social media platforms. Most of us click right through the terms and conditions without thinking about what we are electronically signing and consenting to.

A more concerning aspect of this is the way in which these apps will also pull data from other apps in the background. For instance, when TikTok is downloaded, the app seems to already know who your friends are and will start recommending followers. This occurs because the app was given access to your contact list and has downloaded all your information. It then looks to match you with people who have your phone number stored in their phone. Again, these apps can be very intrusive, but for technology and AI to work, it requires large quantities of data. Even for myself, when I consider the reason, I do not read through the user agreements for these platforms, the answer is that I am volunteering to use the technology and there is no option to change the policy, so in a way, I believe we accept this as it comes. I might cringe over it the ways others do, but it is ultimately a voluntary choice to use these platforms. However, it is my opinion that Big Tech needs to do better with transparency and make it easier for people to customize settings to prevent overreaching. In recent years, public awareness has been raised concerning consumer rights and privacy. Specifically, there have been two recent policies helping consumers gain more control over their data. The first is the "right to be forgotten." The General Data Protection Regulation (GDPR) governs how personal data must be collected, processed, and erased. The "right to be forgotten," which has received a lot of press coverage, has been difficult to implement given the competing interests and the hyperconnected nature of the Internet. The second is the Twenty-First Century Cures Act, which requires vendors to publish their API and patient data directly to the consumer. Health systems now have 72 h to make patient data available online without any restrictions. However, despite these regulations, most developers stand behind the notion that utilizing their platform is a choice we make as consumers and thus view the user agreements as reasonable and imperative to get access to their software.

Another concern that exists about data sourcing and AI technology has been the skepticism behind our devices listening to our conversations. Have you ever had a conversation and soon after, some information related to this discussion appears on a news feed or as a pop-up ad? Tech companies deny eavesdropping through your phone's microphone, but is this true? While I doubt our devices listen to a conversation per se, I do suspect keywords are picked up and the devices may respond accordingly. We also know that there are malicious apps that do listen, so we need to be cautious about what we install on our phones.

So, if these devices are not listening to us, how are these tech companies finding out so much personal information about us, and how will this be used to power AI? As noted above, Google claims to already have access to 70% of credit and debit card transactions in the United States. Facebook and others monitor much of what we are doing across the web. These companies can see many of the pages you and others are visiting by using hidden tracking technologies, allowing them to tailor their ads accordingly. Devices such as Amazon, Echo, Alexa, and Google Home are increasingly popular. The previously mentioned devices do listen, but with the consent of the device owner. What happens when these devices start making their way into exam rooms? At your workplace? Or more private areas? It is one thing for a consumer to knowingly invite an "always-listening" artificial intelligence device into their home, but should we have a right to know when we are being recorded? Under the wire-tap laws, most states prohibit one-party recording, but many companies get around this by having people waive their rights, or they might place a "notice" at the entrance of the building. As an example, have you ever heard the statement, "This call may be recorded or monitored for educational purposes?" Or what about those signs alerting you to surveillance in use. This is your notification, and this is considered an acceptable notice in most states. Some businesses will post signs letting you know the area is under video surveillance, which may have integrated facial recognition, which itself is a whole other world of AI possibilities.

Facial Recognition AI in Healthcare

Another form of AI is facial recognition. Some hospitals are using it to help them detect pain and discomfort based on the patient's facial expressions. There is also technology that can detect emotions in a person's voice, such as stress, depression and anger, to name a few. This technology is extremely helpful for nurse lines or suicide crisis centers. Other uses include allowing a business to know personal information about each consumer walking through the door so they can tailor how they interact with that individual. Some retailers use it to prevent theft by uploading pictures of known shoplifters, while some restaurants can determine which of their customers are high spenders or good tippers. A medical practice may use it to alert the staff about a known hostile patient or for auto check-ins. Yet another example would be protecting sensitive areas such as the maternity wards by only admitting known family members. Again, the possibilities are endless.

Most people respond unfavorably when asked how they feel about facial recognition software alerting other entities to personal information without consent. However, as discussed, we have already forfeited a lot of this personal information by agreeing to communicate on the various social media platforms and search engines that collect enormous amounts of data, including facial images. I am sure many of you have noticed by now that photos uploaded to Facebook are automatically tagged without you making the deci-

sion. The same is true with Instagram, Twitter, LinkedIn, and other platforms. Other data elements can be associated with these images, such as your spending habits, your religious affiliations, your political views, hobbies, and the list goes on. This allows anyone with the software to create customized approaches to how they target you, or worse, treat you differently.

AI in the Exam Room

Today, most healthcare provider organizations have electronic health records (EHRs). However, these tools are static databases with algorithms that complement and support people to complete simple tasks. They do not think of the users; they simply store data and serve as repositories for information. Now, with the advancement of AI, that factor is changing rapidly. AI today can augment human activity with the ability to sense, comprehend, and learn. AI in healthcare represents a collection of technologies enabling machines to comprehend and learn to perform administrative and clinical healthcare functions (see Sect. 35.3 for a list of AI Resources).

AI Resources

The following are a number of online resources (free and paid) that can serve as foundational sources of AI information:

- Udacity's Introduction to AI course and Artificial Intelligence Nanodegree Program.
- Stanford University's online lectures: Artificial Intelligence: Principles and Techniques.
- edX's online AI course, offered through Columbia University,
- Microsoft's open-source Cognitive Toolkit (previously known as CNTK) to help developers master deep-learning algorithms.
- Google's open-source (OS) TensorFlow software library for machine intelligence.
- AI Resources, an open-source code directory from the AI Access Foundation.

- The Association for the Advancement of Artificial Intelligence (AAAI)'s Resources Page.
- MonkeyLearn's Gentle Guide to Machine Learning.
- Stephen Hawking and Elon Musk's Future of Life Institute.
- OpenAI, an open industry, and academia-wide deep-learning initiative.

The primary aim of health-related AI applications should be to analyze relationships between preventative or treatment techniques and patient outcomes. Privacy policies must catch up to AI to ensure there is no overstepping of boundaries. With that said, the most obvious application of AI in healthcare is data management and its compatibility with our existing EHRs. As with all innovations driven by data, collecting, storing, normalizing, and tracing its lineage is the first step in developing an AI strategy. Today, AI programs have already been developed and applied to aid in the diagnosis processes, treatment protocol development, drug development, personalized medicine, and patient monitoring and care. We are now expecting AI to make its way into eliminating repetitive jobs and allowing for predictive automation.

As AI advances, we will need to consider the creation of ethical standards that are applicable any time patient data is used, with a specific emphasis on patient privacy and accountability for data usage. Now is the time to review the patient privacy policies to see how they may need to be updated for changes which include patient messaging, patient portal, text messaging, and other technological considerations.

The Ethics of AI

There are numerous ethical concerns involving AI. Here are some thought-provoking questions and/or considerations:

- Should we allow AI to emulate humans? Bots? Humanoid robots?
- What happens when AI shows bias or acts in a racist manner? (See: Microsoft Tay)

- Inequality—How do we distribute the wealth created by machines?
- The creation of evil AIs (e.g., cures cancer by killing all humans)
- AI Rights: Can non-humans have rights? A: See Corporations
- Humanity: How do machines affect our behavior and interaction?
- IP developed by AI: Who owns it?
- AI's that cause harm: Who is at fault?
- Privacy and Consent (facial recognition, tagging)
- AI prediction of propensity to pay: Are these patients treated differently?
- AI prediction of propensity to commit crimes: Should it be used for employment screening?
- Security: How do we keep AI safe from adversaries?
- Limitation: Requires access to the cloud and an enormous amounts of data
- The right to be forgotten: Can we honestly ensure we can purge all the data we collect on our consumers?

The concerns listed above are yet to be resolved, but they will no doubt need to be confronted at some point in the future.

Moving Forward with an AI Strategy

As you begin the journey towards incorporating AI, it is important to keep expectations in perspective. Despite the advances thus far, there are significant challenges in this field that include:

- The acceptance of AI at the point of care.
- The availability of quality data from which to build and maintain AI applications
- The missing data streams
- The limitations of AI methods in health and healthcare software applications
- From an adoption standpoint, we recommend the following:
- Learn and research AI (See Resource Exhibits)
- Create awareness
- Change mindsets based on responses to awareness campaigns

- Educate leadership
- Start off setting low expectations
- Identify easy wins (*This is most critical)
- Embrace cloud computing
- Form a workgroup
- Identify gaps in data/capabilities
- Consider market-based platforms as opposed to self-developed ones
- Consider enlisting a third-party expert to transfer knowledge.

References

1. Kahn J. 'Sentient' chatbot story shows why it's time for A.I. to retire the Turing test. Forbes; 2022; https://fortune.com/2022/06/14/blake-lemoine-sentient-ai-chatbot-google-turing-test-eye-on-a-i/.

2. Columbus L. 10 charts that will change your perspective on artificial intelligence's growth. Forbes; 2018; https://www.forbes.com/sites/louiscolumbus/2018/01/12/10-charts-that-will-change-your-perspective-on-artificial-intelligences-growth/?sh=3a86ddab4758.

3. Kelleher K. UPS begins using drones to transport medical samples at North Carolina hospitals. Forbes; 2019; http://fortune.com/2019/03/26/ups-matternet-drones-transport-medical-samples-north-carolina-hospitals/.

4. Finnegan J. More patients record doctor visits with or without permission. Fierce Healthcare; 2017; https://www.fiercehealthcare.com/practices/more-patients-are-recording-doctor-visits.

Case Marc

Marc (unrelated to one of the authors of this book) has been in practice with a small group practice for 5 years. Marc was asked to join the quarterly meeting with the practice's accountant. He reviewed the profit and loss statement with the CPA and a few of the doctors. It became apparent to Marc that the doctors had little interest in the trend of rising accounts receivables. When Marc asked about this rising trend, the doctors drew a blank and were like deer caught in headlights. Marc wanted to take more interest in the numbers used to measure the progress and productivity of the practice.

As early career physicians, you have joined a very exclusive club. You are in rare air, and you should celebrate this milestone. Very few professionals have reached your level of success, and you should be applauded and enjoy all the accolades that are sure to come your way. We know that you have heard doctors in the physician's lounges or lunchroom complain about the current state of American medicine and say they wouldn't choose to become a doctor if they were to start all over again. We want you to know that your authors and the colleagues we know are happy and content with their decision to select medicine

as their profession and their life's work. If they had to start over, most physicians would decide to remain in healthcare.

Some of the reasons you should feel reassured that you chose to become a physician:

As a physician, you can care for all age groups, from newborns to geriatric patients. You can care for children, as well as patients in their declining years. You can even delve into the emotional problems of your patients and, with your empathy, can provide them with support and solutions.

Even most medical doctors who care for patients find that our patients do well and get better due to our intervention. We have many skills at our disposal, including prescribing medicines, performing surgery, and using a combination of both treatments to make our patients better off after interacting with us. The knowledge that we can solve many, if not most, of their medical problems is very rewarding and satisfying. Even when we cannot treat or correct a medical problem, we can be understanding and good listeners to provide solace for a patient we cannot cure. As a result, patients continue to hold their doctors in high esteem and are very grateful for our care.

We are fortunate that medicine is a profession where the patient's problem is almost always clearly defined. For example, when a patient presents with a complaint of weight loss, a tremor, or shortness of breath, we can usually locate the problem's locus, discover the defect, and arrive at an accurate diagnosis. With all that information, we then offer a solution. Medicine is not vague, nebulous, or ill-defined where the solution may be cloudy or unclear. We can be exact and narrow the range of diagnoses and options. Patients genuinely appreciate knowing they are in the hands of an expert who can guide them to their treatment or cure.

Let's be thankful that there will always be a demand for our services, and that need will become greater now that the baby boomers are reaching age sixty-five. Ten thousand people reach the age of sixty-five every day. That translates into plenty of work for nearly every American doctor, as most aging baby boomers will eventually need our services. Even pediatricians can care for their grandchildren.

Medicine is broad in scope, although the organ systems we treat are relatively finite. We can focus on a single, defined area of medical conditions. Consequently, if we choose, we can become experts in a single field or subspecialty.

As we read the journals and look at the job boards, we are pleasantly surprised at the wide range of opportunities available for graduating residents and fellows. A newly minted physician can become an academician, join a large group practice, join a small group, or even become a solo practitioner. Young physicians can select from a wide variety of geographic locations. They can always find something that fits their practice style and personal lifestyle. We will always be able to find a job even if the first job does not work out as we have planned.

Our profession offers multiple opportunities for entrepreneurship and creativity. Most of the new devices and interventions in the field are developed by practicing physicians. We can turn our creative juices into developing new ways of treating medical diseases more efficiently and with less pain and discomfort. Our peers and colleagues have advanced mainly the trend of bringing care from the hospital to the office, where the physician is more in control of their schedule. A new trend is providing care for patients in their homes using telemedicine, home testing laboratory tests, and wearables to monitor patients' health between office visits [1].

For those physicians who wish to segue from clinical practice to non-clinical endeavors, there are numerous non-clinical opportunities, such as joining the ranks of pharma, becoming a medical director for an industry or a hospital, and even going into politics, and creating healthcare policy.

Our profession enjoys having a good sense of humor. We have never met a doctor with a cute story or joke to share with colleagues and patients. That may be why we can cope with our career choice; if you are laughing, you cannot be unhappy.

In short, the next time you think about what you would do instead of becoming a physician, stop, and be thankful you chose to become a doctor. You have many reasons to be grateful.

The reality is that only some of us have received the necessary skills to participate in the business side of our practice effectively. However, if we want to be successful, becoming involved in the business will be essential for a successful practice. We are small business professionals regardless of the size or nature of our practice. We must understand the basics of business, and that is what we hope we have given you. We are eager to hear from you, and any ideas you have will be most appreciated when we write the book's second edition.

We want to close this chapter and this book with a few numbers you need to know. Only a few doctors have a business background, an MBA, or a degree in healthcare policy. We recommend that every doctor understand a few metrics or key performance indicators that will impact their practice's success regardless of the practice's size, geographic location, or the organization's hierarchy. Reviewing these five numbers will require less than 10 min each month. Still, it will be an essential barometer of the direction your practice is going to take. These metrics are available in any practice management software and can be viewed in a graphic format to see trends impacting your practice. Also, as a young doctor, you will impress your colleagues and office manager that you are interested in and understand your practice's essential business aspects.

The five essential metrics you need to monitor regularly are (1) charges/receipts, (2) revenue value units (RVUs), (3) accounts receivable, (4) charge lag, and (5) denials.

Charges and Receipts

The total charges of the practice are the gross charges or the total charges for services provided by the practice. This number represents the total work submitted for payment to patients and third-party insurance companies. It would be a wonderful world if we could receive compensation for those gross charges. Guess what? It is not a wonderful world!

The real-world number to know and follow is money *collected* for your services. The net receipts are the most important number to know. These are the *net receipts,* which consist of the gross receipts minus the refunds to patients and insurance companies. It is far easier to collect money at the point of service when the patient is in the office. Why? Every time you try to collect an amount more than 6 months after the service was provided, it will cost the practice about 30 dollars for each collection attempt. You are not very likely to collect amounts owed to you that are older than 180 days.

The gross collection percent is a metric that you will want to compare each month, each quarter, and each year. The gross collection percent is the payments received divided by the charges. For example, if the practice collected $750,000 in revenues and the charges were $1,000,000, that would translate into a 75% gross collection rate.

You will also want to look at charges and net collection percentage (NCP). The net collection percentage is the total payments divided by the charges minus any contractual adjustments. For example, if the payments are $750,000 and the charges are $1,000,000 minus $200,000 in adjustments, the NCP is 93.77%. A well-run practice should have an NCP >97%. This metric compares your practice today to your past performance.

How is the charge data helpful? If you see a decline in gross collections, you need to look into why this metric of gross charges is declining.

Why was there a decrease in gross collections? Was there an increase in Medicaid charges considerably lower than third-party payer charges? Was there an increase in contractual write-offs and an increase in adjustments? If that is the case, do you need to consider renegotiating your contracts with the insurance companies? Was there an increase in costly staff turnover? Staff turnover, especially in the billing departments, is likely to result in a decrease in collections. Therefore, it is incumbent to look for why the staff is leaving the practice and fix that problem.

RVUs

Next, look at the relative value units or RVUs. RVUs measure physician productivity across a period, such as a month, a quarter, or a year. This metric calculates compensation for employed physicians. This number is also helpful for negotiation with hospitals and insurance companies. The calculation of RVUs considers the complexity of the service or the procedure, the time to do the work, the labor involved, the materials or equipment required for the service, the supplies that are needed, and consideration of the malpractice expense. The Centers for Medicare and Medicaid Services (CMS) then multiplies the RVUs for each service or procedure by a "conversion factor," which was $35.89 in 2019. For example, suppose a physician generated 700 RVUs in the last quarter. Their RVU value is 700 times the conversion factor of $35.89 or $25,123. The hospital or the employer will often use this calculation to represent the physician's productivity minus the agreed-upon overhead expense and determine the physician's salary or compensation.

Accounts Receivable

The metric of accounts receivable (AR) is also a necessary metric to monitor. The gross accounts receivable is equal to the charges minus the payments or the receipts. The net AR is the charges minus any contractual allowances or discounts minus the receipts or what has been collected.

This number is what the practice is likely to collect in the future. For example, if the charges are $1,000,000 and the contractual allowances are $200,000, the practice is "owed" $800,000. If the practice has received only $750,000 in payments; then, the net AR is $50,000, representing the fees that are likely to be collected. It is the AR that distinguishes good management from poor financial management.

The aging of AR is also a fundamental metric to review regularly. Most practice management systems will place AR in buckets of 1–60 days, 61–120 days, 121–180 days, and more than 180 days. Ideally, you would like the bulk of the AR to be below 60 days, as these ARs are likely to be collectible. ARs greater than 180 days will seldom be collected. Therefore, it is imperative to monitor these three or four buckets of AR and to keep the majority of the ARs in the 1–60 days category.

Days in AR are part of the AR metric. The days in AR are equal to the total AR divided by the average daily charges (ADC). This latter number is like the quarterly charges divided by 90 days. This metric monitors the efficiency of the practice's billing and collection. The greater the days in AR, the less efficient the practice. Suppose you are watching the trend in ARs and notice rising days in AR. In that case, consider how quickly physicians post charges or how fast the billing staff submits charges to the payor. Another possibility is that a payor is delinquent or delayed in paying the practice, and the payor needs to know that this is unacceptable.

The AR ratio is the ratio of the total accounts receivable divided by the average monthly billings, usually using the last 3 months of charges or billings. For example, if the previous month's AR was $448,000 in uncollected fees and the prior 3 months' billings were $396,000 ($132,000 per month), the AR ratio is $448,000/$132,000 or 3.4 months (102 days). The AR ratio of 3.4 represents 3.4 months of payments due to your practice. The goal for a primary care practice is to maintain an AR ratio of 1.5–2.5, and for a specialty or surgical practice, the goal should be less than 2.0–3.0. The difference between a primary care practice and a surgical practice is that surgi-

cal practices perform more expensive procedures. You have to collect these higher fees from insurance companies who are not as prompt at paying at the time of service when compared with a primary care practice.

Charge Lag

Another important metric is monitoring the charge lag between the date the service is performed and the date the fee is submitted to the insurance company. Ideally, this number should be close to zero or 1 day. A delay means that the practice could better transmit charges to third-party payers. If the charge lag is too long, checking on the process of filing claims in a timely fashion would be appropriate to solve the problem.

Denials

Denial is not a river in Egypt! A claim to an insurance company must be submitted accurately to receive compensation for your services. A "clean claim" refers to a claim that is processed and paid without being returned because of errors. Historically, 10–15% of claims are "dirty" and denied because of errors in submitting the claim. Also, it is of interest that nearly 50% of denied claims are never refiled, which means you are leaving money on the table that is honestly owed to you. The good news is that more than 90% of denied claims are preventable. Denied claims require meticulous attention to detail. For example, the claim will be rejected if the patient's insurance number is not accurately keyed in or if the patient's name is misspelled. The insurance company will deny the claim. And the insurance company will be holding your money, and your practice will spend additional time and expense to refile the claim. Therefore, the billing clerk must be a perfectionist, or you will lose money that honestly belongs to you and your practice.

Bottom Line on Business Metrics

You need to understand these concepts to understand the value of your services. The minimum metrics to follow regularly are charges, receipts, RVUs, accounts receivable, charge lag, and denials. Remember the "buck" starts and stops with the doctor! Finally, medicine is a business; if you want to be a successful doctor, you need to understand business basics. We hope that we have instilled in you the need to be a small business-person and that you will have a very enjoyable and profitable practice.

Don't forget that the "buck" starts and stops with you the doctor! Finally, medicine is a business and if you want to be a successful doctor, you need to understand the basics of business. We hope that we have instilled in you the need for being a small business-person and that you will have a very enjoy- able and profitable practice.

Medicine is a great profession. But, like any other profession, it is a business and proper understanding of business principles and practices is necessary to be successful. We believe that you don't need to be an MBA to understand the principles of business. However, it is necessary to monitor just five metrics to understand the progress and productivity of your practice.

Reference

1. Rhoden PA, Bonilha H, Harvey J. Patient satisfaction of telemedicine remote patient monitoring: a systematic review. Telemedicine and e-Health. 2022;28(9):1332–41. https://pubmed.ncbi.nlm.nih.gov/35041549/

Future of Medicine—The Past Cannot Be Changed. You Can Sculpt Your Future

37

Case @Rayco

@rayco graduated medical school in 2020 and she has been in an equity fund-owned primary care practice since completing her residency with Healthcare American (HA) 15 years ago. HA is the country's largest healthcare conglomerate, being initially formed from the nation's largest independent insurer, a large hospital system, a pharmacy benefits company, and a major retail outlet. @rayco enjoys the coaching aspect of primary care. The group has enrolled eight thousand patients. The patients she sees have already used HA's proprietary software to receive their diagnosis. The software boasts an error rate of less than 5 per 100,000 patients. The software immediately feeds to HA's proprietary electronic health record (EHR) and prescribes a therapeutic plan for each patient. In fact, the EHR feeds information to the on-site pharmacy so that patient's current medications as well as OTC medications and supplements are available prior to the patient's appointment. During residency, @rayco learned how to modify patient behavior and provide healthcare coaching, which are key skills for an effective primary care provider. @rayco is thrilled that her calculated value score, based on both the quality of her care and her costs/patient, places her in the top 10% regarding patient satisfaction, productivity, and cost-effectiveness of all of the primary care providers in her network. As a result, she enjoys a 12% bonus on her base annual salary.

In 1957, three agricultural scientists, Joe M. Bohlen, George M. Beal, and Everett M. Rogers at Iowa State University, published a model of technology adoption that continues to have relevance today. (Ref. Beal, G. M., & Rogers, E. M. (1960). *The adoption of two farm practices in a central Iowa community* (Vol. 26). Agricultural and Home Economics Experiment Station, Iowa State University of Science and Technology.) In this model, the process of technology adoption is defined as a bell curve. The first group to use the product, on the far-left tail of the bell curve, is called *innovators*. The next group, moving left to right, is called *early adopters*. These are followed by *early* and *late majorities*. On the far right are the *laggards*. This model has several limitations, the least of which is that it assumes a linear and continuous model for technology adoption (see Fig. 37.1).

Clayton Christenson, a professor at the Harvard Business School and considered the foremost authority on innovation and technology, in his classic book, *The Innovator's Dilemma*, described "disruptive technologies." (Christensen, C. M. (2013). *The innovator's dilemma: when new technologies cause great firms to fail.* Harvard Business Review Press.). One of the key features of disruptive technologies is that their adoption is not linear, but rather S-shaped such that initial adoption is low, followed by rapid implementation that eventually levels off (see Fig. 37.2). This is because incorporating an innovation is slow and iterative. Initial improvements provide minimal value to the consumer. However, over time, these improvements become drastically better than previous enhancements, leading to rapid product adoption. At the end of the product's lifestyle, the improvements are marginal. For example, consider the mobile phone. Initially those phones were large, expensive, cumbersome, and unreliable. Few people owned them. The Apple's iPhone was dramatically better. Apple has sold more than one billion phones since introduction in 2007! Now consider the most recent iPhone models, they are better than the last model, but not by much. Sales have slowed considerably thus they are on the right of the S-shaped curve.

Disruptive technologies are defined as innovations that interrupt or displace a traditional technology or existing market in order to solve or improve upon a problem that is currently in use. This creates a new market by displacing an older technology. In healthcare, these disruptive innovations will often come at a lower cost, with an enhancement in quality over the product, treat-

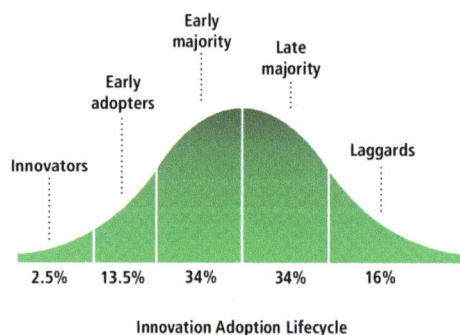

Fig. 37.1 Rogers model of technology adoption

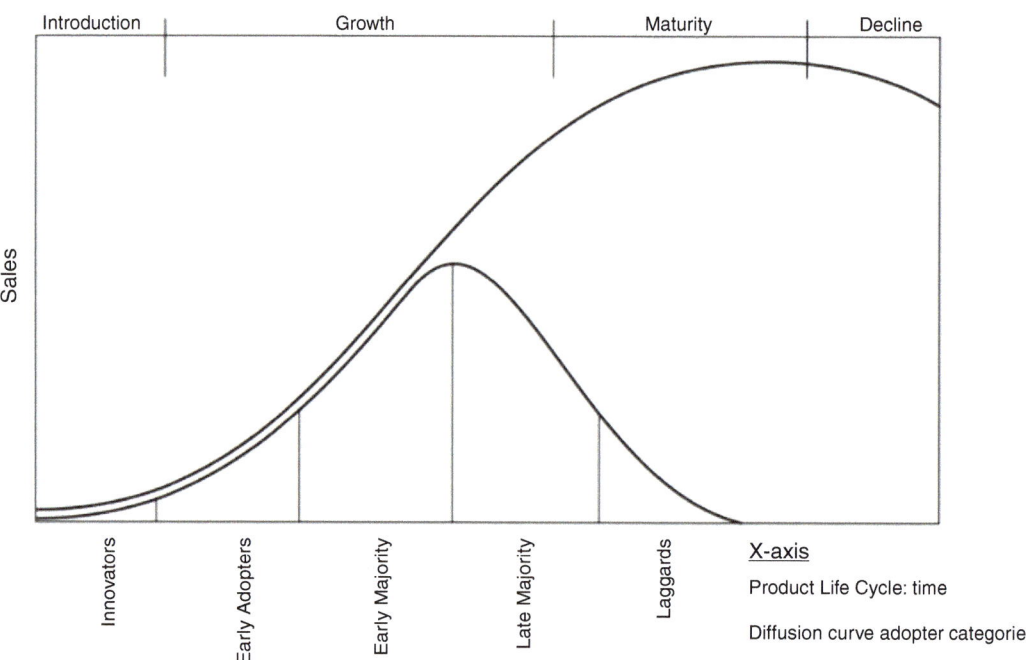

Fig. 37.2 S-shaped model of technology adoption

ment, or technique that it replaces. Over time, these disruptive innovations improve on quality and performance and eventually take over a market. For example, in medicine, ultrasound was originally developed as a less expensive alternative to standard x-rays. Over time, ultrasound technology improved providing enhanced images such that today point of care ultrasound is a necessary skill and requirement in many specialties.

In healthcare, retail outlets such as Walmart have opened urgent care clinics staffed mostly by midlevel providers, i.e., physician assistants, nurse practitioners, or medical assistants. These are cheaper alternatives to hospital-owned clinics or staffing these clinics with medical doctors. Assuming the level of care and the quality of provided to a patient is related to the number of hours of clinical training completed by the provider, the outcomes may be of lower quality. However, looking to the future, assuming these clinics are disruptive innovations, we can predict that they will disrupt the market for primary care services and slowly become the standard of care and become the dominant model. For example, pharmacies are monitoring patients' blood pressure and offering to provide vaccines such as flu and shingles vaccines to patients. This is convenient to patients and is provided at a lower cost than going to a physician's brick and mortar office. And then consider the ease of access for patients seeking medical care at Walmart, Costco, or their local pharmacy compared to the long waits for an appointment to see a doctor in their office. You can easily see why patients are moving in large numbers to these disruptive delivery systems of healthcare.

The danger of disruptive innovation is that established companies typically view the disruptive technology as unattractive, and consequently it is initially ignored. The established market leaders can be blindsided as the technology takes off, leaving them far behind. Remember what happened to Blockbuster video stores with the arrival of Netflix, or observe what is happening to retail stores which are being replaced by Amazon. Fast forward, Amazon is continuing to disrupt the market and is now competing with FedEx, UPS, and the

United States Postal Service by delivering its own packages. Because of the size of the healthcare market, currently more than $3 trillion per year, and the rising cost of medical care and medications, healthcare is ripe for disruption.

What Are the Traditional Forces that Define and Shape US Healthcare?

Healthcare in the United States is distinguished as a predominately private, complex, multipayer system that has focused on scientific and technologic advances. In the recent past, insured patients did not bear the full cost of their medical care due to coverage often paid by the employer, and so patients were not incentivized to consume less services, nor were their providers financially motivated to control the costs of medical care. In addition, competing special interests from physicians, hospitals, insurers, Pharma, and patient advocacy groups have all worked to strengthen their position in the policy landscape, sometimes to the detriment of high value care. Each of these components contributes to the higher costs, with little accountability regarding quality or outcomes.

Although the rate of healthcare growth has slowed somewhat in recent years [1–3], it has not reached a ceiling. As more of the economy's resources are devoted to healthcare, less is available for other goods and services. While jobs within the healthcare sector are generally higher paying, if the overall growth of healthcare outpaces that of the rest of the economy, Americans will find themselves less able to access and afford the medical care they need. American businesses are also faced with the burden of growing healthcare costs as they struggle to provide benefits to their employees and remain competitive internationally [4].

Future Changes in Reimbursement

The fee-for-service (FFS) model often results in over-utilization of low-value and unnecessary care [5]. FFS impedes coordination of care for patients across the healthcare system [6]. The FFS model is not sustainable, especially with an increase in the baby boomer population as 10,000 boomers turn 65 every day [7], and those with chronic and complex health needs [8, 9] are also increasing. As long as providers are rewarded for the volume of care delivered, as in FFS arrangements, instead of the value provided, they are pressured to deliver more care, and population healthcare costs will continue to rise without regard to improvement in patient outcomes. Both private and public payers of healthcare have recognized this and have begun to shift their payment models that are soon going to be tied to outcomes and to quality of care. Newer payment models are intended to reduce the cost of care and improve the quality of care.

The previous paradigm was for doctors to provide a service, perform a procedure, or order a test. The more tests and procedures that the doctor did, the greater the compensation. That payment method, fee for service (FFS), worked for many decades but the future of that model is no longer tenable. There is probably no greater disruption to modern healthcare than the movement from payment for the volume of care provided to the value of care delivered.

Multiple changes are occurring every day making it difficult for young or new physicians to navigate.

For employed physicians, FFS may be computed as the Relative Value Unit (RVU) metric, but it is still based on "you get what you kill." (Isn't that a moronic term applied to the healthcare profession where we take an oath "to do no harm" and to restore health and certainly not to kill patients?)

In addition to changes in physician reimbursement, employers have recently started shifting costs to employees by requiring employees to contribute a percentage of their insurance premiums and offering employees a high deductible health plans (HDHP) which reduces the annual insurance premiums [10]. In 2021, enrollment in HDHPs is 28% of insured workers, up from a 4% in 2006 [11]. As more patients are enrolled in HDHPs and responsible for their initial care,

these patients are more likely to demand transparency of healthcare costs as well see better results or outcomes. Ultimately, today's employees want to understand what they are receiving for their increased payments.

The Department of Health and Human Services is striving to have 90% of all Medicare FFS payments tied to quality or value by 2020 [12]. Value is defined as quality divided by cost. Medicare's new payment reform system, The Medicare Access and CHIP Reauthorization Act (MACRA), will help the organization to reach that goal. MACRA consolidates previous quality reporting systems to streamline tracking and reporting, and thus further encouraging value-based care over volume of care provided (see Chap. 12 on MACRA). If previous policy changes are any indication, as Medicare goes, so too will private insurance also follow very quickly.

Indeed, the future of medicine is moving from volume to value. If a young physician can demonstrate that they can adapt to new incentives by improving costs while maintaining and enhancing their quality and their outcomes, these young physicians will be more competitive in the changing marketplace.

Future Importance of Medical Quality Assessment

The importance of quality in healthcare may seem obvious. It is emphasized by the Hippocratic Oath that physicians take attesting *primum non nocere,* or, first, to do no harm. Poor quality of care can also mean higher costs—whether it is through providing unnecessary care that results in iatrogenic disease or forgoing important preventive care that ultimately results in greater disease burden requiring more expensive medical care. Of course, quality matters to patients as well. Patients want to receive quality healthcare even if it is difficult to assess. To this end, providers are likely to face competition based on the quality they provide. As the forces at play continue to transition incentives from volume to value, quality of care will be tied to provider payment, and properly measuring quality will be of primary importance.

Defining quality in healthcare is not a simple task, because quality holds different meanings to different stakeholders [13]. However, the widely-used Institute of Medicine (IOM) definition of quality encapsulates a broad understanding of quality as, "the degree to which health services for individuals and populations increase the likelihood of desired health outcomes and are consistent with current professional knowledge." [14] The IOM further specifies that high-quality care should be safe, effective, patient-centered, timely, efficient, and equitable [15].

How Will We Improve Outcomes in the Future?

Proper measurement is the first step to improve outcomes. Tracking how patients fare can largely be achieved through electronic medical records. Many physicians overestimate their performance on quality measures until they are provided with their performance data [16]. To this end, continuous feedback on improvement also needs to be available to providers. From this feedback, payers can reward providers not only for achieving specific quality standards but also for incremental improvements. By providing ongoing feedback for progressively better results, instead of continuing to penalize for not meeting a benchmark, providers are encouraged to find innovative ways to improve.

Other approaches to improve quality include public reporting of outcomes, although research is mixed on the effectiveness of this method [17, 18]. If patients see comparisons between providers, it may promote competition or at last an incentive to improve quality. One of the problems with this method is that providers may find ways to game the measurement process.

How can we continuously improve quality?

- Continuously assess and revise metrics to accurately reflect quality that matters to stakeholders.
- Assess whether process measures continue to accurately reflect outcomes.

- Revise standards and clinical practice guidelines concurrent with new evidence.
- Promote a learning atmosphere—less punitive, more encouraging of success.
- Promote effective communication within and between organizations.
- Maintain and improve IT systems to accurately and efficiently capture care and outcomes.
- Use outcomes that are easiest to track and difficult to manipulate.

The healthcare profession is about to experience a tsunami regarding payment models that focus on value and quality. No longer will volume of patients seen or number of services provided be the metric for payment and reimbursement. Providers, payers, patients, and also the government will have to make a big adjustment by moving from volume to value. We believe that the success of a medical practice is going to depend on the speed at which the healthcare profession can make these transitions.

Future Outcome Metrics

In the past outcomes consisted of measuring survival, length of stay, or readmission rates. Those certainly are metrics that are important but now it will be necessary to go beyond those basic outcome measurements and start recording and documenting additional data that will clearly demonstrate superior outcomes.

Outcome measurement plays a pivotal role in medical decision making for physicians, payors, and for patients who are searching for high-quality medical care. It is outcome measurements which quantify components of quality such as clinical outcomes, patient satisfaction, and the functional status of our patients.

The end results of outcome measurement identify patterns and trends and provide the healthcare profession with the effectiveness, or even the lack of effectiveness, of our medical interventions. By recording outcomes, we can maximize favorable outcomes, and can minimize poor outcomes. As result of obtaining and recording outcomes, we can demonstrate quality of care and will hopefully lead to improved medical care and a lower cost.

The benefits of outcome measurements prevent overuse, underuse, and misuse of healthcare services as well as enhancing patient safety. Outcome measurements also drive innovation and research and development which enhance disease control and improvement in patient's quality of life. By tracking outcomes payors and providers are held accountable for providing high-quality care. When the outcomes are transparent, patients can make informed choices regarding their care and can select providers who have stellar outcome data. Also, when outcomes are measured, there is competition among payers and providers, and with increased competition, prices are certainly going to decrease. Finally, patients with improved outcomes are more engaged in their care, more committed to treatment plans, and more receptive to medical advice.

Back to Case

@rayco continued on with Healthcare American. She participated in seminars and workshops offered by her specialty society and improved her coaching skills. Because she was able to significantly modify some of the high-risk behavior evident in her patient panel, she continued to receive bonuses for her outstanding care. In addition to improving the quality of her care, she also learned more about the cost structure of her care through participation in several hologram-based learning exercises. This led to further improvement in her value scores. @rayco went on to produce several hologram-based exercises on her own so that her colleagues could benefit from her innovations.

Bottom Line

Yogi Berra said, "You've got to be very careful if you don't know where you're going because you might not get there." The future of medicine will include alterations in payment with a focus on value rather than volume. Quality measurement and assessment will be critically important features of these newer models. You need to know that the quality train is leaving the station….all aboard!

References

1. Hartman M, Martin AB, Lassman D, et al. National health spending in 2013: growth slows, remains in step with the overall economy. Health Aff. 2015;2015(34):150–60.
2. Martin AB, Hartman M, Whittle L, Caitlin A. National health expenditures accounts team. National health spending in 2012: rate of health spending growth remained low for the fourth consecutive year. Health Aff. 2014;33:67–77.
3. Cutler DM, Sahni NR. If slow rate of health care spending growth persists, projections may be off by $770 billion. Health Aff. 2013;32(5):841–50.
4. Sood N, Ghosh A, Escarce JJ. Employer-sponsored insurance, health care cost growth, and the economic performance of U.S. industries. Health Serv Res. 2009;44(5p1):1449–64.
5. Shen J, Andersen R, Brook R, Kominski G, Albert PS, Wenger N. (2004). The effects of payment method on clinical decision-making. Med Care. 2004;42(3):297–302.
6. Institute of Medicine. Rewarding provider performance: aligning incentives in Medicare. Washington, DC: National Academies Press; 2006.
7. Ortman JM, Velkoff VA, Hogan H. An aging nation: the older population in the United States. Washington, DC: US Census Bureau; 2014; https://www.census.gov/prod/2014pubs/p25-1140.pdf. Accessed 24 Apr 2017.
8. Wu S, Green A. Projection of chronic illness prevalence and cost inflation. Washington: DC RAND Health; 2000.
9. Centers for Disease Control and Prevention. About chronic diseases. CDC; 2022; https://www.cdc.gov/chronicdisease/about/index.htm.
10. Claxton G, Rae M, Long M, et al. Health benefits in 2016: family premiums rose modestly, and offer rates remained stable. Health Aff. 2016;35:1908–17.

11. Dolan R. Health policy brief: high-deductible health plans. Health Aff. 2016; http://www.healthaffairs.org/healthpolicybriefs/brief.php?brief_id=152. Accessed 24 Apr 2017.

12. Burwell SM. Setting value-based payment goals--HHS efforts to improve U.S. health care. New Engl J Med. 2015;372(10):897–9.

13. McGlynn EA. Six challenges in measuring the quality of health care. Health Aff. 1997;16(3):7–21.

14. Institute of Medicine. Medicare: a strategy for quality assurance. Washington, DC: National Academies Press; 1990.

15. Institute of Medicine. Crossing the quality chasm: a new health system for the 21st century. Washington, DC: National Academies Press; 2001.

16. Donabedian A. Evaluating the quality of medical care. Milbank Mem Fund Q. 1966;44(3):166–206.

17. Hibbard JH, Stockard J, Tusler M. Hospital performance reports: impact on quality, market share, and reputation. Health Aff. 2005;24(4):1150–60.

18. Fung CH, Lim YW, Mattke S, Damberg C, Shekelle PG. Systematic review: the evidence that publishing patient care performance data improves quality of care. Ann Intern Med. 2008;148(2):111–23.

Index